AF352152

Contributors

MASAAKI ARAKAWA, M.D.

Professor of Medicine
Director of Division of Nephrology
Department of Medicine
Kawasaki Medical School
Kurashiki, Japan

MASANOBU EDANAGA

Senior Research Scientist
Research Laboratory
Yoshitomi Pharmaceutical Industry
Yoshitomi-cho, Fukuoka-ken, Japan

TERUO FUJIMOTO, M.D.

Professor, Department of Pathology
Osaka City University Medical School
Osaka, Japan

YOICHIRO KONDO, M.D.

Professor, Department of Pathology
School of Medicine, Chiba University
Chiba, Japan

YOZO MASUGI, M.D.

Professor, Department of Pathology
Nippon Medical School, Tokyo, Japan

ATSUSHI OKABAYASHI, M.D.

Professor Emeritus
Department of Pathology
School of Medicine, Chiba University
Chiba, Japan

MASAAKI OKADA, M.D.

Chief, Division of Pathology
Clinical Research Institute
National Medical Center Hospital
Tokyo, Japan

SEIICHI SHIBATA, M.D.

Associate Professor
Third Department of Internal Medicine
Faculty of Medicine, University of Tokyo
Tokyo, Japan

HIDEKAZU SHIGEMATSU, M.D.

Associate Professor
Department of Pathology
School of Medicine, Chiba University
Chiba, Japan
Present address: Professor, Department of
Pathology, School of Medicine
Shinshu University, Matsumoto, Japan

TOMIO TADA, M.D.

Professor, Laboratories for Immunology
School of Medicine, Chiba University
Chiba, Japan
Present address: Professor, Department of
Immunology, Faculty of Medicine
University of Tokyo, Tokyo, Japan

JUNICHI TOKUNAGA, M.D.

Professor, Department of Microbiology
Kagoshima University Dental School
Kagoshima, Japan

HIROKI TSUCHIDA, M.D.

Department of Internal Medicine
Chiba Shakai Hoken Hospital
Chiba, Japan

MASAFUMI WAKASHIN, M.D.

Assistant Professor
First Department of Internal Medicine
School of Medicine, Chiba University
Chiba, Japan

YOKO WAKASHIN, M.D.

First Department of Internal Medicine
School of Medicine, Chiba University
Chiba, Japan

Preface

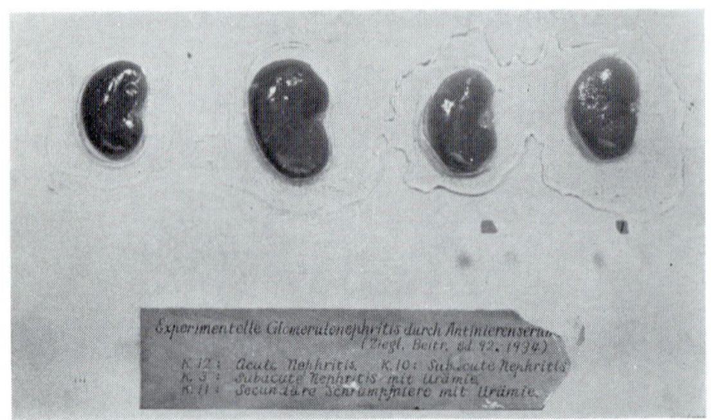

Original Specimens of Rabbit Masugi Nephritis (1934)*
Department of Pathology, School of Medicine, Chiba
University, Chiba, Japan

Matazo Masugi graduated from Faculty of Medicine, University of Tokyo, Tokyo in 1921 and entered its Department of Pathology (Prof. M. Nagayo and Prof. T. Ogata). Following further study, from 1925 to 1927, in Europe (under Prof. L. Aschoff and Prof. R. Rössle) and the U.S.A., in 1927 he was appointed Professor of Pathology at the Chiba Medical College, Chiba, where he conducted extensive research on renal as well as allergic diseases.

A new era for autoimmunity and autoimmune disease was developing to break through Ehrlich's doctrine of horror autotoxicus when in 1931 Masugi produced nephrotoxic nephritis and believed its pathogenesis should theoretically be reverse anaphylaxis. It is not surprising that, as is usual, contemporary investigators did not know the true implications of Masugi's highly artificial but highly sophisticated experiment (see Chapters 1 and 6).

This Masugi's model characterized by its high reproducibility was the subject of numerous further investigations for several decades.

Subsequent studies have revealed that nephrotoxic serum or Masugi nephritis comprises a direct effect of heterologous antikidney antibodies to renal glomeruli and their subsequent interaction with autologous antibodies produced. Although the underlying mechanisms are complicated and rather unique, the results of investigation on this experimental model have stimulated the performance of further studies on hetero- as well as autoimmune experimental models. And careful examinations have greatly contributed to establishing our current concept concerning immunopathology of glomerulonephritis in general. Advances in the studies of immunologically induced experimental glomerulonephritis have been reviewed by Unanue and Dixon (1967) and other authors (see Chapters 5 and 6).

---

* See also Masugi, M.: Über die experimentelle Glomerulonephritis durch das spezifische Antinierenserum. Ein Beitrag zur Pathogenese der diffusen Glomerulonephritis. *Beitr. path. Anat. 92*: 429–466, 1934.

Chapters 1–6 in this book delineate a survey of previous and recent studies on Masugi nephritis and some other immunologically induced experimental models. Especially, in Chapter 2, a new concept accounting for the pathogenesis of nephrotoxic nephritis is introduced.

It is believed that the unifying concept for diverse experimental models is so important that in every model of nephritis it is essential to search for a possible coherent underlying pathogenic mechanism. Various animal models of glomerulonephritis established until now are claimed to develop on the basis of more or less different mechanisms. These, however, are mostly, if not entirely, connected by a subtle tie with the immune response. If possible, a unifying concept from the immunologic aspect should therefore be introduced to realize a coherent process operating in diverse nephritis models. Though the work is difficult, the effort must still be made. Our attempt in this respect may be seen especially in Chapter 6.

Chapters 7 and 8 concern some of the clinical implications of experimental nephritides at the present time.

We are deeply grateful to those contributors who have found time to prepare these chapters and are highly appreciative of their enthusiasm for this book. Also, the cooperation and assistance of the publishers in the production of this book are gratefully acknowledged.

Atsushi OKABAYASHI, M.D.
Yoichiro KONDO, M.D.

Department of Pathology
School of Medicine, Chiba University
Chiba, Japan

Contents

Chapter 3
Immunohistochemistry of Nephrotoxic Nephritis

Chapter 4
Scanning Electron Microscopy of the Glomerulus in Masugi Nephritis of Rabbits

Chapter 6
Nephrotoxic Serum Nephritis and Some Other Immunologically
Induced Experimental Models: A Coherent View

Chapter 7
Renal Tissue Antigens and Antikidney Antibodies in the Serum and
Urine of Patients with Glomerular, or Tubular and Interstitial Renal
Diseases

Chapter 8
Clinical Implications of Masugi and Other Immunologically Induced Experimental Glomerulonephropathies

Chapter 1

Pathology of Masugi Nephritis
Forty years' progress and present status

Teruo FUJIMOTO

I. Introduction

In 1931 and 1932 Masugi et al. [86, 87] in the Department of Pathology, Chiba University succeeded in inducing experimentally renal lesions closely resembling human diffuse glomerulonephritis by means of injections of heterologous anti-kidney sera into rats and rabbits. Since that time the experimental renal disease, so-called Masugi nephritis, has been reinvestigated and confirmed by many investigators. The nature of Masugi nephritis, however, has not been completely elucidated in spite of the numerous contributions to this field of experimental pathology. This has probably been due to the lack of knowledge concerning the role of anti-kidney antibody in the pathogenesis of glomerulonephritis until recent years. But, since the recent proposal of the concepts of autoimmunization, the significance of autoantibody in the pathogenesis of immunopathologic processes has been progressively a matter of common knowledge. Another obstacle in the first 20 years to the elucidation of the pathology of Masugi nephritis was lack of adequate analytical methods in this field except for conventional serological and morphological techniques. Recent advances in the methods of immunopathological analyses including radioisotope labeled or fluorescent antibody techniques, immunochemical analysis, ultrastructural study employing electron microscopy, etc. have been offering much promise in the solution of the still unsettled problems.

II. Early Investigations

There have been two controversial opinions regarding the pathogenesis of diffuse glomerulonephritis, one is the theory of inflammation of the glomeruli and the other is that of contraction of the afferent arteriole followed by anemia of the glomeruli. One of the reasons appeared to be the lack of knowledge about the initial lesions of glomerulonephritis even though there have been some reports about war nephritis. Accordingly, considerable effort has been devoted to elucidate the pathology of glomerulonephritis, but many investigators were not able to succeed in the induction of diffuse glomerulonephritis except for some sporadic occurrence of glomerulonephritis in a very small proportion of experimental animals treated with bacterial infection or injection of heterologous protein.

III. Experimental Glomerulonephritis Induced by Anti-Kidney Serum (Masugi Nephritis)

Before Masugi et al. [86, 87] succeeded in inducing glomerulonephritis by means of injection of heterologous anti-kidney serum there had been many studies on the specific pathogenic action of heterologous anti-kidney antibody upon the kidney since Lindemann [78]. In these studies the urinary tubular epithelium was considered to be the target of the nephrotoxic action. In 1931 and 1932 Masugi et al. [86, 87] were able to produce renal lesions, closely resembling human glomerulonephritis, in rats and rabbits by means of injections of heterologous anti-kidney sera. When anti-rat-kidney rabbit serum was injected intravenously into rats the animals developed a glomerulonephritis characterized by thickening of loop walls immediately after the administration of the serum and by endothelial proliferation 9 to 15 days after injection of the serum [88]. The initial glomerular lesion exhibited a picture of circulatory disturbance such as plasma stasis, fibrin thrombosis, or stasis roughly proportional to the low, medium, or high titers of the anti-kidney antibody. In the rabbits injected with anti-rabbit-kidney duck serum a glomerulonephritis characterized by anemic capillaritis was induced 4 to 11 days after injection [89]. The experimental glomerular lesions were accompanied with clinical features of glomerulonephritis such as albuminuria, hematuria, hypertension, increase of nonprotein nitrogen, etc. Masugi [89] produced various types and phases of glomerulonephritis, i.e., acute, subacute glomerulonephritis, secondarily contracted kidneys, and fulminant glomerulonephritis with stasis or fibrin thrombosis of glomeruli. Masugi [90, 91] stated that the mechanism involved in the glomerulonephritis induced in rats and rabbits lies in the action of anti-kidney antibody upon kidney, a reverse anaphylaxis, and the latent period observed in the rabbit nephritis is the time needed for the fixation of anti-kidney antibody to the antigenic kidney tissue. Ogawa and Sato [111] pointed out that serum complement levels of the rabbits injected with anti-rabbit-kidney duck serum decreased when glomerulonephritis was induced in these animals.

IV. Further Progress in the Researches for Masugi Nephritis

1. Fundamental pathologic processes in Masugi nephritis

a. Renal lesions

1) Masugi nephritis induced in rats by injections of anti-rat-kidney rabbit serum. Smadel [141, 143], Smadel and Farr [142], and Swift and Smadel [153], repeating Masugi's experiment, interpreted the renal lesions as glomerulonephritis as Masugi had. Heymann et al. [50, 51, 52] were the first to point out that the experimental renal disease in rats more colsely resembles the nephrotic syndrome of infants and children than it does glomerulonephritis. Lippman et al. [80, 81] described mild proliferative glomerulitis with moderate tubular degeneration appearing as early as 30 minutes after administration of a single dose of anti-kidney gammaglobulin and reaching a maximum damage at one week. Lippman and Jacobs [82] demonstrated that the administration of nephrotoxic globulin into the rat does not result in tubular ischemia. Ehrich et al. [28] stated that the renal disease caused by anti-kidney serum in rats varies with the dose and potency of the serum. According to this study, large doses or potent sera caused lipid nephrosis commencing immediately after injection, whereas in smaller doses, or if potent, anti-kidney serum produced intracapillary glomerulonephritis after a latent period of one week. The lipid nephrosis in rats was characterized morphologically by fibrinoid degeneration of the glomerular membrane which was not proceeded by or associated with proliferation of endothelium. The interpretation of the dissimilarities in the pathologic processes to be dependent upon the potencies of the anti-kidney serum as stated here was later supported by Fisher and Gruhn [34]. Weinreb et al. [170], through quantitative studies of Masugi nephritis in rats, concluded that (a) the acute disease produced in rats can resemble either nephritis or "pure" lipid nephrosis depending on the severity of the process, (b) glomerular changes can be relatively slight at this stage and yet proteinuria may be present, and (c) the chronic disease induced by the same procedure resembles chronic glomerulonephritis with nephrotic clinical manifestations.   Piel et al. [122], first introducing electron microscopy into the study of the experimental renal disease in rats, described osmiophilic material lining the foot processes of epithelial cells at 1 hour after injection and prominent thickening of the basement membrane by 6 hours.   The latter change persisted throughout 10 weeks of their observations.   Bohle et al. [15] and Miller and Bohle [95] observed early predominant thickening of lamina densa 1 to 6 hours after injection and swelling of the endothelial cells with increase in numbers of mitochondria and endoplasmic reticulum 72 to 96 hours after injection.   According to Hackel and Heymann [44] chronic renal disease leading to severe uremia was produced in 65 rats following injection of rabbit anti-rat-kidney serum, and in the arterial walls there were calcified medial lesions in 39 rats and lipid deposits in 18 rats. In these animals the existence of secondary hyperparathyroidism was also noticed.   Churg et al. [21] described intimal swelling and vacuolization of the endothelium which subsided later, and swelling, distortion, and disappearance of the foot processes which were most evident 1 to 3 days after injection.   They also noticed thickening and splitting of the capillary basement membrane with fragmentation of the outer split layer, widening of the intercapillary spaces with mild cellular proliferation, increase in basement membrane branches and deposition of fine fibrils.   According to the study of Feldman et al. [33] rabbit nephrotoxic serum or gammaglobulin induced an immediate proteinuria.   In this primary phase glomerular basement membranes were thickened by fine deposits (a complex of rabbit gammaglobulin and host complement).   There were also endothelial cell hyperplasia and swelling, and mesangial zone dilatation.   The primary phase was limited and reversible, because rats tolerant to rabbit gammaglobulin recovered morphologically and their proteinuria disappeared.   A second phase began 5 to 7 days after injection of nephrotoxin, in normal untreated rats only, and was signaled by persistence or increase of proteinuria.   Between basement membrane and endothelial cells appeared dense, nonhomogeneous deposits which were probably complexes of host gammaglobulin, rabbit gammaglobulin and complement. During the ensuing weeks the deposits were incorporated into the basement membranes, which became thickened and distorted.   There were also progressive alterations of endothelial, mesangial and epithelial cells, which, with the distorted basement membranes, resulted in glomerular destruction.   Phase 2 alterations did not occur in tolerant rats unable to make an antibody response to the rabbit gammaglobulin bound to basement membranes.   There was, therefore, no evidence that an autoimmune anti-kidney antibody was a component of nephrotoxic serum nephritis.   Fujimoto et al. [38] observed a biphasic course of the renal disease by means of follow-up studies employing repeated renal biopsies.   They described thickening of lamina densa and subendothelial deposition of electron dense fibrinoid substance not infrequently associated with capillary thrombosis of glomeruli in the first phase (Fig. 1-1), and swelling and proliferation of capillary endothelial cells in the swollen glomerular loops 4 to 7 days after injection and formation of basement membrane-like structures along these proliferated cells thereafter (Fig. 1-2).   In the anti-kidney serum nephritis of rats animals with arteritis (32 of 51 rats with necrotizing arteritis, and 11 with acute arteritis) showed moderately advanced glomerular disease and comparatively little tubular atrophy, whereas 21 animals with calcific medial necrosis had advanced glomerular lesions and extensive tubular atrophy [22].

According to Cochrane et al. [23], in acute nephrotoxic nephritis induced in rats by injection of anti-rat-kidney rabbit globulin, polymorphonuclear leukocytes (polymorphs)

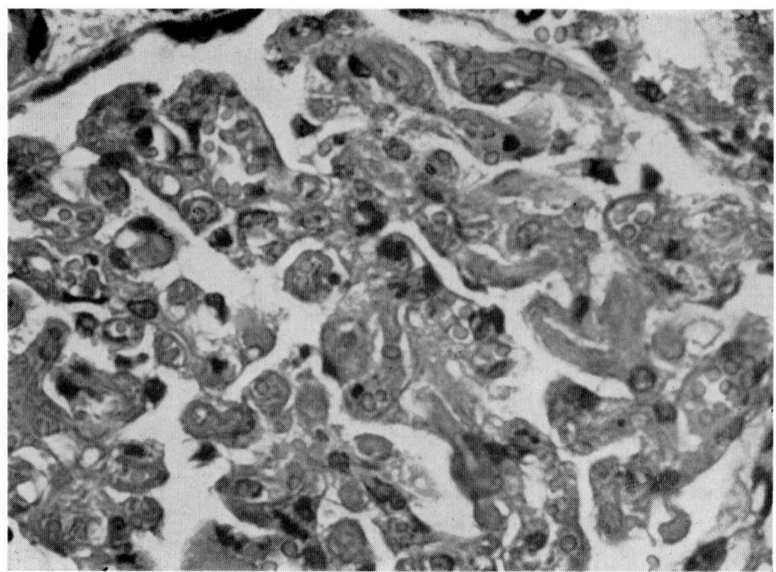

Fig. 1-1 Glomerulitis with thickening and fibrinoid degeneration of loop walls, comparable to "wire-loop" lesions, accompanied by some thrombi. HE stain. 19.30 hours after injection of anti-rat-kidney rabbit gammaglobulin. Autopsy. Rat R16. (From the work of Fujimoto, T., Okada, M., Kondo, Y., and Tada, T.)

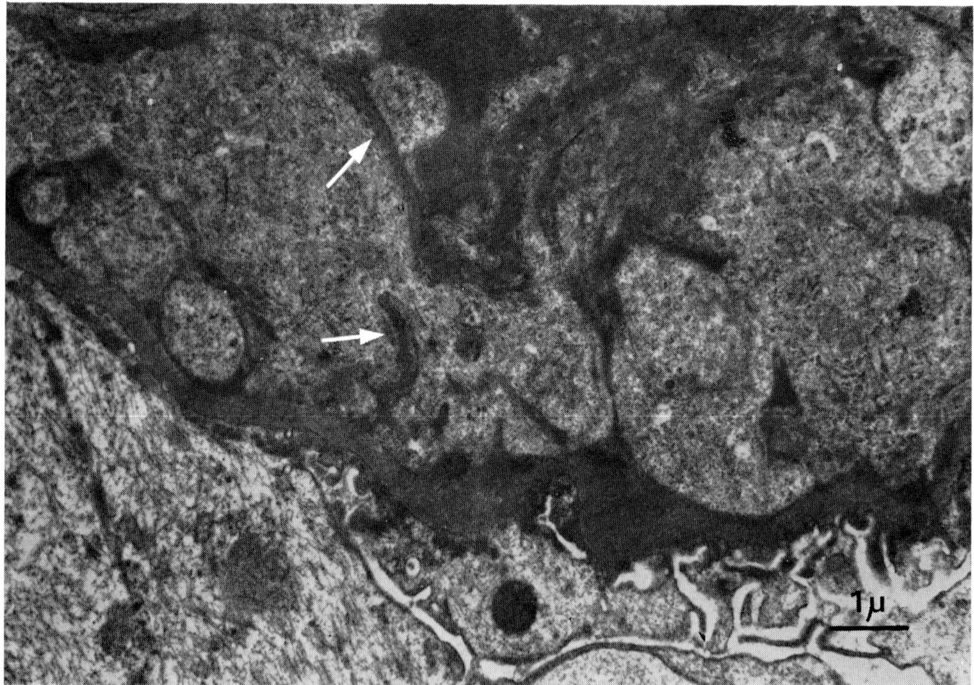

Fig. 1-2 Subendothelial deposition of fibrinoid substance and thickening of lamina densa of glomerular loop associated with swelling and proliferation of endothelial cells. Formation of basement membrane-like materials as indicated with arrows along these proliferated cells is seen. 7 days after exacerbation (14 days after injection of anti-rat-kidney rabbit gammaglobulin). Autopsy. Rat R70. (From the work of Fujimoto, T., Okada, M., Kondo, Y., and Tada, T.)

accumulated in large numbers in the glomeruli during the first 12 hours.   The endothelial cells were dislodged by the polymorphs which caused them to lie immediately adjacent to the glomerular basement membranes.   Depletion of polymorphs in rats prevented the development of proteinuria.   Elimination of polymorphs from the circulation was only partially effective in preventing glomerular damage when large doses of nephrotoxic globulins were used.   This indicated that under these circumstances, a polymorph-independent glomerular injury may also take place during the first stage of nephrotoxic nephritis.   Shigematsu [136] reported that in the initial phase of Masugi nephritis of rats induced by a single intravenous injection of rabbit nephrotoxic gammaglobulin, neutrophil infiltration and mononuclear cell (monocyte) accumulation were noted.   From 2 to 12 hours there was a prominent infiltration of neutrophils and platelets together with an enhanced formation of fibrin thrombi in the capillary lumen.   At the ultrastructural level the endothelial layer was dislodged on the neutrophils attached to the denuded basement membrane.   Degranulation and destructive changes were observed in the neutrophils.   From 12 to 72 hours neutrophil infiltration and clotting substances were rapidly diminished and a large number of monocytes accumulated in the lumen.   These monocytes were transformed into macrophages and giant cells.   Within 72 hours both thrombotic changes and monocytic reaction disappeared, and then the injured endothelial layer was gradually repaired by elongation of the cytoplasm and by mitosis of the endothelial cells.   Kobayashi [64], on the basis of the study of Masugi nephritis induced in rats by injection of rabbit γM antibody, concluded that rabbit γM antibody against the glomerular basement membrane has nephritogenic properties in rats similar to that of γG antibody, although the activity of the former antibody appeared to be somewhat less than that of the latter. Shigematsu and Kobayashi [137] studied the glomerular changes in the secondary phase of Masugi nephritis induced in rats by injection of weak anti-rat-kidney rabbit gammaglobulin.   In the secondary phase, rabbit gammaglobulin, autologous gammaglobulin and complement were usually observed along the glomerular basement membrane with a characteristic linear pattern by the fluorescent antibody technique.   Moreover, they clarified the point that prominent granular localization of the fluorescence of each component is also confirmed electron microscopically as subepithelial deposits.   They also observed abundant accumulations of migrant monocytes (macrophages) in the glomerular capillary loops, which were supposed to be concerned with the removal of the subendothelial deposits.   Irreversible glomerular injury in the secondary phase of rat Masugi nephritis was studied by Shigematsu and Kobayashi [139].   According to them the simplification of the glomerular tufts initiated from mesangiolysis resulted in glomerular intracapillary disorganization, and the extracapillary exudation often associated with the rupture of glomerular basement membrane caused crescent formation or periglomerular graunlomatous inflammation.

2) Masugi nephritis induced in rabbits by injections of anti-rabbit-kidney duck serum.   Since the earlier works of Masugi et al. [87, 89], Hemprich [49], Weiss [171], Tsuji [157], Ehrich et al. [27, 28], Asano [5], etc. it has been well established that the renal disease induced in rabbits by injections of anti-rabbit-kidney duck serum closely resembles human diffuse glomerulonephritis.   It has been also a characteristic feature that the disease begins after a latent period of 4 to 11 days following the injection.   Fujimoto [35], Fujimoto and Akashi [36], and Fujimoto and Yamanaka [37] first ascertained the mode of development of the glomerular changes in the same individual animals on the basis of the findings of biopsy materials surgically resected on consecutive days.   According to the study it was clarified that the glomerular alterations appeared simultaneously with the onset of albuminuria. The typical changes accompanied by marked endothelial proliferation of glomerular loops were summarized and expressed as the transformation of glomerular capillary and its intercapillary connective tissue into enmeshed structure, or disorganization of the glomerular architecture following histolysis (Fig. 1-3). The subsequent course was characterized by total or axial fibrosis of a new structural material. In the case of milder proliferative glomerulitis the initial stage was characterized by edematous swelling of capillary walls and the subsequent course by diffuse (axial and peripheral) or axial sclerosis in the swollen capillary walls, whereas in the severer or more extreme case the initial phase was characterized by necrosis of glomerular loops following thrombosis or stasis and the subsequent stage by organization of the necrotic area by granulation tissue formed from the adjacent Bowman's capsule and its surrounding tissue. In 1957 Sakaguchi et al. [128] first introduced electron microscopy into the study of Masugi nephritis of rabbits, and interpreted the hypercellularity of glomeruli to be caused by proliferation of mesangial cells on the basis of the findings in individual animals at autopsy. By means of repeated biopsies in the same individual animals, Fujimoto et al. [38] clarified the pathologic processes of rabbit nephritis. According to this study, there were no lesions consistent with glomerulitis or glomerular inflammation in the latent period. The characteristic findings appeared simultaneously with the onset of albuminuria. They were characterized by swelling, hypercellularity, and anemia of glomeruli produced by swelling and proliferation of capillary endothelial cells with enmeshed or reticular arrangement in the earlier stage of the disease, and subsequently there appeared an increase of basement membrane-like materials along these proliferated cells (Fig. 1-4) followed by crowding of proliferated cells toward the axial portion of the loops and recirculation in the peripherally arranged blood space a few days later. According to the study of Matsuura [93] with vital staining of renal glomeruli of Masugi nephritic rabbits, there were found phagocytic endothelial cells, commom endothelial cells, mesangial cells, and endothelium-like cells. The large "endothelial cells" (syncytial and frequently transformed into multinuclear giant cells) appearing in the nephritic glomeruli were not a single kind of cells. In the stages soon before and after the onset of the nephritis, the majority of them consisted of the common endothelial cells, and in the severest stage, of the endothelium-like cells. In the latent stage and thereafter, they were composed of miscellaneous, namely degenerating endothelium-like cells, regenerating common and phagocytic endothelial cells, and mesangial cells reconstructing the mesangial tissue. According to Kondo and Shigematsu [67] severe proliferative glomerulonephritis was induced, after a latent period, by the single injection of a small amount of anti-rabbit-kidney duck gammaglobulin, and the glomerular lesions recovered within 27 days. In this study it was concluded that the glomerular hypercellularity was mainly caused by the prominent accumulation of monocytes in contrast to some contribution of endothelial and mesangial cells. Kondo et al. [68] also revealed that injection of large amounts of nephrotoxic duck antibody caused crescentic glomerulonephritis in rabbits. In glomeruli, proliferation of endothelial and mesangial cells, infiltration of polymorphonuclear leukocytes, marked accumulation of monocytic clear cells (epithelioid cells), fibrin deposition, and local necrosis of the tufts were observed from an early stage of the disease process. In these lesions disorganization of the glomerular structure, in particular rupture of the glomerular basement membrane leading to disappearance of some lobuli was distinct. The proliferation of glomerular and capsular epithelial cells appeared around the necrotic area. The authors stressed that the so-called epithelial crescent consisted of proliferated epithelial cells as well as monocytic-epithelioid cells which migrated from the glomerular capillaries into the Bowman's capsular spaces. Throughout the conclusions of these two reports [67, 68], it appears that not only detailed electron microscopic observations but also

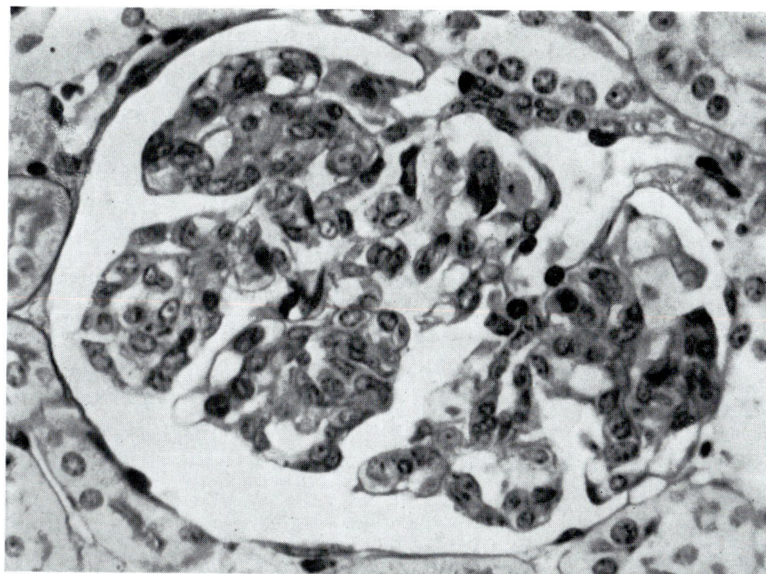

Fig. 1-3   Proliferative glomerulitis with transformation of glomerular loop architecture into enmeshed structure. PAS stain. One day after onset of albuminuria (7 days after injection of anti-rabbit-kidney duck serum). 3rd biopsy. Rabbit R283. (From Fujimoto, T.: *Acta Path. Jap. 4*: 1–19, 1954, Fig. 7)

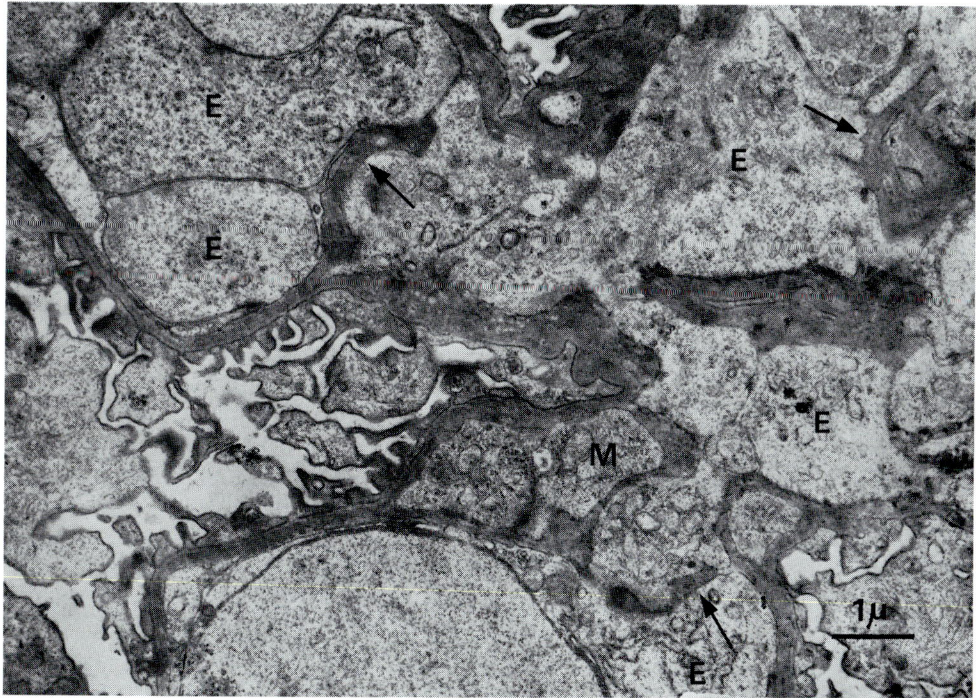

Fig. 1-4   Formation of basement membrane-like materials with similar electron density to that of lamina densa as indicated with arrows along the proliferated endothelial cells (E). 3 days after onset of albuminuria (9 days after injection of anti-rabbit-kidney duck serum). 3rd biopsy. Rabbit S651. (From Fujimoto, T., Okada, M., Kondo, Y., and Tada, T.: *Acta Path. Jap. 14*: 275–310, 1964, Fig. 18)

further insights into histologic organization are necessary in order to determine the origin of proliferated cells in glomeruli more correctly. For instance, knowledge of the difference between behavioristic features both of proliferated cells facing the blood stream and those existing intramurally is at least required for the correct understanding of the origin of proliferated cells.

3) Masugi nephritis induced in rats by injections of anti-rat-kidney duck serum. Heymann et al. [52] first injected nephrotoxic sera obtained from ducks into rats and induced diffuse proliferative glomerulonephritis with a latent period varying from 3 to 21 days. Stavitsky et al. [149] reported development of renal disease without a latent period in 10 to 20 per cent of rats following injection of duck anti-rat-kidney serum. Hasson et al. [47] also reported induction of an immediate or delayed nephritis by injections of anti-rat-kidney duck serum and suggested that the latent period often seen following injection of duck anti-rat-kidney serum results from the low titer of nephrotoxic antibody and not from a peculiar property of the duck serum. Fujimoto et al. [38] described the development of renal disease characterized by proliferative glomerulitis 4 to 7 days after injection through follow-up studies by repeated renal biopsies.

In acute nephrotoxic nephritis induced in rats by injection of anti-rat-kidney duck globulin Cochrane et al. [23] observed accumulation of polymorphonuclear leukocytes (polymorphs) in glomeruli in the first 12 hours, and following dislodgement of endothelial cells caused by attachment of polymorphs to the glomerular basement membranes. It was also revealed that depletion of polymorphs in rats prevented the development of proteinuria.

4) Masugi nephritis induced in rats by injections of anti-rat-kidney sheep serum. According to Winemiller et al. [172] potent nephrotoxic anti-rat-glomerular basement membrane sheep serum injected into rats produced early proteinuria. Electron microscopic study revealed focal exfoliation of the endothelial cytoplasm, occlusion of capillary lumina with leukocytes and platelets, penetration of neutrophils through the endothelial cell layer, fibrin thrombi, foot process fusion 4 to 12 hours after injection, and endothelial cell proliferation and basement membrane changes of greater severity on 4th and 9th days.

5) Masugi nephritis induced in a rabbit by injection of anti-rabbit-kidney guinea pig serum. Fujimoto et al. [38] recognized early proteinuria 3 hours after injection of anti-rabbit-kidney guinea pig gammaglobulin into a rabbit and were able to observe a glomerulonephritis characterized by thickening and fibrinoid degeneration of glomerular loop walls at autopsy 3 days later.

6) Masugi nephritis induced in rabbits by injections of anti-rabbit-kidney sheep serum. According to Vassalli and McCluskey [165] injections of anti-rabbit-kidney sheep serum resulted in induction of a severe proliferative glomerulonephritis with frequent fibrinoid deposits in glomeruli, crescent formation and progressive diffuse glomerular sclerosis. Immunofluorescent studies with anti-fibrinogen serum showed positive staining, not only within fibrin deposits but also diffusely within proliferating intracapillary cells. It was shown that these cells were highly phagocytic for circulating colloidal carbon and by electron microscopy that they ingested fibrin. When rabbits were given injections of rabbit anti-sheep-gammaglobulin antibodies shortly after the administration of sheep nephrotoxic serum, massive intraglomerular fibrin deposition occurred rapidly. Treatment with anti-coagulant Warfarin resulted not only in the prevention or suppression of intracapillary cell swelling and proliferation, but also in complete prevention of crescent formation and glomerular sclerosis.

Cochrane et al. [23] revealed that in acute nephrotoxic nephritis induced in rabbits by injection of anti-rabbit-kidney sheep globulin polymorphonuclear leukocytes (polymorphs) accumulated in glomeruli in the first 12 hours, causing dislodgement of endothelial cells and attachment of polymorphs to glomerular basement membranes. Depletion of polymorphs in rabbits resulted in prevention of the development of proteinuria.

7) Masugi nephritis induced in dogs by injections of anti-dog-kidney rabbit serum. Hayasi [48] reported that development of glomerulonephritis was observed in dogs sacrificed on the day when anti-dog-kidney rabbit serum was injected through 11th day. Movat and Steiner [99] and Movat et al. [100] described early proteinuria 3 to 4 days after injection. In the first phase the dog glomeruli showed swelling and fragmentation of glomerular basement membrane, whereas there appeared intracapillary (endothelial and mesangial) cellular proliferation, deposition of electron dense substance between endothelial cells and basement membrane as well as in proliferated cells in the second phase (after 7 days). Swollen and proliferated intracapillary cells were provided with numerous organelles in their cytoplasms, and the epithelial cells exhibited increase of mitochondria and granular endoplasmic reticulum, vacuolization, formation of hyaline droplet, and fusion of foot processes.

8) Masugi nephritis induced in monkeys by injections of anti-monkey-kidney rabbit serum. Experimental renal disease simulating the nephrotic syndrome as observed in children was produced in 5 Taiwan monkeys (*Macaca cyclopsis*) by the intravenous injection of nephrotoxic serum obtained from rabbits, while attempts to produce experimental renal disease by the intravenous injection of anti-monkey-kidney serum obtained from ducks failed in Taiwan monkeys [56]. Battifora and Markowitz [8] reported the sequential studies of nephrotoxic nephritis in monkeys, in which electron dense deposits of variable appearance became prominent after 4 weeks and were virtually restricted to the subepithelial space, increasing progressively thereafter. From the findings they postulated that these deposits may be species-related and have been overlooked in other species by previous investigators because of their shorter follow-up periods.

b. Lesions of various other organs

1) Rats injected with anti-rat-kidney rabbit serum. Fujimoto et al. [38] reported that hyperplasia of bone marrow, spleen, liver (Glisson's capsules), and lymph nodes with plasma cellular reaction took place in 8 of 10 rats which survived more than 4 days after injection of anti-rat-kidney rabbit serum. Besides these changes of antibody-forming organs occurrence of diffuse or focal pneumonitis (33 of 38 rats), interstitial myocarditis (10 rats including one with myocarditis of rheumatic type), congestion, hemorrhage, and necrosis of liver (24 rats), and interstitial rhabdomyositis with myofiber lesions (2 rats) was recognized. Shigematsu and Kobayashi [138] studied the pulmonary involvement in the initial phase of rat Masugi nephritis using light, fluorescent and electron microscopes. According to their studies, the animals which received large doses of anti-rat-kidney rabbit gammaglobulin died of acute pulmonary edema soon after the injection, and the rabbit gammaglobulin and rat β_{1c}-globulin were seen to be bound diffusely along the alveolar capillary wall, while the other animals that survived showed focal binding of these two components along the alveolar wall and focal transient and recoverable pneumonitis characterized by hypercellularity attributed to the accumulation of neutrophils and monocytes in the interalveolar septa and alveolar hemorrhage. From their experiment they concluded that there are similar pathogenetic mechanisms in the development of the lesions of both the kidney and the lung.

2) Rabbits injected with anti-rabbit-kidney duck serum. Rabbits that were sacrificed or died 5 to 29 days after injection showed hyperplasia with plasma cellular reaction of bone marrow, spleen, and lymph nodes [38]. Seven, 2, and 3 of 11 animals demonstrated proliferative pneumonitis, interstitial myocarditis, and interstitial rhabdomyositis with myofiber damages respectively.

3) Rats injected with anti-rat-kidney duck serum. Eight of 9 rats autopsied 4 to 18 days after injection had hyperplasia and plasma cellular reactions of bone marrow, spleen, liver (Glisson's capsules), and lymph nodes [38]. Moreover, all except 2 of these 9 rats showed proliferative pneumonitis and interstitial myocarditis.

4) Rabbit injected with anti-rabbit-kidney guinea pig serum. Focal necrosis of myocardium and diffuse pneumonitis developed in the rabbit when autopsied 3 days after injection [38].

Addendum.   Serum and urinary protein patterns in Masugi nephritis

Sumiyoshi [152] reported early increase of total protein and marked diminution after onset of albuminuria, marked decrease of serum albumin after onset of albuminuria, and increase of globulin after injection of anti-rabbit-kidney duck serum into rabbits and especially after the onset of the disease. Urinary protein consisted largely of albumin. Maeda [85] noted increase of gammaglobulin in the urine when glomerulonephritis was predominant.

2. Immunological response against anti-kidney serum

1) Masugi nephritis induced in rats by injections of anti-rat-kidney rabbit serum. Pressman and Keighley [124], utilizing 131I-labeled method, clarified that anti-rat-kidney serum iodinated, upon inoculation into rats, localized in the kidney with the greatest activity per gram of tissues among various organs. Takeda [154] supported Masugi's view that the nature of the nephrotoxic nephritis in rats is a reverse anaphylaxis in the kidney, and stated that no further exacerbation of rat nephritis is probable in the later stage. Pfeiffer et al. [118] pointed out that mode of development of Masugi nephritis in rats is monophasic, immediate, and accompanied by lowered serum complement levels, and here antibody against rabbit serum is not contributory. Stavitsky et al. [148] concluded that complement may be reduced in vivo as a result of extrarenal tissue antigen-antibody reactions from the study of the experiment in which anti-rat-kidney rabbit serum was injected into normal or bilaterally nephrectomized rats or after antibodies to rat plasma and rat red cells had been removed. Mellors et al. [94] and Ortega and Mellors [116], applying fluorescent antibody technique to the elucidation of immunohistochemical events in rat Masugi nephritis, observed that autologous antibody localized primarily in the membrane of glomerular tufts in a pattern that corresponded closely to that of nephrotoxins from 6 to 9 days to 3 months. They considered these findings to be consistent with the pathogenesis of nephrotoxic nephritis, as postulated in rabbit Masugi nephritis by Kay [60]. According to Goodman and Baxter [41] injection of the blue dye into nephrotic rats with proteinuria due to administration of nephrotoxic anti-rat-kidney serum was followed by blue staining of the cortex of the kidneys. This was thought to indicate that protein reabsorption by the tubular cells was greater than normal, and that the proteinuria was a result of increased glomerular permeability and not of decreased tubular reabsorption of normally filtered protein. Seegal [130] observed the localization and retention of nephrotoxic rabbit serum in the glomeruli of rats for at least 10 months. Localization in extrarenal sites particularly in cells of red pulp of spleen and in cells lining capillaries of adrenals was also recognized. Evidence for the presence of nephrotoxic sera in the liver and lung was not obtained. Klein and Burkholder [62], by means of fluorescent antibody technique, demonstrated fixation of guinea pig complement to glomeruli of rats injected with anti-rat-kidney rabbit serum and sacrificed 2 hours later. Hiramoto et al. [55] studied the in vivo localization of anti-rat-kidney rabbit antibody 18 hours after injection by immunohistochemical procedures. Fixation to a high concentration was observed in ovary, spleen, kidney, and adrenal. A lower concentration was seen in thyroid, lymph nodes, and liver, while none was observed in testis, lung, skin, brain, and heart. Vogt and Kochem [166], using histoserologic technique, revealed immediate fixation of anti-rat-kidney rabbit serum to the basement membrane of the glomerulus, and the simultaneous complement fixation at the site of localization of anti-kidney serum. Burkholder [18] also demonstrated by means of immunohistochemical technique that the sites of rabbit globulin fixation in glomerular capillary walls of rat kidney were the same sites at which guinea pig complement was fixed in vitro. Andres et al. [1] demonstrated the localization of anti-rat-kidney rabbit gammaglobulin in basement membrane of glomerular loops and basement membrane-like substance of dilated epithelial cisternae by means of ferritin-conjugated antibody techniques. Seegal et al. [131] observed the persistence of anti-kidney gammaglobulin in rat glomeruli 291 days after injection as far as examined. Hammer and Dixon [45] presented the following idea about pathogenesis of nephrotoxic rabbit serum nephritis in rats: The primary phase of nephrotoxic nephritis appears to be dependent to a great extent, but not completely upon the participation of serum complement, while the secondary phase appears to depend largely or entirely upon the host's antibody response to the heterologous gammaglobulin fixed in the glomeruli. No evidence could be available for the existence of an autoimmune antibody response by the host in their study. Unanue and Dixon [159] clarified the localization of rat β_{1c}-globulin as well as an ability to fix guinea pig complement in the glomerular basement membrane in the first and second phases by fluorescent antibody technique. Fujimoto et al. [38] and Fujimoto [39] mentioned that anti-rat-kidney rabbit antibody which fixes to glomerular membrane plays a pathogenic role in the occurrence of a degenerative glomerulitis (fibrinoid degeneration of loop walls) in the first phase, and an exacerbation characterized by proliferative glomerulitis takes place in the second phase due to the reaction between rabbit gammaglobulin already localized in the glomerular loop walls and rat antibody against rabbit gammaglobulin (Fig. 1-5). ^{131}I-labeled method and fluorescent antibody technique revealed localization of anti-kidney rabbit gammaglobulin in alveolar walls, liver, spleen, lymph nodes, etc. in addition to kidneys. Nagasawa et al. [103] recognized early localization of fluorescent labeled anti-rat-kidney rabbit gammaglobulin in the proper basement membrane of rat glomeruli immediately after its intravenous injection. According to Okuda et al. [114] diffuse staining of glomerular capillary loops appeared in rats 7 to 10 days after injection of rabbit anti-rat-kidney serum, and persisted for 6 months. Unanue and Dixon [160] showed that in order to produce immediate proteinuria an amount of rabbit gamma-2 kidney-fixing antibody capable of occupying approximately 45 per cent or more of the capillary filtration

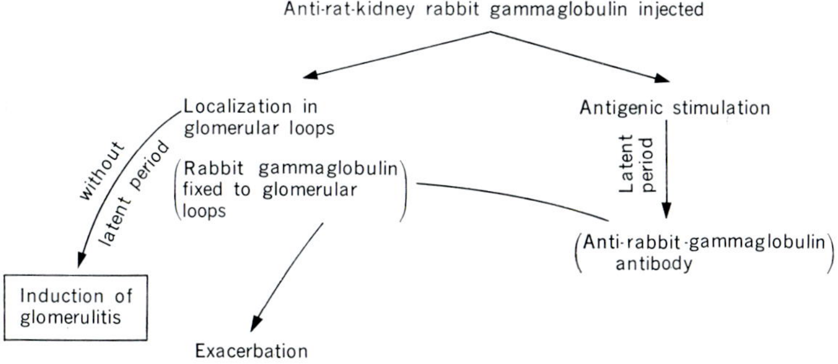

Fig. 1-5 Mechanism of Masugi nephritis induced in rats by injections of anti-rat-kidney rabbit serum. (From Fujimoto, T., Okada, M., Kondo, Y., and Tada, T.: *Acta Path. Jap. 14*: 275–310, 1964, Fig. 10)

surface was needed. All nephrotoxic antibodies in hyperimmune rabbit nephrotoxic sera were of the gamma-2 variety. Mercaptoethanol had no effect on rabbit gamma-2. They also postulated, on the basis of their studies of experimental glomerulonephritis induced in rats by injection of anti-rat-kidney antibody and immunization to the heterologous rabbit gammaglobulin supplying the nephrotoxic antibody, that in the presence of excess circulating antibody, antigens occupying at most a small percent of the glomerular capillary surface can provide an antigen-antibody interaction which will over a period of time cause detectable morphologic and functional alterations of the glomerulus [161]. Nakanoin and Vogt [106] reported that if quantities of rabbit anti-rat-kidney sera sufficient to cause nephritis in all animals of the test group were injected, the proteinuria appeared without a latent period, which may be attributed to the ability of rabbit anti-kidney antibody to fix mammalian complement. Vogt et al. [168] reported that electron microscopy revealed a heavy accumulation of the basement membrane-fixed ferritin-conjugated rabbit antibodies almost exclusively at the endothelial side after intravenous injection into rats. At least 40 basement membrane-fixed antibody molecules from the rabbit per 3,000 mμ^2 of filtration surface were needed to cause immediate nephritis. Ooami [115] clarified that sites of antigen-antibody reaction in the nephrotoxic nephritis lie in lamina rara interna on the basis of ultrastructural study of Masugi nephritis induced by injection of anti-rat-kidney rabbit gammaglobulin using immunoferritin technique. Warnatz et al. [169] pointed out that lymphocytes do not play a role in the pathogenesis of nephrotoxic serum nephritis on the basis of the experimental results that neither autologous kidney extract nor nephrotoxic rabbit serum and normal rabbit serum caused an increased transformation of lymphocytes obtained from rats with nephrotoxic serum nephritis, while cultures of lymphocytes from these rats showed a depression of blast cell formation after being exposed to nephrotoxic serum in comparison with lymphocytes of normal rats. Chow and Drummond [20] reported that there is increased incorporation of proline into glomerular basement membrane and conversion of proline to hydroxyproline in nephrotoxic nephritic rats. Masugi [92] stated, on the basis of immunoelectron microscopic studies of nephrotoxic nephritis in rats, that the mechanisms involved in the beginning and progression of the nephritis are the initial binding of heterologous anti-kidney antibodies to the intrarenal antigenic determinants, which are supposed to be concentrated mainly along the laminae densae of the glomerular basement membranes and partially in the mesangial matrices, and followed by gradually increased corporation of complement β_{1c}-components; appearance of the hitherto formed immune complexes in the lamina rara interna of the basement membranes and in the mesangial areas by non-immunological transportation and deposition; and the successive interactions between the immune complexes and the mesangial cells. According to Beregi and v. Mayersbach [11] the nephrotoxic anti-rat-kidney antibodies of rabbits were organ-specific and caused nephritis in mice and gerbils as well. The antibody localized in these animals as in rats. The pathologic alterations in the early stage of nephritis in young animals were characterized by cellular proliferation, while those in older animals by a thickening of the glomerular basement membrane. In the later stages no difference was noticed between the age groups.

  2) Masugi nephritis induced in rabbits by injections of anti-rabbit-kidney duck serum. Sarre and Wirtz [129] concluded, from their experiment in which an injection of anti-rabbit-kidney duck serum during the first several minutes of clamping of one renal artery for 15 minutes resulted in induction of glomerulonephritis only in the contralateral kidney the artery of which was not clamped, that the anti-kidney antibodies fix rapidly, at least within 15 minutes to kidney. Kay [60] presented a new hypothesis, suggested from his analysis of the experimental nephritis based on conventional serological analytical methods, that nephrotoxic nephritis is not produced by direct interaction between anti-kidney antibody and the kidney but by reaction between rabbit antibody against duck serum and duck anti-kidney antibody fixed to kidney immediately after injection.   Kay [61] reported that in rabbits injected with duck serum, either normal or nephrotoxic, several days or weeks prior to the injection of nephrotoxic serum, antibodies to duck serum reappeared rapidly and the duration of the latent period was shortened.   Spühler et al. [147] also pointed out the significance of rabbit antibody against injected anti-kidney duck serum in the pathogenesis of Masugi nephritis.   Tsuji [158], on the basis of biphasic skin reaction due to direct injection of anti-kidney serum into the skin, concluded that the nature of Masugi nephritis lies in periangitis caused by the reaction between anti-kidney serum which is rich in the pericytotrope antibody and overlying cells of the glomeruli.   Oka-bayashi et al. [112] confirmed the results of Sarre-Wirtz's experiment on the basis of follow-up histopathologic study of bilateral kidneys in the unilateral Masugi nephritis similarly induced during the period up to 96 days after injection.   Lange et al. [74] were not able to induce glomerulonephritis by means of injections of the serum of ne-phritic rabbits into normal rabbits.   Lange et al. [74], and Seegal [130] who first in-troduced fluorescent antibody technique into the analysis of Masugi nephritis in rabbits demonstrated independently that rabbit gammaglobulin localized in the glomeruli when disease appeared but not during the delay period, while duck serum localized immediately after anti-rabbit-kidney duck serum was administered.   Rother and Sarre [126] could not demonstrate formation of autoantibody against kidney throughout their observation over several months of unilateral chronic glomerulonephritis induced by injection of anti-kidney serum during the temporary clamping of contralateral renal artery for 20 minutes.   Fujimoto et al. [38] and Fujimoto [39] reported that anti-rabbit-kidney duck antibody localizes in the glomerular loop walls promptly after injection without development of glomerulitis and initiates proliferative glomerulitis when host antibody against duck gammaglobulin fixes to glomerular loops where duck gammaglo-bulin has already fixed (Fig. 1-6).   According to their studies the glomerular loop walls in which antigen-antibody complexes are localized have a property of complement fixation. They also confirmed that preceding sensitization with normal duck gammaglobulin or passive transfer of anti-duck gammaglobulin rabbit serum into rabbits, when combined with injection of anti-rabbit-kidney duck gammaglobulin, induced glomerulonephritis without a latent period (Table 1-1).   They also recognized that anti-kidney gamma-globulin localized in bone marrow, spleen, lymph nodes, liver, lungs, etc. several hours,

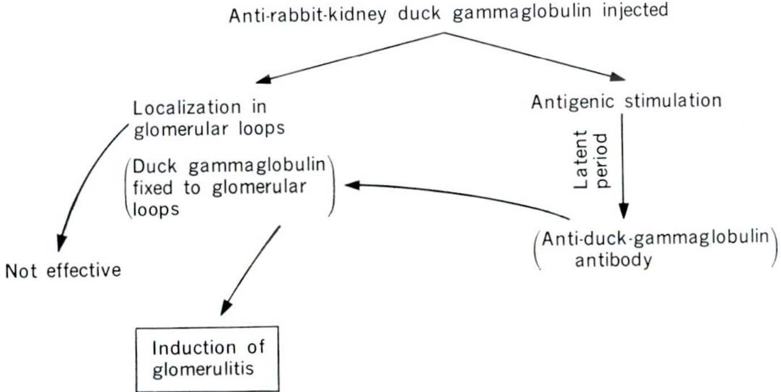

Fig. 1-6 Mechanism of Masugi nephritis induced in rabbits by injections of anti-rabbit-kidney duck serum. (From Fujimoto, T., Okada, M., Kondo, Y., and Tada, T.: *Acta Path. Jap.* 14: 275–310, 1964, Fig. 9)

Table 1-1 Various modes of induction of Masugi nephritis in rabbits.

Procedures	Localization of RabGG in glomerulus		Latent period of Masugi nephritis
	within 2 days	after 4 to 10 days	
Injection of AKDGG	−	+	+
Sensitization with DGG+Injection of AKDGG	+	+	−
Injection of soluble complex of AKDGG and anti-DGG	+	+	−
Injection of anti-DGG+Injection of AKDGG	+	+	−
Injection of AKDGG+Injection of anti-DGG	+	+	−
Injection of AKDGG+Injection of pepsin-digested anti-DGG	+	+	+

AKDGG=Anti-rabbit-kidney duck gammaglobulin
DGG=Duck gammaglobulin
Anti-DGG=Anti-duck-gammaglobulin rabbit gammaglobulin
RabGG=Rabbit gammaglobulin
(From Fujimoto, T., Okada, M., Kondo, Y., and Tada, T.: *Acta Path. Jap. 14*: 275–310, 1964, Table 4)

4, 6, 10, 15, 17, and 29 days after injection employing ^{131}I-labeled method and fluorescent antibody technique. Shibata [133] postulated that anti-rabbit-kidney duck serum localizes in and injures rabbit glomerular basement membrane, being followed by production of anti-kidney autoantibody which is significant for the occurrence and progress of glomerulonephritis. According to the study of Nagasawa et al. [104] duck gammaglobulin was found to localize selectively in the glomerular basement membrane within 20 minutes following injection of duck anti-rabbit-kidney serum and there was no remarkable loss of its intensity until the end of four weeks; subsequently the amount of duck gammaglobulin in glomeruli decreased very slowly and on 210th day it was barely perceptible as a specific fluorescence in glomeruli. In contrast, rabbit gammaglobulin appeared in the glomerular basement membrane 6 days after injection and its localization in the glomerular basement membrane corresponded closely to that of duck gammaglobulin. Its intensity reached a maximum on the 8th or 10th day and persisted for 210 days until the end of the experiment.

Lehmann et al. [76] reported that kidneys from rabbits with nephrotoxic serum nephritis demonstrated a significant increase in the incorporation of ^{14}C-amino acids into soluble protein and immunoglobulin when compared with kidneys from normal rabbits. The antibody synthesis persisted in the kidney for 33 days following the injection of the serum.

3) Masugi nephritis induced in rats by injections of anti-rat-kidney duck serum. Pressman et al. [125] showed the presence of kidney-localizing antibodies in nephrotoxic anti-rat-kidney sera prepared in ducks. Stavitsky et al. [149] pointed out that there was no correlation between the time of complement fixation and onset of renal disease in rats injected with anti-rat-kidney duck serum. In a few rats studied by them there was some correlation between the time of appearance of antibodies to duck serum and onset of disease, while in none of the rats which developed disease immediately was complement fixed concurrently. Vogt and Kochem [166] reported an early fixation of anti-rat-kidney duck serum to rat glomerular loop walls without the development of glomerulonephritis until 6 to 7 days after injection. Complement fixation was not demonstrated until the 3rd day. Seegal et al. [131] demonstrated the persistence of localization of anti-kidney duck gammaglobulin in glomeruli as far as the observation for 291 days was concerned. Hammer and Dixon [45] mentioned that duck nephrotoxic serum produces, occasionally if ever, its primary renal injury without detectable utilization of or dependence upon serum complement, while the secondary phase appears to be caused by antibody response of the host to heterologous gammaglobulin fixed to glomeruli.   Fujimoto et al. [38] and Fujimoto [39] detected localization of anti-kidney duck gammaglobulin and fixation of guinea pig complement 4 to 7 days after injection when serum complement levels were also decreased. They also demonstrated by fluorescent antibody technique and ^{131}I-labeled method, localization of the anti-kidney duck gammaglobulin in the kidneys, lungs, liver, spleen, lymph nodes, etc. 1, 7, and 13 days after injection.

Unanue and Dixon [160] revealed that in order to induce immediate proteinuria an amount of duck gamma-2 kidney-fixing antibody capable of occupying approximately 45 per cent or more of the capillary filtration surface was necessary.   Nephrotoxic antibodies in potent duck nephrotoxic sera were found in gamma-2 and gamma-1M fractions. Gamma-1M duck nephrotoxic antibody was 60 times more potent a nephritogen than gamma-2 duck nephrotoxic antibody on a molecular basis.   Mercaptoethanol abolished the nephrotoxicity of gamma-1M duck antibody, and reduced that of gamma-2 duck antibodies.

According to Nakanoin and Vogt [106], when quantities of duck antisera which cause nephritis in all of the animals of test group were used, poteinuria did not appear until after a latent period of a few days to several weeks.   This was thought to be due to the inability of duck antibody to fix mammalian complement.   Kozima et al. [70] reported that the glomeruli of all rats which were injected with strong duck nephrotoxic serum were capable of fixing complement in capillary pattern within the first day, when the proteinuria started immediately.   The staining for host β_{1c} or guinea pig β_{1c} was generally weaker than that observed in rats which had been injected with comparable amounts of rabbit nephrotoxic serum.   Fujita [40] clarified the mechanism of immediate development of nephrotoxic nephritis using duck anti-rat-kidney sera.   The deposition of the complement of the host on the glomerulus was demonstrated but only mildly.   The effective factor for prompt onset was contained in γG fraction but not in γM fraction.   The nephritogenic potency of duck nephrotoxic serum was markedly weakened by 2-mercaptoethanol.   According to the study of Vogt et al. [168] on the experimental nephritis due to injection of ferritin-conjugated duck anti-rat-kidney globulin it was revealed that a heavy accumulation of the basement membrane-fixed antibody occurred almost exclusively at the endothelial side. The once-fixed antibody remained at the site of reaction though decreasing with time. To induce nephritis using duck antibody, a larger amount of basement membrane-fixed antibody seemed to be necessary [168].

4) Masugi nephritis induced in a rabbit by injection of anti-rabbit-kidney guinea pig gammaglobulin.   Fujimoto et al. [38] and Fujimoto [39] observed early decrease of serum complement levels a few hours after injection and fixation of guinea pig complement to rabbit glomeruli in the rabbit which received anti-rabbit-kidney guinea pig gammaglobulin.

5) Masugi nephritis induced in dogs by injections of anti-dog-kidney rabbit serum.   Hayasi [48] noted the decrease of serum complement levels at the onset of glomerulonephritis, and their recovery when the nephritis subsided.

6) Masugi nephritis induced in rats by injections of anti-rat-kidney guinea pig gammaglobulin. Kobayashi et al. [65] paid attention to the non-complement mediated glomerular injury in the initial phase of Masugi nephritis through the observation that nephrotoxic guinea pig IgG$_1$ antibody, when injected into rats, was capable of inducing glomerulonephritis, which was characterized by an immediate massive proteinuria, marked intraluminal fibrin formation, subendothelial fibrinoid deposition, phagocytic accumulation of small numbers of neutrophils and monocytes, and only weak deposition of rat β_{1c}-globulin, while injected

IgG$_2$ did not cause a significant proteinuria in spite of the localization of rat β_{1c} in glomeruli.   They [66] also pointed out that the fixation of pepsin-digested divalent fragments of nephrotoxic guinea pig IgG$_1$ antibody to glomerular basement membrane is able to cause damage of endothelial cells and a transient proteinuria without detectable participation of complement and neutrophils.

7) Nephritogenicity of the protein fractions of various anti-kidney sera.   Smadel [141] first pointed out that the nephrotoxic principle of anti-rat-kidney rabbit serum was present in the globulin fractions.   Lippman et al. [81] further showed that nephrotoxic activity of rabbit anti-rat-kidney serum resides wholly in the gammaglobulin.   Lange et al. [74] were able to produce glomerulonephritis in rabbits by injecting only the globulin fraction of anti-rabbit-kidney duck serum just as when injecting whole serum.   Powell [123] mentioned that the localizing activity of labeled anti-rat-kidney gammaglobulin was strongly concentrated by gradient elution from kidney sediment, and the material so obtained was about 20 times more active and, with respect to cross localization in liver, was 4 times as specific for rat kidney as was the original unpurified gammaglobulin.   Yagi and Pressman [117], by electrophoresis on starch of anti-rat-kidney rabbit antibody, clarified the gammaglobulin nature of kidney-localizing antibody, and by ultracentrifugation revealed that the antibody lies in alpha-chain.   Fujimoto et al. [38] also confirmed that nephritogenicity of both anti-rabbit-kidney duck serum and anti-rat-kidney rabbit serum was present in their gammaglobulins.   Nephritogenicity of anti-rabbit-kidney guinea pig serum and of anti-rat-kidney duck serum was also revealed to be present in their gammaglobulins.

3. Immunochemical properties of anti-kidney serum

Smadel [141] could not correlate nephritogenicity of anti-rat-kidney rabbit serum with its precipitin titer for kidney extracts.   The anti-rat-kidney rabbit serum had relative organ specificity and was hardly susceptible for desensitization.   Izumi [58] demonstrated that guinea pig complement does not fix to anti-kidney duck serum combined with rabbit kidney, liver, muscle, or extracts in vitro.   Lippman et al. [79] reported that rabbit anti-rat-kidney gammaglobulin inhibits the growth in tissue culture of rat heart muscle as well as rat kidney, chick brain, chick heart muscle and chick mesonephros.   Korngold and Pressman [69] mentioned that antibodies from anti-lung, anti-liver, and anti-spleen sera localized in the greatest concentration in the homologous organ when the purification was carried out with the cellular fractions of lung, liver and spleen respectively, whereas with the anti-kidney serum the best results were obtained with the kidney blood vessel fraction. Cruickshank and Hill [25] demonstrated that globulin from antiserum prepared against whole rat kidney and conjugated with a fluorescein derivative has been shown by fluorescence microscopy to react with basement membrane and reticulin in many rat organs and with sarcolemma and neurilemma, and a more limited study has shown that anti-rat-glomerulus and anti-rat-lung globulins react similarly.   According to Bale and Spar [6] antibodies prepared against rat kidney localized strongly in adrenal and ovary as well as in kidney.   Antibodies against rat ovary localized strongly in adrenal and ovary, and to a lesser degree in spleen and kidney.   Lange and Wenk [73] demonstrated that when small amounts of anti-rat-kidney rabbit serum were added to the perfusate recirculated through isolated rat kidneys from artery to vein the complement titer of the perfusate fell to zero after passage through the kidney, whereas anti-rat-kidney duck sera did not produce a fall in complement activity of the perfusate circulating through the isolated rat kidney.   According to Bale et al. [7] anti-kidney antibodies showed specificity for kidney compared with other rat tissues, and anti-Walker rat carcinoma 256 antibodies showed specificity for this tumor tissue. Spar et al. [146] reported that eluates from the rabbit kidneys immunized against rat kidneys and those for a normal rabbit when injected into rats and rabbits showed preferential kidney localization persisting for days. Localization was greater for preparation made from immunized kidney, but the difference has not been demonstrated to be statistically significant. One preparation of immunized kidneys showed a concentration of ^{131}I in the kidney of injected rabbits 15 times higher than in the spleen, the next highest organ of 13 organs studied, in rabbits sacrificed 3 days and a week after injection. Liu et al. [84] reported that rabbit antisera to both rat kidney saline homogenate and the trypsin digest of rat kidney adsorbed on streptococci caused cytotoxic effects upon rat kidney cells in tissue culture as well as renal lesions in vivo following intravenous injection into rats. Blau et al. [12] revealed that the major fraction (80%) of rabbit anti-rat-kidney sera localized quite rapidly, probably in antigens located in the vascular bed, while the remainder of the antibody localized more slowly either because of the low concentration or inaccessibility of the antigen. They [13] also showed that rabbit antibodies against rat kidney injected into rats directly, after passage through nephrectomized rats, or after passage through normal rats localized in the liver and other tissue as well as in the kidney. De Oliveira [26] showed that rat kidney and lung extracts, diffusing against duck anti-rat-kidney serum in the same plate, gave bundles of precipitation lines that joined, forming typical "reactions of identity", and that rat lung extract incorporated in the gel inhibited all the reaction between kidney extract and rabbit anti-rat-kidney serum. Hiramoto et al. [54] demonstrated that anti-rat-kidney rabbit antibody, when injected into rats, localized along the vessels and sinusoids of the adrenal cortex but not in the medulla although the medulla did contain antigen capable of reacting with the antibody in vitro. Fujimoto et al. [38] and Fujimoto [39] pointed out that anti-kidney gammaglobulins capable of inducing glomerulonephritis were generally provided with the property of precipitin reaction and antigen-combining capacity, whereas anti-rabbit-kidney guinea pig gammaglobulin and anti-rat-kidney rabbit gammaglobulin having the potentialities of inducing immediately glomerulonephritis in rabbits and rats respectively were provided with properties of complement fixation and induction of passive cutaneous anaphylaxis (Table 1-2). In addition, it was shown that anti-duck-gammaglobulin and anti-rabbit-gammaglobulin rat gammaglobulins also had the above four properties (Table 1-2).

Stelos et al. [150], by digesting rabbit antibodies against rat kidney with papain and trace labeling of the fragments with radioiodine, observed the following properties: The kidney-localizing activity was found in fractions I and II of anti-rat-kidney gammaglobulin; and the adsorption of fractions with kidney sediment indicated the presence of antibody activity in fractions I and II. Baxter and Small [10] mentioned that whereas intact antibody to rat kidney (7S) produced immediate and sustained proteinuria in rats, univalent fragments (papain digests) of the antibody did not, and divalent fragments (pepsin digests) produced only transitory proteinuria. The antibody fragments differed from the intact antibody in fixing little, if any, complement in vitro, which may explain why they did not cause serious renal damage. Fujimoto et al. [38] and Fujimoto [39] were able to induce glomerulonephritis characterized by proliferative glomerulitis in rats 5, 6 to 7, or 7 days after injection of fractions I and II of papain-digested anti-rat-kidney rabbit gammaglobulin, soluble preparation, fractions I and II of pepsin-digested one, or mercaptoethanol-iodoacetamide-treated one respectively (Table 1-2). They could not induce glomerulonephritis by injection of fraction III of digested anti-kidney gammaglobulins (Table 1-2). They also observed localization of antibody fractions capable of inducing glomerulitis in glomerular loops immediately after injection, but early fixation of

Table 1-2 Serological and biological properties of anti-kidney gammaglobulins and related antibody gammaglobulins.

Gammaglobulins (GG)		Precipitin reaction	Antigen-combining capacity	Complement fixation	Passive cutaneous anaphylaxis	Mode of development of Masugi nephritis		Recipient animals
						1st phase	2nd phase	
Anti-rabbit-kidney duck GG		+	+	−	−	−	+	
Anti-rabbit-kidney guinea pig GG		+	+	+	+	+	?+	Rabbits
Anti-rat-kidney rabbit GG								
Untreated		+	+	+	+	+	+	
Pepsin-digested	Fraction I	+	+	−	−	−	+	
	Fraction II	+	+	−	−	−	+	
	Fraction III	−	−	−*	−*	−	+	
	Soluble (I+II)	+	+	−	−	−	−	
Papain-digested	Fraction I	−	+	−	−	−	+	Rats
	Fraction II	−	+	−	−	−	+	
	Fraction III	−	−	−*	−*	−	−	
Mercaptoethanol-iodoacetamide-treated		+	+	+	−	−	+	
Anti-rat-kidney duck GG		+	+	−	−	−	+	
Anti-duck-gammaglobulin rabbit GG								
Untreated		+	+	+	+			
Pepsin-digested, soluble		+	+	−	−			
Anti-rabbit-gammaglobulin rat GG		+	+	+	+			

*Aggregated +
(From Fujimoto, T., Okada, M., Kondo, Y., and Tada, T.: *Acta Path. Jap. 14*: 275–310, 1964, Table 5)

guinea pig complement to these sites was not recognized except when mercaptoethanol-iodoacetamide-treated anti-kidney gammaglobulin was injected (Table 1-2).   Injection of fraction III did not elicit any immunological effects in the glomeruli (Table 1-2).   In a rabbit injected with anti-rabbit-kidney duck gammaglobulin and with pepsin-digested, soluble preparations of anti-duck-gammaglobulin rabbit gammaglobulin 3 hours later glomerulonephritis developed only 7 days after injection in contrast to the case in which non-treated anti-duck-gammaglobulin rabbit gammaglobulin was injected following injection of anti-kidney duck gammaglobulin (Tables 1-1 and 1-2).   Small and Baxter [144] reported that digestion of anti-rat-kidney rabbit antibody to produce univalent and divalent fragments greatly reduced its nephrotoxicity and ability to fix complement in vivo, suggesting that the nephrotoxicity may be in large part dependent on complement fixation. The univalent fragments produced no significant proteinuria, and neither type of fragment fixed quantities of complement large enough to be regarded as definite.   However, the divalent fragments retained the ability to produce early proteinuria to a greater degree than they retained the ability to fix complement.   It was suggested from this that the antibody may be able to cause some damage independent of complement fixation but requires divalent molecules.   In the study of Osaka [117] it was demonstrated that rats given fraction I (fraction C of nephrotoxic gammaglobulin fractionated by CM cellulose chromatography according to the method of Palmer, and then refractionated by DEAE cellulose chromatography) intravenously showed proliferative glomerular lesions and immediate and severe proteinuria, while those given fraction II demonstrated slight renal lesions and moderate proteinuria after the latent period.   Katz and Unanue [59] showed that at least 150 to 200 μg of rabbit anti-rat-kidney antibody must fix in a rat's kidneys to induce immediate nephritis.   Vogt et al. [167] mentioned that in optimally sensitized rats a nephritis could be initiated when about 400 γ antibody-N or more of an antiserum (directed against the monovalent fragments) was injected.   The complement-fixing antibody from the rat induced immediately a nephritis without exception, whereas the nephritis induced by duck antibody always appeared after a latent period.   The duck antibody was not able to fix significant amounts of rat complement.

4. Antigenic substance responsible for production of anti-kidney serum

Heymann and Lund [50] reported that anti-kidney rabbit serum produced by injection of renal cortex or whole kidney of rats was nephritogenic, while half of the specimens of anti-kidney serum produced by injection of renal medulla were not effective.   Solomon et al. [145] demonstrated that nephritogenicity of anti-rat-kidney rabbit serum was absorbed by saline extract of rat glomeruli but not by suspensions of other components of kidneys and other organs.   Greenspon and Krakower [42] considered that the antigenic substance of renal cortex responsible for the production of anti-kidney serum resides in the glomeruli because of the data that injection of dog glomeruli into rabbits was able to produce potent anti-dog-kidney rabbit serum but injection of renal cortical tissue freed of glomeruli was ineffective.   Krakower and Greenspon [71] also showed that basement membranes of dog glomeruli were more antigenic than epithelial and endothelial elements by ultracentrifugation.   Cole et al. [24] pointed out that trypsin digestion of rat kidney at pH 8 can produce a soluble substance which combines with anti-kidney antibody of anti-rat-kidney rabbit serum and absorbs nephritogenic antibody from the anti-kidney serum.   Greenspon et al. [43] postulated that the nephrotoxic antigen obtained from canine renal glomeruli is an integral part of the collagen which forms the glomerular basement membrane and specifically, its protein moiety.   Hill et al. [53] demonstrated, by the fluorescent antibody technique, that anti-rat-kidney rabbit globulins reacted with glomeruli, basement membranes of pars convoluta of urinary tubules and cytoplasm of tubular epithelium of normal rats, while anti-lung or anti-glomerular antibody globulin also reacted with basement membranes but not with tubular epithelial cells. According to the study of Hill et al. [53] it was concluded that kidney tissue contains at least two distinct antigens — one in the basement membrane and the other in the cytoplasm of convoluted tubules. By injection of the anti-glomerulus serum into rats it has been shown that an antibody specific for the former of these antigens is capable of producing nephritis. Cruickshank and Hill [25] postulated that the nature of the antigenic substance with which the anti-rat-glomerular globulins react is possibly a mucopolysaccharide. Krakower and Greenspon [72] clarified that the concentration of "nephrotoxic" antigen(s) in the glomerular basement membrane of the developing kidney in dog increases commensurate with the maturation of the glomeruli. The concentration is presumably very low in developing glomeruli of the nephrogenic zone. It rises abruptly when the glomeruli become capable of functioning as filters in the midzone of the neonatal cortex and has apparently not quite reached adult levels in the larger glomeruli of the juxtamedullary zone. The concentration of "nephrotoxic" antigen(s) in adult canine glomerular basement membrane is apparently increased more than three- to fivefold by venous congestion and in the presence of marked hydronephrosis. It is decreased two- to threefold, or more, in association with compensatory renal hypertrophy. There is only slight reduction in concentration with marked ischemia, induced by clamping the renal artery. Baxter and Goodman [9] noted that the antigenic substance responsible for the production of anti-rat-kidney rabbit serum resides in renal cortex and medulla, and soluble inhibitory factor which is able to absorb nephritogenic antibody from anti-kidney serum is obtained in high concentration by trypsin digestion of rat kidney homogenate. The factor is stable at 60 °C, is nondialyzable, and is precipitated by ammonium sulphate. Studies of Yagi et al. [175] revealed that a soluble material capable of inhibiting the localization of kidney-localizing anti-kidney antibodies was isolated from a trypsin digest of rat kidney. The material left after further digestion with ribonuclease and desoxyribonuclease was able to neutralize only about 75 per cent of the kidney-localizing antibodies. Yagi and Pressman [176] showed that heating and treatment with 60% trichloroacetic acid were shown to affect various rat kidney antigens differently, and heated or unheated trypsin digest of kidney sediment neutralized localizing antibodies differently in a qualitative manner, which suggested the multiple nature of kidney antigens responsible for fixing antibodies in vivo. Shibata [133] found that ultrasupernatants of trypsin-digested rat and rabbit kidney contain complete antigens in the serological sense, and the antisera produced against the supernatants are nephritogenic. He also clarified by chemical purification that the antigenic substance in the supernatants lies in polysaccharide. Naruse [107] reported that zone electrophoresis is effective for removing contaminated nucleic acid and reducing nitrogen level from the antigenic substance contained in the ultrasupernatant of trypsin digested kidney homogenate. According to Miyakawa [96] the active antigenic factor (polysaccharide) in the supernatant of kidney cortex emulsion, not treated with trypsin, was assumed to be found with a protein. And so, the protein extraction techniques were introduced to purify this protein bound antigen. Only the fraction precipitating between 50 per cent and 67 per cent saturated ammonium sulfate solution was proved to posess complete nephrotoxic serum antigenicity. The active antigenic principle in this precipitate was further purified by starch block electrophoresis. The nephrotoxic serum antigenicity was found in the fraction in which the highest protein and hexose levels were observed. Takuma et al. [155] showed that when more than 30 mg of trypsin was used with an incubation time of 3 hours at 37 °C, the chemical compositions of the ultrasupernatants were nearly identical with those of samples extracted by the original method for extracting active antigenic substance from kidney cortex homogenate in which 50 mg trypsin and 3 hours incubation at 37 °C for the digestion of 6 g kidney homogenate were used.   Shibata et al. [134] reported that almost all the antigenic activity responsible for the production of nephrotoxic antibody after purification by starch block electrophoresis was found in fraction 3 free of nucleic acid.   Fluorescent antibody technique revealed that this purified antigen (fraction 3) is derived from the glomerular basement membranes.   Active principle of this antigenic substance is closely related to the polysaccharide moiety.   Nagasawa et al. [105] clarified that rabbit antisera against trypsin-digested ultrasupernatant of rat renal medulla have an ability to produce nephrotoxic nephritis in rats, and the nephrotoxic antigen in medulla exists in tubular and/or capillary basement membranes.   According to them [105] staining of normal rat kidney with fluorescein labeled nephrotoxic sera (anti-rat-kidney cortex, -glomerulus, -glomerular basement membrane, -lung, -aorta, -heart, -muscle, and -liver rabbit antisera) has demonstrated that all these antisera react with glomerular basement membrane, tubular basement membrane including Bowman's capsule and media of blood vessels.   In the antisera against kidney cortex, and liver, specific fluoresecnce was found in tubular cytoplasms as well as in glomerular basement membrane, tubular basement membrane, and blood vessels.   According to Shibata et al. [135] water-soluble antigen that induces nephrotoxic antiserum was isolated and purified from rat glomerular basement membrane, which had the character of a glycoprotein.   Naruse and Shibata [108] reported that not only the separation of glomerular basement membrane from cells, but the effective nephrotoxic glomerular basement mcmbrane antigen can be obtained in a water-soluble form mechanically by sonic disruption of rat glomeruli.

5. Masugi nephritis in young animals

Erdmann [30, 31] considered that immature glomeruli do not entirely or sufficiently combine with anti-kidney serum on the basis of the findings that inflammatory changes took place only in the differentiated juxtamedullary glomeruli of young rabbits after injection of anti-rabbit-kidney duck serum.   He also noted that young animals did not produce sufficient amounts of precipitating antibody against duck serum.   Moriuchi [98] studied the age difference of rat Masugi nephritis induced by anti-rat-kidney rabbit serum. According to him, young animals presented florid changes earlier than adult animals when injected with the same amount of anti-kidney serum.   The fully developed lesions in the young animals were characterized by fibrinoid thrombosis, whereas those in the adult exhibited a tendency to cellular proliferation.   A nephrotic syndrome developed in young rats after injection of smaller amonuts of anti-kidney serum than to adult animals.   Rabbit anti-rat-kidney serum injected into newborn rats at birth promptly produced acute proliferative glomerulonephritis associated with proteinuria, and rabbit gammaglobulin and rat complement localized promplty in the basement membranes of the more mature glomeruli in the inner part of the renal cortex but not in the glomeruli of the peripheral renal cortex [46].   Calcagno et al. [19] also reported the induction of glomerular lesions in the inner cortex by injection of anti-rat-kidney serum into newborn rats.

6. Masugi nephritis in pregnant animals

Brent et al. [16] mentioned that injection of a prescribed dosage of rabbit anti-rat-kidney sera into pregnant rats on the 8th day of gestation, resulted in severe congenital malformations in 100 per cent of the fetuses, and larger doses caused complete fetal re-sorption.   Brent [17] also reported that rabbit anti-rat-kidney serum, when injected into rats 7, 8, 9, and 10 days pregnant, resulted in embryonic death, growth retardation and malformations.   Irino [57], on the basis of data suggesting that severe anaphylaxis is more exaggerated in pregnant rabbits injected with anti-rabbit-kidney guinea pig serum than in non-pregnant rabbits injected with anti-kidney serum, pointed out an important role of inner secretion in the pathogenesis of Masugi nephritis.   Yagi [174] reported that anti-rabbit-renal medulla guinea pig antibody, when injected into pregnant rabbits, was able to produce diffuse glomerulonephritis as in the case when anti-renal cortex antibody was employed.

7. Influence of hormone, radiation, etc. upon Masugi nephritis

Knowlton et al. [63] showed that in rats rendered nephritic with a rabbit anti-rat-kidney serum DOCA given concurrently with NaCl greatly intensified the nephritic process and gave rise to striking arterial hypertension.   Winternitz and Hackel [173] reported that intensive administration of Pyribenzamine was ineffective for the modification of acute nephritis produced in rabbits by the injection of duck anti-rabbit-kidney serum, but there was a slight delay in the onset of albuminuria.   Bohle and Hieronymi [14] observed an exaggeration of the nephrotic syndrome in rats given DOCA 24 hours prior to injection of anti-rat-kidney rabbit serum and died within 10 days.   Rats that survived after 4 weeks demonstrated glomerulonephritis and panarteritis in kidneys, myocardium, pancreas, and small intestine, which was especially conspicuous in the animals given sodium choloride in drinking water, and bilaterally adrenalectomized.   Shibata and Kurisu [132] mentioned that a large dose of cortisone was effective in inhibiting rabbit Masugi nephritis, but ACTH was much less effective.   According to Lippman et al. [83] cortisone and hydrocortisone given subcutaneously in the male increases the severity of the nephritis by all criteria, while cortisone given intraperitoneally in the male or given subcutaneously had little or no effect.   DOCA given subcutaneously in the male produced an increase in proteinuria and in blood pressure elevation, while DOCA given intraperitoneally in the male had effects which simulated incompletely those of cortisone given simultaneously.   Adrenalectomy in the male after nephrotoxic globulin administration greatly reduced the rate of protein excretion.   According to Yokoyama [178], administration of DOCA prior to injection of anti-rabbit-kidney duck serum into rabbits led to an increase in glomerulitis, but that of cortisone, or ACTH was not able to inhibit the occurrence of glomerulonephritis.   Rabbits given cortisone had mild glomerulitis, and the two groups given cortisone and ACTH demonstrated a serum protein pattern of the nephrotic syndrome.   According to Huang et al. [56] the experimental renal disease appeared to be intensified by the administration of ACTH or predonisolone before or during heteronephrotoxic serum injections into Taiwan monkeys.

Nishimori [109] noted the development of more severe hypertension and vascular alterations in rats injected with anti-rat-kidney rabbit serum 1 week after adrenalectomy and foregoing administration of 1% saline solution than in Masugi nephritis of control animals.

Kay [60] was able to inhibit the occurrence of nephrotoxic nephritis by depressing antibody formation with x-ray irradiation of rabbits.   According to the study of Arhelger et al. [2] simultaneous injection of nephrotoxic serum and minute amounts of gram-negative bacterial endotoxin resulted in acute death in a high percentage of rats and renal lesions resembling those of the generalized Shwartzman reaction.   They [3] also reported that simultaneous or spaced injections of heterologous hyperimmune anti-kidney serum and minute amounts of *E. coli* endotoxin resulted in similar pathological events to those previously reported [2].   Renal lesions in surviving animals showed a marked progression toward chronic changes as compared to rats given nephrotoxic serum alone.   Arhelger et al. [4] reported on the inhibition of occurrence of Masugi nephritis due to x-ray irradiation of the rabbit abdomen which caused poor localization of anti-rabbit-kidney duck serum in glomerular capillaries and diminished the reaction between this antiserum and the autologous antibody against duck serum.

Shibata and Kurisu [132] noted that administration of the same amount of Strong Neo Minophagen C (S. N. M. C.) prior to injection of anti-kidney duck serum inhibited the occurrence of Masugi nephritis, whereas the administration of S. N. M. C. after the onset of nephritis palliated nephritis itself.

8. Masugi nephritis in previously sensitized animals

Nogiwa [110] succeeded in inducing a diffuse glomerulonephritis characterized by severe degenerative glomerulitis with fibrinoid degeneration and thickening of loop walls resembling wire-loop lesions 4 to 6 days after injection of anti-rabbit-kidney duck serum into rabbits which had previously been sensitized with egg albumin for 120 to 140 days.   It was worthy of note that in these animals histologic manifestations were characterized by degenerative glomerulitis in contrast to the usual proliferative glomerulitis in Masugi nephritis in rabbits.   Okada [113] was able to induce prolonged glomerulonephritis characterized by thickening of glomerular loop walls 3 to 6 days after injection of anti-rabbit-kidney duck serum into rabbits previously sensitized with egg albumin for 56 days. It was interesting that serum protein patterns of the nephrotic syndrome had developed during the course of this renal disease.

9. Unilateral Masugi nephritis

Sarre and Wirtz [129], by intravenous injection of anti-rabbit-kidney duck serum into rabbits during unilateral clamping of their renal arteries for 15 minutes, were able to induce glomerulonephritis in the contralateral kidneys, whereas little or no renal lesion was produced in the homolateral kidneys.   Clamping of unilateral renal arteries prior to injection or that of bilateral renal arteries during injection did not induce unilateral Masugi nephritis.   They postulated from these data that anti-kidney antibody combines with kidney within 15 minutes after injection.   Sugai [151] ascertained the persistence of unilateral Masugi nephritis induced by injection of anti-rabbit-kidney duck serum during the clamping of unilateral renal arteries for 15 minutes by means of repeated biopsies of bilateral kidneys during the period of 96 days after injection.   Shiina [140] was able to induce unilateral subacute glomerulonephritis or secondarily contracted kidney by repeated injections of anti-kidney serum during short-term unilateral clamping of the renal arteries.   Nagasawa [102] was also capable of inducing unilateral contracted kidneys by a single injection of anti-kidney serum into rabbits according to the method of Sarre-Wirtz.   In this experiment hyaline thickening and elastosis of arterioles were induced, but the typical picture of contracted kidneys following glomerulonephritis was not obtained.   Rother and Sarre [126] pointed out that autologous antibody against rabbit kidneys was not demonstrated throughout the course of unilateral Masugi nephritis of rabbits for several months.   On the basis of unilateral Masugi nephritis in rats, Federlin et al. [32] postulated that the nephrotoxic antibody at first precipitates in one kidney only, and it also reaches the other "free" kidney with increasing survival time.   This was thought to be due to an ablution of transiently precipitated nephrotoxin from extrarenal vessels as well as from the primarily affected kidney.   Tsuchida [156] reported, on the basis of electron microscopic study of unilateral Masugi nephritis in rabbits, that the endothelium-like cells originate from mesangial cells and that the former represent the various features of the latter caused by the conditions of the environment around them.   In the latent stage, the majority of the proliferated intracapillary cells were endothelial cells.   In the initial and severest stages the endothelium-like cells played an important role in the destruction and distortion of the glomerular structure.   Miyakawa et al. [97] reported that in rabbits with a contracted kidney of right side which had previously been induced by injection of anti-rabbit-kidney duck serum during clamping of the left renal artery, when the contralateral left kidney was attacked by the same anti-kidney serum with or without protection of the right kidney by clamping the right renal artery, renal failure occurred with chronic, subacute and slowly progressive course.

10. Masugi nephritis in parabiotic animals

Pfeiffer et al. [119] reported that healthy rats parabiotic with rats injected with anti-rat-kidney rabbit serum 3 to 5 days before developed nephritis accompanied by dysproteinemia and albuminuria.   Pfeiffer et al. [120] reported that they could transfer nephrotoxic nephritis into genetically identical rats and they considered that blood of nephritic rats was pathogenic in this case.   On the basis of the experiment on transfer of chronic nephritis they suspected the role of tissue destructing factor produced by chronic nephritis. Lange et al. [75] reported that parabiosis of rats made nephritic by anti-rat-kidney rabbit serum to healthy rats leads to a mild but clear-cut nephritis in the healthy partner with proteinuria and typical histologic changes.   Rat gammaglobulin, presumably antibody, but not rabbit gammaglobulin could be shown on the glomeruli of such secondarily diseased animals.   They postulated that the primary nephritic partner forms an autoantibody against its own altered tissue, which is then in turn able to attack the healthy kidney tissue of the secondary partner.   Pfeiffer [121] disclosed that the nephritis of parabiotic rats was not induced by the action of anti-rat-kidney rabbit serum, and was transferable with leukocytes of peripheral blood 70 to 80 per cent of which consisted of lymphocytes, and postulated that a transfer factor was combined with lymphocytes.   In their experiment serum, blood plasma or suspension of kidney substance was not able to induce nephritis in animals, and no substance combining with rat kidney was demonstrated in the serum globulin of nephritic animals.   It was indeed a very interesting finding but renal lesions induced in the second animals were very mild, and it was difficult to consider these renal lesions as equivalent to the nephritis in the original animals.   According to Unanue et al. [162], neither functional nor morphological abnormalities were noted in the normal kidneys in the experiments consisting of transplantation of a normal isologous kidney to a nephritic rat and parabiosis of a normal rat to a nephritic rat.   In the study of Müller-Ruchholtz et al. [101] some of the rats treated with anti-rat-kidney rabbit antibody were allowed to live parabiotically.   Among these animals fluorescence following treatment with anti-rabbit globulin was observed only in the primarily nephritic rats (15 animals). Fluorescence was absent both in the primarily healthy parabiotic partner animals and in the rats treated with control serum (ovalbumin, horse serum, and normal rat serum) (13 animals).   Unanue et al. [163] performed two experimental procedures.   In the first, radioiodine labeled nephrotoxic gammaglobulin was injected into rats which were then united by parabiosis to non-injected isologous rats.   These experiments showed a continuous transfer of labeled antibody from the injected rat to the kidneys and other viscera of the normal partner. By nephrectomizing and/or hepatectomizing the injected rat it could be shown that virtually all the transferred antibody dissociated from the injected rat's non-renal antigens and that this antibody had a low specificity for renal versus non-renal antigens as well as a low avidity for all tissue antigens. In the second, a kidney from a rat injected with labeled nephrotoxic antibody was transplanted to a non-injected isologous rat. The rate of decline of labeled antibody in the transplanted kidney was four times more rapid than that observed in intact rats receiving labeled antibody in which loss of kidney-fixed antibody and transfer of antibody from non-renal sites to kidney were occurring simultaneously. The antibody fixed in the kidney had a high specificity.

11. Masugi nephritis in complement-deficient animals

According to Unanue et al. [164], during the heterologous or early phase the rabbit anti-mouse-kidney gammaglobulin fixed to both glomerular and tubular basement membranes, but induced very mild disease in all mice, some of which lacked hemolytic complement activity. Glomeruli of all strains of mice had little or no fixation of β_{1c}-globulin, no leukocytic infiltration and no proliferative lesions. However, a membranous glomerulonephritis developed as part of the autologous or delayed phase in all strains. They assumed that since a partial fixation of C' to C'3 occurred in the C'-deficient mice, these results do not exclude the participation of the first components of C' as a mediator of glomerular injury. Rother et al. [127] observed nephritis induced by injection of anti-rabbit-kidney sheep serum capable of producing only the second phase in C'6-deficient rabbits. In this study no information concerning a possible role of components of complement activated earlier than C'6. Since β_{1c} is demonstrable in glomeruli of defective rabbits with glomerulonephritis, it could be concluded that all of the steps up to C'3 fixation occur. Lindberg and Rosenberg [77] reported that complement-containing progeny from the hybridization of B10.D2-old line females with B10.D2-new line males were used to study the role of the complement system in immune tissue injury. In this experiment, small differences in the severity on nephrotoxic serum nephritis were found following the injection of nephrotoxic serum which would implicate the late acting complement components as intensifiers of tissue injury.

V. Pathological Significance of Masugi Nephritis

Masugi and Tomizuka [86] and Masugi et al. [87] succeeded in reproducing renal lesions closely resembling human glomerulonephritis by injecting heteronephrotoxic serum into rats and rabbits. Not only the animal disease was entirely comparable in its histogenesis to that of human glomerulonephritis but it was also produced with 100 per cent incidence. Accordingly, it is highly probable that the most essential point of pathogenesis of human glomerulonephritis lies in the pathogenesis of Masugi nephritis. Pathologic processes of Masugi nephritis, however, are not so uniform as simply interpreted to be equivalent to human glomerulonephritis. Masugi nephritis of rats induced by injection of anti-rat-kidney rabbit serum was characterized by an immediate occurrence of the nephrotic syndrome, while Masugi nephritis of rabbits induced by injection of anti-rabbit-kidney duck serum was initiated by nephritic processes after a latent period of from 4 to 11 days. The difference of the pathologic processes as well as the biological significance of the latent period has long been waiting for a proper explanation.

In the early investigations the pathogenesis of Masugi nephritis was considered as reverse

through careful follow-up studies of glomerular lesions in the same individual rats.

It is worthy of note that the pathology of Masugi nephritis suggests there are two modes of development of glomerulitis produced by antigen-antibody reaction: One is the induction of proliferative glomerulitis by heterologous antigen-antibody reaction localized in glomeruli as in the case of classic Masugi nephritis of rabbits or in the second phase of that of rats, and the other is the induction of degenerative glomerulitis by direct reaction between glomerular loops and antibody against them as in the first phase of classic Masugi nephritis of rats.

It is especially noteworthy that the latter process is consistent with autoimmunization because of the direct reaction of anti-kidney antibody and the corresponding antigenic glomerular basement membrane. The mode of development of glomerulitis suggested from the study of Masugi nephritis will offer clues to the understanding of the nature of glomerulonephritis, lupus nephritis, and allied conditions. Why different glomerular inflammatory processes are produced by different antigen-antibody systems awaits further elucidation.

REFERENCES

1. Andres, G.A., Morgan, C., Hsu, K.C., Rifkind, R.A., and Seegal, B.C.: Electron microscopic studies of experimental nephritis with ferritin-conjugated antibody. The basement membranes and cisternae of visceral epithelial cells in nephritic rat glomeruli. *J. Exp. Med. 115*: 929–936, 1962.

2. Arhelger, R., Smith, F., Brunson, J., Good, R., and Vernier, R.: Effect of gram-negative endotoxin on nephrotoxic serum nephrosis in rats. *Proc. Soc. Exp. Biol. Med. 96*: 424–428, 1957.

3. Arhelger, R.B., Brunson, J.G., Good, R.A., and Vernier, R.L.: Influence of gram-nagative endotoxin on the pathogenesis of nephrotoxic serum nephritis in rats. *Lab. Invest. 10*: 669–687, 1961.

4. Arhelger, R.B., Smith, P.N., Walker, B.S., Fant, W.M., and Brunson, J.G.: Influence of local abdominal radiation on response of rabbits to nephrotoxic serum. *Amer. J. Path. 39*: 631–642, 1961.

5. Asano, S.: Experimental nephritis induced by injection of anti-kidney serum (in Japanese). *J. Jap. Soc. Intern. Med. 26*: 71–104, 1938–1939. Ibid. *27*: 109–125, 1939–1940.

6. Bale, W.F. and Spar, I.L.: In vivo localization of rat organ antibodies in ovaries, adrenals, and other tissues. *J. Immunol. 73*: 125–133, 1954.

7. Bale, W.F., Spar, I.L., Goodland, R.L., and Wolfe, D.E.: In vivo and in vitro studies of labeled antibodies against rat kidney and Walker carcinoma. *Proc. Soc. Exp. Biol. Med. 89*: 564–568, 1955.

8. Battifora, H.A. and Markowitz, A.S.: Nephrotoxic nephritis in monkeys. Sequential light, immunofluorescence, and electron microscopic studies. *Amer. J. Path. 55*: 257–281, 1969.

9. Baxter, J.H. and Goodman, H.C.: Nephrotoxic serum nephritis in rats. I. Distribution and specificity of the antigen responsible for the production of nephrotoxic antibodies. *J. Exp. Med. 104*: 467–485, 1956.

10. Baxter, J.H. and Small, P.A., Jr.: Antibody to rat kidney: In vivo effects of univalent and divalent fragments. *Science 140*: 1406–1407, 1963.

11. Beregi, E. und v. Mayersbach, H.: Immunohistologische Untersuchungen experimenteller Nephritiden. I. Die Masugi-Nephritis. *Virchows Arch. Abt. B Zellpath. 4*: 225–245, 1970.

12. Blau, M., Day, E.D., and Pressman, D.: The rate of localization of anti-rat kidney antibodies. *J. Immunol. 79*: 330–333, 1957.

13. Blau, M., Day, E.D., Planinsek, J., and Pressman, D.: Specificity and cross-localization of anti-kidney antibodies. *J. Immunol. 79*: 334–336, 1957.

14. Bohle, A. und Hieronymi, G.: Über die Wirkung von Desoxycorticosteronacetat auf die Niere und das Gefässsystem der Ratte bei Bestehen einer Masugi-Nephritis. *Frankf. Ztschr. Path. 64*: 261–284, 1953.

15. Bohle, A., Miller, F., Sitte, H., und Yolac, A.: Frühveränderungen bei der Masugi-Nephritis der Ratte. Elektronenmikroskopische Untersuchungen. *In* Grabar, P. and Miescher, P. (eds.): *Immunopathology (Ist International Symposium)*, 70–81, Benno Schwabe, Basel-Stuttgart, 1958.

16. Brent, R.L., Averich, E., and Drapiewski, V.A.: Production of congenital malformations using tissue antibodies. I. Kidney antisera. *Proc. Soc. Exp. Biol. Med. 106*: 523–526, 1961.

17. Brent, R.L.: The production of congenital malformations using tissue antisera. II. The spectrum and incidence of malformations following the administration of kidney antiserum to pregnant rats. *Amer. J. Anat. 115*: 525–542, 1964.

18. Burkholder, P.M.: Complement fixation in diseased tissues. I. Fixation of guinea pig complement in sections of kidney from humans with membranous glomerulonephritis and rats injected with anti-rat kidney serum. *J. Exp. Med. 114*: 605–616, 1961.

19. Calcagno, P.L., Rubin, M.I., Mukherji, P.K., and Terplan, K.L.: Response to nephrotoxic serum in the newborn rat. *Proc. Soc. Exp. Biol. Med. 114*: 124–130, 1963.

20. Chow, A.Y.K. and Drummond, K.N.: Incorporation and hydroxylation of proline-3-4-H^3 as an index of glomerular basement membrane synthesis in normal and nephrotoxic nephritic rats. *Lab. Invest. 20*: 213–218, 1969.

21. Churg, J., Grishman, E., and Mautner, W.: Nephrotoxic serum nephritis in the rat. Electron and light microscopic studies. *Amer. J. Path. 37*: 729–749, 1960.

22. Churg, J. and Sakaguchi, H.: Vascular lesions in anti-kidney serum nephritis of the rat. *Amer. J. Path. 47*: 953–963, 1965.

23. Cochrane, C.G., Unanue, E.R., and Dixon, F.J.: A role of polymorphonuclear leukocytes and complement in nephrotoxic nephritis. *J. Exp. Med. 122*: 99–116, 1965.

24. Cole, L.R., Cromartie, W.J., and Watson, D.W.: A specific soluble substance involved in nephrotoxic nephritis. *Proc. Soc. Exp. Biol. Med. 77*: 498–501, 1951.

25. Cruickshank, B. and Hill, A.G.S.: The histochemical identification of a connective-tissue antigen in the rat. *J. Path. Bact. 66*: 283–289, 1953.

26. De Oliveira, H.L.: Analysis of rat kidney and lung extracts by gel diffusion against anti-rat-kidney serum. *Int. Arch. Allergy 12*: 356–360, 1958.

27. Ehrich, W.E., Wolf, R.E., and Bartol, G.M.: Acute experimental glomerular nephritis in rabbits: a correlation of morphological and functional changes. *J. Exp. Med. 67*: 769–790, 1938.

28. Ehrich, W.E., Forman, C.W., and Seifer, J.: Diffuse glomerular nephritis and lipid nephrosis. Correlation of clinical, morphological, and experimental observations. *Arch. Path. 54*: 463–503, 1952.

29. Ehrlich, P.: Die Schutzstoffe des Blutes. *In* Himmelweit, F., Marquart, M., and Dale, H. (eds.): *The Collected Papers of Paul Ehrlich 2*, 298–315, Pergamon Press, London, 1957.

30. Erdmann, G.: Experimentelle Nephritis des Jungtieres. *Monatschr. Kinderheilk. 106*: 151–155, 1958.

31. Erdmann, G.: Altersunterschiede der immunopathologischen Befunde bei experimenteller Nephritis. *In* Grabar, P. and Miescher, P. (eds.): *Immunopathology (Ist International Symposium)*, 82–98, Benno Schwabe, Basel-Stuttgart, 1958.

32. Federlin, K., Marx, K.H., Crespin, S., Ostner, K.H., Menzel, W., und Pfeiffer, E.F.: Studien zur "Übertragung" der Masugi-Nephritis der Ratte. XI. Versuche zur Erzeugung einer einseitigen Nephritis bei der Ratte und zum Problem der Nierenfixation des heterogen Antikörpers. *Z. Immun. -Forsch. 131*: 480–502, 1966.

33. Feldman, J.D., Hammer, D., and Dixon, F.J.: Experimental glomerulonephritis. III. Pathogenesis of glomerular ultrastructural lesions in nephrotoxic serum nephritis. *Lab. Invest. 12*: 748–763, 1963.

34. Fisher, E.R. and Gruhn, J.: Histochemical observations concerning some renal enzymes in nephrotoxic nephrosis in the rat. *Arch. Path. 64*: 664–672, 1957.

35. Fujimoto, T.: Histopathologic study of Masugi nephritis. The mode of development of the glomerular changes. *Acta Path. Jap. 4*: 1–19, 1954.

36. Fujimoto, T. and Akashi, S.: Mode of development of the edematous-sclerosing processes in glomeruli. Histopathologic study of Masugi nephritis. *Osaka City Med. J. 2*: 7–20, 1955.

37. Fujimoto, T. and Yamanaka, H.: Mode of development of the necrotizing processes in glomeruli. Histopathologic study of Masugi nephritis. *Osaka City Med. J. 2*: 21–31, 1955.

38. Fujimoto, T., Okada, M., Kondo, Y., and Tada, T.: The nature of Masugi nephritis. Histo- and immunopathological studies. *Acta Path. Jap. 14*: 275–310, 1964.

39. Fujimoto, T.: Serum sickness nephritis and Masugi nephritis. Histo- and immunopathological analyses. *Acta Path. Jap. 15*: 421–424, 1965.

40. Fujita, T.: Role of complement in immediate nephrotoxic nephritis of rats induced by duck anti-rat-kidney sera. *Kobe J. Med. Sci. 14*: 327–342, 1968.

41. Goodman, H.C. and Baxter, J.H.: Tubular reabsorption of protein in experimentally produced proteinuria in rats. *Proc. Soc. Exp. Biol. Med. 93*: 136–140, 1956.

42. Greenspon, S.A. and Krakower, C.A.: Direct evidence for the antigenicity of the glomeruli in the production of nephrotoxic serums. *Arch. Path. 49*: 291–297, 1950.

43. Greenspon, S.A., Bollinger, F.W., and Krakower, C.A.: Some chemical properties of nephrotoxic antigen. *Feder. Proc. 11*: 416–417, 1952.

44. Hackel, D.B. and Heymann, W.: Vascular lesions in rats with nephrotoxic renal disease. Relation to secondary hyperparathyroidism. *Arch. Path. 68*: 431–437, 1959.

45. Hammer, D.K. and Dixon, F.J.: Experimental glomerulonephritis. II. Immunologic events in the pathogenesis of nephrotoxic serum nephritis in the rat. *J. Exp. Med. 117*: 1019–1034, 1963.

46. Hammer, D.K., Vazquez, J.J., and Dixon, F.J.: Nephrotoxic serum nephritis in newborn rats. *Lab. Invest. 12*: 8–15, 1963.

47. Hasson, M.W., Bevans, M., and Seegal, B.C.: Immediate or delayed nephritis in rats produced by duck anti-rat-kidney sera. *Arch. Path. 64*: 192–204, 1957.

48. Hayasi, D.: Forschungen über den Komplementtiter des Serums im Verlaufe der diffusen Glomerulonephritis des Menschen und der experimentellen Nephritis des Hundes (japanisch). *Chiba Igakkai Zasshi 18*: 833–877, 1940.

49. Hemprich, R.: Zur Frage der experimentellen Glomerulonephritis. *Ztschr. ges. exper. Med. 95*: 304–321, 1935.

50. Heymann, W. and Lund, H.Z.: Lipemic nephrosis in rats. *Science 108*: 448–449, 1948.

51. Heymann, W. and Lund, H.Z.: Nephrotic syndrome in rats. *Pediatrics 7*: 691–706, 1951.

52. Heymann, W., Lund, H.Z., and Hackel, D.B.: The nephrotic syndrome in rats; with special reference to the progression of the glomerular lesion and to the use of nephrotoxic sera obtained from ducks. *J. Lab. Clin. Med. 39*: 218–224, 1952.

53. Hill, A.G.S., Cruickshank, B., and Crossland, A.: A study of antigenic components of kidney tissue. *Brit. J. Exp. Path. 34*: 27–34, 1953.

54. Hiramoto, R., Yagi, Y., and Pressman, D.: In vivo fixation of antibodies in the adrenal. *Proc. Soc. Exp. Biol. Med. 98*: 870–874, 1958.

55. Hiramoto, R., Jurandowski, J., Bernecky, J., and Pressman, D.: Precise zone of localization of anti-kidney antibody in various organs. *Proc. Soc. Exp. Biol. Med. 101*: 583–586, 1959.

56. Huang, C.C., Chang, S.C., Lin, Y.C., Chen, K.H., and Hsu, I.K.: Nephrotoxic serum renal disease in the Taiwan monkey. *J. Lab. Clin. Med. 62*: 201–215, 1963.

57. Irino, T.: Electron microscopic studies on antigen-antibody reaction in the kidney and its similar reaction. 1) Glomerular changes caused by anti-kidney serum in pregnant rabbits (in Japanese). *Jap. J. Allergy 13*: 452–468, 1964.

58. Izumi, F.: Experimentelle Studien über Glomerulonephritis. 1) Serologische Untersuchung des nephrotoxischen Immunserums, des Hämolysins und des Präcipitins (gegen Kaninchenserum gerichtetes Immunserum) (japanisch). *Folia Endocr. Jap. 16*: 532–555, 1940.

59. Katz, D.H. and Unanue, E.R.: Nephrotoxic properties of various anti-tissue antibodies in rats. *Feder. Proc. 25*: 660–660, 1966.

60. Kay, C.F.: The mechanism by which experimental nephritis is produced in rabbits injected with nephrotoxic duck serum. *J. Exp. Med. 72*: 559–572, 1940.

61. Kay, C.F.: The mechanism of a form of glomerulonephritis. Nephrotoxic nephritis in rabbits. *Amer. J. Med. Sci. 204*: 483–490, 1942.

62. Klein, P. und Burkholder, P.: Ein Verfahren zur fluoreszenzoptischen Darstellung der Komplementbindung und seine Anwendung zur histo-immunologischen Untersuchung der experimentellen Nierenanaphylaxie. *Dtsch. med. Wschr. 84*: 2001–2004, 1959.

63. Knowlton, A.I., Loeb, E.N., Stoerk, H.C., and Seegal, B.C.: Desoxycorticosterone acetate. The potentiation of its activity by sodium chloride. *J. Exp. Med. 85*: 187–198, 1947.

64. Kobayashi, Y.: Induction of Masugi nephritis with rabbit M antibody in rats (in Japanese). *JJN 12*: 493–512, 1970.

65. Kobayashi, Y., Shigematsu, H., and Tada, T.: Nephritogenic properties of nephrotoxic guinea pig antibodies. I. Glomerulonephritis induced by guinea pig IgG_1 antibody in rats. *Virchows Arch. Abt. B Zellpath. 14*: 259–271, 1973.

66. Kobayashi, Y., Shigematsu, H., and Tada, T.: Nephritogenic properties of nephrotoxic guinea pig antibodies. II. Glomerular lesions induced by $F(ab')_2$ fragments of nephrotoxic IgG_1 antibody in rats. *Virchows Arch. Abt. B Zellpath. 15*: 35–44, 1973.

67. Kondo, Y. and Shigematsu H.: Cellular aspects of rabbit Masugi nephritis. I. Cell kinetics in recoverable glomerulonephritis. *Virchows Arch. Abt. B Zellpath. 10*: 40–50, 1972.

68. Kondo, Y., Shigematsu, H., and Kobayashi, Y.: Cellular aspects of rabbit Masugi nephritis. II. Progressive glomerular injuries with crescent formation. *Lab. Invest. 27*: 620–631, 1972.

69. Korngold, L. and Pressman, D.: The in-vitro purification of tissue localizing antibodies. *J. Immunol. 71*: 1–5, 1953.

70. Kozima, K., Nakanoin, K., and Vogt, A.: Immediate and delayed nephrotoxic nephritis in the rat induced by duck antibody. Correlation between onset of proteinuria and complement fixation in the glomeruli. *Int. Arch. Allergy 32*: 404–415, 1967.

71. Krakower, C.A. and Greenspon, S.A.: Localization of the nephrotoxic antigen within the isolated renal glomerulus. *Arch. Path. 51*: 629–639, 1951.

72. Krakower, C.A. and Greenspon, S.A.: Factors leading to variation in concentration of "nephrotoxic" antigen(s) of glomerular basement membrane. *Arch. Path. 58*: 401–432, 1954.

73. Lange, K. and Wenk, E.J.: Investigations into the site of complement loss in experimental glomerulonephritis. *Amer. J. Med. Sci. 228*: 454–460, 1954.

74. Lange, K., Wenk, E.J., Wachstein, M., and Noble, J.: The mechanism of experimental glomerulonephritis produced in rabbits by avian antikidney sera. *Amer. J. Med. Sci. 236*: 767–778, 1958.

75. Lange, K., Wachstein, M., and McPherson, S.E.: Immunologic mechanism of transmission of experimental glomerulonephritis in parabiotic rats. *Proc. Soc. Exp. Biol. Med. 106*: 13–16, 1961.

76. Lehmann, J.D., Smith, J.W., Miller, T.E., Barnett, J.A., and Sanford, J.P.: Local immune response in the kidneys of rabbits with nephrotoxic serum nephritis. *Brit. J. Exp. Path. 50*: 371–377, 1969.

77. Lindberg, L.H. and Rosenberg, L.T.: Nephrotoxic serum nephritis in mice with a genetic deficiency in complement. *J. Immunol. 100*: 34–38, 1968.

78. Lindemann, W.: Sur le mode d'action de certains poisons rénaux. *Ann. Inst. Pasteur 14*: 49–59, 1900.

79. Lippman, R.W., Cameron, G., and Campbell, D.H.: The specificity of anti-kidney antibody determined by its effect upon tissue culture explants. *Proc. Nat. Acad. Sci. 36*: 576–580, 1950.

80. Lippman, R.W., Marti, H.U., and Campbell, D.H.: Nephrotoxic globulin nephritis. I. Course after a single intravenous injection. *Arch. Path. 53*: 1–14, 1952.

81. Lippman, R.W., Marti, H.U., and Jacobs, E.E.: Nephrotoxic globulin nephritis. II. Relation of severity to adrenal size. *Arch. Path. 54*: 169–184, 1952.

82. Lippman, R.W. and Jacobs, E.E.: Nephrotoxic globulin nephritis. III. Prompt death after administration of nephrotoxic globulin to the rat. *Proc. Soc. Exp. Biol. Med. 81*: 586–590, 1952.

83. Lippman, R.W., Marti, H.U., Jacobs, E.E., and Campbell, D.H.: Nephrotoxic globulin nephritis. V. Effects of adrenal steroid administration or adrenalectomy. *Arch. Path. 57*: 405–416, 1954.

84. Liu, C.T., McCrory, W.W., and Flick, J.A.: Cytotoxic effect of nephrotoxic serum on rat tissue culture. *Proc. Soc. Exp. Biol. Med. 95*: 331–335, 1957.

85. Maeda, T.: Experimental study on albuminuria caused by Masugi nephritis and some other renal damages (mercuric, uran- and synthalin-nephrosis) (in Japanese). *Tr. Soc. Path. Jap. 48*: 446–458, 1959.

86. Masugi, M. und Tomizuka, Y.: Über die spezifischen zytotoxischen Veränderungen der Niere und der Leber durch das spezifische Antiserum (Nephrotoxin und Hepatotoxin). Zugleich ein Beitrag zur Pathogenese der Glomerulonephritis. *Tr. Jap. Path. Soc. 21*: 329–341, 1931.

87. Masugi, M., Sato, Y., Murasawa, S., und Tomizuka, Y.: Über die experimentelle Glomerulonephritis durch das spezifische Antinierenserum. *Tr. Jap. Path. Soc. 22*: 614–628, 1932.

88. Masugi, M.: Über das Wesen der spezifischen Veränderungen der Niere und der Leber durch das Nephrotoxin bzw. das Hepatotoxin. Zugleich ein Beitrag zur Pathogenese der Glomerulonephritis und der eklamptischen Lebererkrankung. *Beitr. path. Anat. 91*: 82–112, 1933.

89. Masugi, M.: Über die experimentelle Glomerulonephritis durch das spezifische Antinierenserum. Ein Beitrag zur Pathogenese der diffusen Glomerulonephritis. *Beitr. path. Anat. 92*: 429–466, 1934.

90. Masugi, M.: Über die Grundvorgägne der Allergie und ihre Bedeutung für die Auffassung der menschlichen Erkrankungen. *Jap. J. Med. Sci. V. Path. 4*: 1–24, 1939.

91. Masugi, M.: Referat. Die Allergie und ihre pathologische Bedeutung. *Tr. Soc. Path. Jap. 29*: 603–631, 1939.

92. Masugi, Y.: Immunoelectron microscopic studies on local vascular changes after immunological tissue injuries — especially on the mechanism of nephrotoxic nephritis. *Acta Path. Jap. 19*: 265–281, 1969.

93. Matsuura, T.: Vital staining of renal glomerulus of normal and Masugi nephritic rabbits, with special reference to the origin of "endothelial cells" in nephritic glomerulus (in Japanese). *JJN 8*: 421–440, 1966.

94. Mellors, R.C., Siegel, M., and Pressman, D.: Analytical pathology. I. Histochemical demonstration of antibody localization in tissues, with special reference to the antigenic components of kidney and lung. *Lab. Invest. 4*: 69–89, 1955.

95. Miller, F. und Bohle, A.: Elektronenmikroskopische Untersuchungen am Glomerulum bei der Masugi-Nephritis der Ratte. *Virchows Arch. 330*: 483–497, 1957.

96. Miyakawa, Y.: Demonstration and purification of nephrotoxic serum antigenic substance contained in the supernatant of kidney cortex emulsion (in Japanese). *JJN 8*: 195–206, 1966.

97. Miyakawa, Y., Nagasawa, T., and Shibata, S.: Experimental chronic glomerulonephritis (in Japanese). *JJN 11*: 499–512, 1969.

98. Moriuchi, M.: Age difference in nephrotoxic nephrosis in rats (in Japanese). *JJN 4*: 263–290, 1962.

99. Movat, H.Z. and Steiner, J.W.: Studies of nephrotoxic nephritis. I. The fine structure of the glomerulus of the dog. *Amer. J. Clin. Path. 36*: 289–305, 1961.

100. Movat, H.Z., McGregor, D.D., and Steiner, J.W.: Studies of nephrotoxic nephritis. II. The fine structure of the glomerulus in acute nephrotoxic nephritis of dogs. *Amer. J. Clin. Path. 36*: 306–321, 1961.

101. Müller-Ruchholtz, W., Kraus, E., Federlin, K., Mosler, J., und Pfeiffer, E.F.: Studien zur "Übertragung" der Masugi-Nephritis der Ratte VII. Weitere fluoreszenzmikroskopische Untersuchungen an Parabionten und nephritischen Einzeltieren. *Z. Immun. -Forsch. 128*: 137–160, 1965.

102. Nagasawa, T.: Studies on experimental chronic nephritis (in Japanese). *JJN 3*: 193–209, 1961.

103. Nagasawa, T., Naruse, T., and Shibata, S.: Studies on the rat nephrotoxic nephritis by use of fluorescent antibody technique — especially using intravenous injection of fluorescein labeled nephrotoxic antibody (in Japanese). *Jap. J. Allergy 14*: 44–53, 1965.

104. Nagasawa, T., Miyakawa, Y., and Shibata, S.: Studies on nephrotoxic serum nephritis by means of fluorescent antibody technique. III. Duck- and rabbit-gamma globulin in glomeruli during the course of rabbit nephritis induced by the injection of duck anti-rabbit kidney serum (in Japanese). *Jap. J. Allergy 15*: 595–603, 1966.

105. Nagasawa, T., Miyakawa, Y., Naruse, T., and Shibata, S.: Studies on rat nephrotoxic serum nephritis by means of fluorescent antibody technique. VI. Ability of the antiserum against tryptic digested ultrasupernatant of rat inner medulla for the production of nephrotoxic serum nephritis (in Japanese). *Jap. J. Allergy 18*: 46–55, 1969.

106. Nakanoin, K. und Vogt, A.: Speciesbedingte Unterschiede im Ablauf der experimentellen Nephritis der Ratte nach Injektion von Kaninchen- und Enten-Antirattennierenserum. *Virchows Arch. 340*: 177–184, 1965.

107. Naruse, T.: The purification of nephrotoxic serum antigen — Studies with starch zone electrophoresis (in Japanese). *JJN 8*: 181–194, 1966.

108. Naruse, T. and Shibata, S.: Extraction of the water-soluble nephrotoxic antigen from rat glomerular basement membrane by means of the ultrasonic treatment (in Japanese). *Jap. J. Allergy 19*: 239–242, 1970.

109. Nishimori, I.: The production of hypertension and cardiovascular lesions by nephrotoxic nephritis combined with adrenal regeneration in rats. *Acta Path. Jap. 10 (Suppl.)*: 409–417, 1960.

110. Nogiwa, H.: Histopathological studies of Masugi nephritis in rabbits by prolonged sensitization with egg white (in Japanese). *J. Chiba Med. Soc. 35*: 1850–1861, 1960.

111. Ogawa, S. und Sato, Y.: Über das Verhalten des Komplementgehaltes im Serum im Laufe der experimentellen Glomerulonephritis. *Tr. Soc. Path. Jap. 28*: 212–218, 1938.

112. Okabayashi, A., Fujimoto, T., and Sugai, M.: Asymmetrical nephritis (I). Induction of unilateral Masugi nephritis in rabbits. *Acta Path. Jap. 7*: 408–409, 1957.

113. Okada, M.: Kidneys in prolonged sensitization. An experimental histopathological study (in Japanese). *J. Chiba Med. Soc. 38*: 396–416, 1963.

114. Okuda, R., Kaplan, M.H., Cuppage, F.E., and Heymann, W.: Deposition of autologous gamma globulin in kidneys of rats with nephrotoxic renal disease of various etiologies. *J. Lab. Clin. Med. 66*: 204–215, 1965.

115. Ooami, H.: Immunelectron microscopic studies of nephrotoxic nephritis using ferritin antibody method (in Japanese). *Nippon-Ika-Daigaku Zasshi 35*: 263–276, 1968.

116. Ortega, L.G. and Mellors, R.C.: Analytical pathology. IV. The role of localized antibodies in the pathogenesis of nephrotoxic nephritis in the rat. *J. Exp. Med. 104*: 151–170, 1956.

117. Osaka, S.: Studies on nephrotoxic nephritis. 4. Studies on fractionation of anti-rat kidney rabbit serum (nephrotoxin) (in Japanese). *JJN 8*: 513–527, 1966.

118. Pfeiffer, E.F., Schöffling, K., Bruch, H.E., und Spielmann, W.: Masugi-Nephritis und Serumkomplement der Ratte. (Speziesgebundene Unterschiede im pathogenetischen Mechanismus der Masugi-Nephritis von Ratte und Kaninchen). *Ztschr. ges. exper. Med. 122*: 446–464, 1954.

119. Pfeiffer, E.F., Schöffling, K., Sandritter, W., Schröder, J., Steigerwald, H., und Wolf L.: Studien zur "Übertragung" der Masugi-Nephritis der Ratte: Die "Übertragung" durch kurzdauernde Parabiose. *Ztschr. ges. exper. Med. 124*: 471–480, 1954.

120. Pfeiffer, E.F., Sandritter, W., Schöffling, K., Treser, G., Kraus, E., Menk, W., und Hermann, M.: Studien zur "Übertragung" der Masuginephritis der Ratte. II. Die Übertragung durch Parabiose genetisch gleichartiger Partner. *Ztschr. ges. exper. Med. 132*: 436–452, 1960.

121. Pfeiffer, E.F.: Demonstration of and evidence for the lymphocyte bound nature of a secondary nephritis producing factor in nephrotoxic glomerulonephritis in rats. *In* Grabar, P. and Miescher. P. (eds.): *Immunopathology 3 (IIIrd International Symposium)*, 220–239, Benno Schwabe, Basel-Stuttgart, 1963.

122. Piel, C.F., Dong, L., Modern, F.W.S., Goodman, J.R., and Moore, R.: The glomerulus in experimental renal disease in rats as observed by light and electron microscopy. *J. Exp. Med. 102*: 573–580, 1955.

123. Powell, A.E.: Purification of antikidney globulins on a cellulose columns. *J. Immunol. 81*: 161–171, 1958.

124. Pressman, D. and Keighley, G.: The zone of activity of antibodies as determined by the use of radioactive tracers; the zone of activity of nephrotoxic antikidney serum. *J. Immunol. 59*: 141–146, 1948.

125. Pressman, D., Korngold, L., and Heymann, W.: Localizing properties of anti-rat-kidney serum prepared in ducks. *Arch. Path. 55*: 347–348, 1953.

126. Rother, K. und Sarre, H.: Untersuchungen zur pathogenetischen Bedeutung der Autoantikörper: Einseitige experimentelle chronische Glomerulonephritis. *Klin. Wschr. 40*: 429–434, 1962.

127. Rother, K., Rother, U., Vassalli, P., and McCluskey, R.T.: Nephrotoxic serum nephritis in C′6-deficient rabbits. I. Study of the second phase of the disease. *J. Immunol. 98*: 965–971, 1967.

128. Sakaguchi, H., Suzuki, Y., and Yamaguchi, T.: Electron microscopic study of Masugi nephritis. I. Glomerular changes. *Acta Path. Jap. 7*: 53–66, 1957.

129. Sarre, H. und Wirtz, H.: Geschwindigkeit und Ort der "Nephrotoxin"-bindung bei der experimentellen Glomerulonephritis. *Klin. Wschr. 18*: 1548–1550, 1939.

130. Seegal, B.C.: In vivo localization of specific antiorgan sera: Relation to occurrence of renal lesions. *In* Shaffer, J.H., LoGrippo, G.A., and Chase, M.W. (eds.): *Henry Ford Hospital International Symposium—Mechanisms of Hypersensitivity*, 143–154, Little, Brown, Boston-Toronto, 1958.

131. Seegal, B.C., Hsu, K.C., Rothenberg, M.S., and Chapeau, M.L.: Studies of the mechanism of experimental nephritis with fluorescein-labeled antibody. II. Localization and persistence of injected rabbit or duck anti-rat-kidney serum during the course of nephritis in rats. *Amer. J. Path. 41*: 183–203, 1962.

132. Shibata, S. and Kurisu, A.: The influence of S.N.M.C., cortisone and A.C.T.H. on Masugi nephritis (in Japanese). *Jap. J. Allergy 3*: 197–203, 1954.

133. Shibata, S.: Purification of nephrotoxic antigenic factor. Its significance in the elucidation of the mechanism of Masugi nephritis. *Acta Path. Jap. 15*: 419–420, 1965.

134. Shibata, S., Naruse, T., Nagasawa, T., Takuma, T., and Miyakawa, Y.: Purification by starch block electrophoresis of renal antigen that induces nephrotoxic antibody. *J. Immunol. 99*: 454–464, 1967.

135. Shibata, S., Miyakawa, Y., Naruse, T., Nagasawa, T., and Takuma, T.: A glycoprotein that induces nephrotoxic antibody: Its isolation and purification for rat glomerular basement membrane. *J. Immunol. 102*: 593–601, 1969.

136. Shigematsu, H.: Glomerular events during the initial phase of rat Masugi nephritis. *Virchows Arch. Abt. B Zellpath. 5*: 187–200, 1970.

137. Shigematsu, H. and Kobayashi, Y.: The development and fate of the immune deposits in the glomerulus during the secondary phase of rat Masugi nephritis. *Virchows Arch. Abt. B Zellpath. 8*: 83–95, 1971.

138. Shigematsu, H. and Kobayashi, Y.: Pulmonary involvements in the initial phase of rat Masugi nephritis. *Virchows Arch. Abt. B Zellpath. 11*: 111–123, 1972.

139. Shigematsu, H. and Kobayashi, Y.: The distortion and disorganization of the glomerulus in progressive Masugi nephritis in the rat. *Virchows Arch. Abt. B Zellpath. 14*: 313–328, 1973.

140. Shiina, I.: Histopathologic study of recurrent Masugi nephritis in rabbits (in Japanese). *J. Chiba Med. Soc. 35*: 739–755, 1959.

141. Smadel, J.E.: Experimental nephritis in rats induced by injection of anti-kidney serum. I. Preparation and immunological studies of nephrotoxin. *J. Exp. Med. 64*: 921–942, 1936.

142. Smadel, J.E. and Farr, L.E.: Experimental nephritis in rats induced by injection of anti-kidney serum. II. Clinical and functional studies. *J. Exp. Med. 65*: 527–540, 1937.

143. Smadel, J.E.: Experimental nephritis in rats induced by injection of anti-kidney serum. III. Pathological studies of the acute and chronic disease. *J. Exp. Med. 65*: 541–555, 1937.

144. Small, P.A. and Baxter, J.H.: Digestion of anti-kidney antibody: Effects on its nephrotoxicity and ability to fix complement. *J. Immunol. 95*: 282–287, 1965.

145. Solomon, D.H., Gardella, J.W., Fanger, H., Dethier, F.M., and Ferrebee, J.W.: Nephrotoxic nephritis in rats. Evidence for the glomerular origin of the kidney antigen. *J. Exp. Med. 90*: 267–272, 1949.

146. Spar, I.L., Bale, W.F., Wolfe, D.E., and Goodland, R.L.: Organ specificity of I^{131} labeled rabbit kidney eluates in rats and rabbits. *J. Immunol. 76*: 119–129, 1956.

147. Spühler, O., Zollinger, H.U., und Enderlin, M.: Zum Mechanismus der Masugi-Nephritis. *Schweiz. med. Wschr. 81*: 904–908, 1951.

148. Stavitsky, A.B., Hackel, D.B., and Heymann, W.: Reduction of serum complement following in vivo tissue antigen-antibody reactions. *Proc. Soc. Exp. Biol. Med. 85*: 593–596, 1954.

149. Stavitsky, A.B., Heymann, W. and Hackel, D.B.: Relation of complement fixation to renal disease in rats injected with duck antikidney serum. *J. Lab. Clin. Med. 47*: 349–356, 1956.

150. Stelos, P., Yagi, Y., and Pressman, D.: Localization properties of radioiodinated fragments of antirat kidney antibody. *J. Immunol. 87*: 106–109, 1961.

151. Sugai, M.: Histopathologic study of unilateral Masugi nephritis in rabbits (in Japanese). *Tr. Soc. Path. Jap. 46*: 722–737, 1957.

152. Sumiyoshi, M.: An electrophoretical study in Masugi-nephritis. An electrophoretical study of serum protein and urinary protein in various kinds of Masugi-nephritis (in Japanese). *Jap. Circul. J. 21*: 332–341, 1957.

153. Swift, H.F. and Smadel, J.E.: Experimental nephritis in rats induced by injection of anti-kidney serum. IV. Prevention of the injurious effects of nephrotoxin in vivo by kidney extract. *J. Exp. Med. 65*: 557–564, 1937.

154. Takeda, K.: Allergy and reverse allergy. Allergy and immunity (in Japanese). *Jap. J. Allergy 1*: 23–28, 1952.

155. Takuma, T., Miyakawa, Y., and Shibata, S.: Studies on the method to prepare the ultra-supernatant of trypsin digested dog-kidney homogenate (in Japanese). *Jap. J. Allergy 15*: 491–496, 1966.

156. Tsuchida, H.: An electron microscopic study of the endothelium-like cells in the glomerular tufts of Masugi-nephritic rabbits (in Japanese). *JJN 9*: 351–366, 1967.

157. Tsuji, S.: Ein Beitrag zur Frage der immun-cytotoxischen Glomerulonephritis. *Beitr. path. Anat. 98*: 425–482, 1937.

158. Tsuji, S.: Über das Wesen der Glomerulonephritis (japanisch). *Folia Endocr. Jap. 17*: 603–629, 641–652, 1941–1942. Ibid. *18*: 702–751, 1942–1943.

159. Unanue, E. and Dixon, F.J.: Experimental glomerulonephritis. IV. Participation of complement in nephrotoxic nephritis. *J. Exp. Med. 119*: 965–982, 1964.

160. Unanue, E.R. and Dixon, F.J.: Experimental glomerulonephritis. V. Studies on the interaction of nephrotoxic antibodies with tissues of the rat. *J. Exp. Med. 121*: 697–714, 1965.

161. Unanue, E.R. and Dixon, F.J.: Experimental glomerulonephritis. VI. The autologous phase of nephrotoxic serum nephritis. *J. Exp. Med. 121*: 715–725, 1965.

162. Unanue, E.R., Lee, S., Dixon, F.J., and Feldman, J.D.: Experimental glomerulonephritis. VII. The absence of an autoimmune antikidney response in nephrotoxic serum nephritis. *J. Exp. Med. 122*: 565–578, 1965.

163. Unanue, E.R., Dixon, F.J., and Lee, S.: Experimental glomerulonephritis. VIII. The in vivo fixation of heterologous nephrotoxic antibodies to, and their exchange among, tissues of the rat. *Int. Arch. Allergy 29*: 140–150, 1966.

164. Unanue, E.R., Mardiney, M.R., Jr., and Dixon, F.J.: Nephrotoxic serum nephritis in complement intact and deficient mice. *J. Immunol. 98*: 609–617, 1967.

165. Vassalli, P. and McCluskey, R.T.: The pathogenic role of the coagulation process in rabbit Masugi nephritis. *Amer. J. Path. 45*: 653–677, 1964.

166. Vogt, A. and Kochem, H.G.: Immediate and delayed nephrotoxic nephritis in rats. The role of complement fixation. *Amer. J. Path. 39*: 379–392, 1961.

167. Vogt, A., Reich, L., und Nakanoin, K.: Die passive nephrotoxische Nephritis. *Virchows Arch. 341*: 224–236, 1966.

168. Vogt, A., Bockhorn, H., Kozima, K., and Sasaki, M.: Electron microscopic localization of the nephrotoxic antibody in the glomeruli of the rat after intravenous application of purified nephritogenic antibody-ferritin conjugates. *J. Exp. Med. 127*: 867–878, 1968.

169. Warnatz, H., Scheiffarth, F., and Hagel, F.: Studies on lymphocyte transformation in nephrotoxic serum nephritis of the rat. *J. Immunol. 103*: 364–368, 1969.

170. Weinreb, M.S., Soules, K.H., and Wissler, R.W.: Quantitative studies of acute nephrotoxic nephritis in rats. *Amer. J. Path. 30*: 311–335, 1954.

171. Weiss, A.: Weitere Beiträge zur Frage der experimentellen Glomerulonephritis. *Beitr. path. Anat. 96*: 111–128, 1935.

172. Winemiller, R., Steblay, R., and Spargo, B.: Electron microscopy of acute anti-basement membrane serum nephritis in rats. *Feder. Proc. 20*: 408–408, 1961.

173. Winternitz, W.W. and Hackel, D.B.: Effect of anti-histaminics on experimental nephritis in rabbits. *Proc. Soc. Exp. Biol. Med. 78*: 294–295, 1951.

174. Yagi, T.: Studies on the antigen-antibody reaction in the kidney. 1. Influence of anti-renal medulla serum on pregnant rabbit (in Japanese). *Jap. J. Allergy 17*: 141–152, 1968.

175. Yagi, Y., Korngold, L., and Pressman, D.: Purification of kidney components capable of neutralizing kidney localizing anti-rat kidney antibodies. *J. Immunol. 77*: 287–293, 1956.

176. Yagi, Y. and Pressman, D.: Multiplicity of the components of rat kidney antigen responsible for the localization of antirat kidney antibodies. *J. Immunol. 81*: 7–13, 1958.

177. Yagi, Y. and Pressman, D.: Properties of specifically purified kidney localizing antikidney antibody. *J. Immunol. 86*: 431–439, 1961.

178. Yokoyama, H.: The influence of pituitary-adrenocortical hormone on Masugi-nephritis (in Japanese). *Jap. Circul. J. 21*: 342–350, 1957.

Note added in proof: Clear-cut evidence for delayed hypersensitivity mechanism in the pathogenesis of Masugi nephritis had scarcely been presented before preparation of this manuscript, but most recently there has appeared in the Journal of Experimental Medicine, Vol. 148, pp. 246–260, issued in 1978 a report entitled "Evidence for a pathogenic role of a cell-mediated immune mechanism in experimental glomerulonephritis" by Bhan, A.K., Schneeberger, E.E., Collins, A.B., and McCluskey, R.T.

Chapter **2**

Nephrotoxic Serum Antigen
Immunochemical purification and schematic demonstration of its location on the endothelial aspects of the glomerular basement membrane

Seiichi SHIBATA

I. Release of Nephrotoxic Serum Antigen into Solution

Experimental glomerulonephritis induced in rats, rabbits or dogs by the injection of anti-rat (-rabbit, -dog) kidney serum has been studied by many investigators since it was first described by Masugi in 1929 [23–25]. Little information has been obtained, however, about the precise nature of the kidney antigen which gives rise to the nephrotoxic antibody, because attempts to extract a pure nephrotoxic serum antigen from whole kidney homogenate have been unsuccessful. The reason for this is that the extraction of the kidney with water, saline, alkaline and acid solutions, alcohol, diethylen glycol and many other solvents failed to bring the antigen into solution.

Thus, animals were injected intraperitoneally with saline suspensions (not the supernatant) of whole kidney tissue homogenate (later, of isolated glomeruli or glomerular basement membrane, GBM), for the production of nephrotoxic antiserum.

In 1951, Cole et al. [6] did not detect the antigen in saline extract of the kidney, but found that trypsin digestion of rat kidney homogenate released a substance into solution which had the ability to absorb the nephrotoxic antibody from nephrotoxic antiserum. However, their attempts to produce rabbit antisera nephrotoxic for rat kidney, by injecting this substance repeatedly into rabbits, were unsuccessful.

Thus, kidney (cortex)-ST (the ultrasupernatant substance of trypsin-digested rat kidney homogenate) has been heretofore considered a hapten, but not a complete antigen [6]. This hypothesis had been supported by several investigators [8, 12].

About 15 years later, this ultrasupernatant substance, kidney (cortex)-ST, has been found, in our laboratory, to be a potent antigenic substance which is contained in the GBM [33]: that is, 1) antisera against this kidney (cortex)-ST were found to have an ability to produce a strong precipitin reaction, on Ouchterlony plates, with kidney (cortex)-ST; 2) immunodiffusion and immunoelectrophoretic studies demonstrated that both antisera against kidney (cortex)-ST and antisera against renal cortex homogenate have a common antibody (i.e. antibody against kidney (cortex)-ST. Identical results were obtained in rats, dogs and rabbits; and 3) in rats, rabbits and dogs receiving a single intravenous injection of these antisera against corresponsing kidney (cortex)-ST, clinical and histological manifestations of typical glomerulonephritis were induced without any latent period [33].

On the other hand, kidney (cortex)-PT (the precipitate substance of trypsin-digested kidney homogenate) did not even absorb the nephrotoxic antibody from nephrotoxic antiserum. These results clearly indicate that the water-soluble kidney (cortex)-ST is the antigen responsible for the production of nephrotoxic antisera, regardless of species.

Moreover, immunodiffusion and immunoelectrophoretic studies demonstrated that both antisera against kidney (cortex)-ST and antisera against kidney (glomerulus)-ST have a common antibody (i.e. antibody against kidney (glomerulus)-ST). And, glomerulonephritis was also induced by a single intravenous injection of antisera against kidney (glomerulus)-ST. Thus, it seems clear that this antigenic substance is contained in kidney (glomerulus)-ST: that is, the active principle of the antigenic substance, kidney (cortex)-ST, is located in the glomerulus. A new fluorescent antibody technique (in vivo method) was introduced in this study, for the purpose of demonstrating that the antigenic substance, kidney (cortex)-ST, is present in the renal glomerulus or GBM.

Previous to our study, Ortega and Mellors [29] have reported that by the fluorescent antibody technique (in vitro method) the renal location of the nephrotoxic antibody (anti-whole kidney serum) is primarily — and perhaps exclusively — in the "membrane" of the glomerular tufts (although, they do not specify the basement membrane). However, it appears that this method is too indirect for the demonstration of antiGBM sera which are capable of inducing clinical and histological changes of glomerulonephritis.

On the contrary, using our in vivo method, the intravenous injection of FITC (fluorescent isothiocyanate)-labeled gamma-globulin fraction of nephrotoxic antiserum (anti-rat renal cortex homogenate rabbit serum) resulted in the uptake of the fluorescent antibody exclusively in the GBM.

Identical results were obtained by the intravenous injection of FITC-labeled gamma-globulin fraction of antisera against kidney (cortex)-ST and antisera against kidney (glomerulus or GBM)-ST.

Thus, it appears that the results obtained by the use of this in vivo method prove a direct connection between antigen-antibody interaction in the GBM and the histological manifestation of glomerulonephritis, and that all of these antisera are antiGBM sera, — that is, the active antigenic principle is most probably derived from the GBM.

II. Chemical Properties of Nephrotoxic Serum Antigen

When animals were immunized with kidney (cortex)-ST, kidney (cortex) homogenate and kidney (glomerulus)-ST, many antibodies which are not harmful to animal kidneys (that is, not nephrotoxic) were always produced, along with the specific nephrotoxic antibody. Therefore, the antigenic substance effective for the production of nephrotoxic antibody needs further purification.

In the next step of the investigation, further attempts were made to purify this specific antigenic substance [34].

1. Chemical composition of kidney (cortex)-ST from rabbit, rat and dog

The chemical properties of kidney (cortex)-ST were examined, at first, qualitatively. One per cent solution of kidney (cortex)-ST gave strongly positive Molisch reaction, whereas the Bial reaction was almost negative (green color appeared). The biuret reaction was negative. This substance retained its activity by heating at 65 °C for 30 minutes or at 70 °C for 15 minutes. It was non-dialyzable and proved to be lyophilized without any decrease in its activity. Thus, dialyzed and lyophilized samples were used for chemical analysis. As shown in Table 2-1, similar results on the chemical composition were obtained, regardless of species.

(Fig. 2-2). We have not seen any previous reports of such typical chronic glomerulo-nephritis in rats (so-called contracted kidney) being induced by a single intravenous in-jection of nephrotoxic antiserum (antiserum against whole kidney homogenate).

Experiments using the fluorescent antibody technique proved that in rats injected with antisera against fraction-3, uptake of the fluorescent antibody occurred only in the GBM. This fact may provide direct evidence that the active principle in the purified fraction -3 was derived from the GBM (Fig. 2-3).

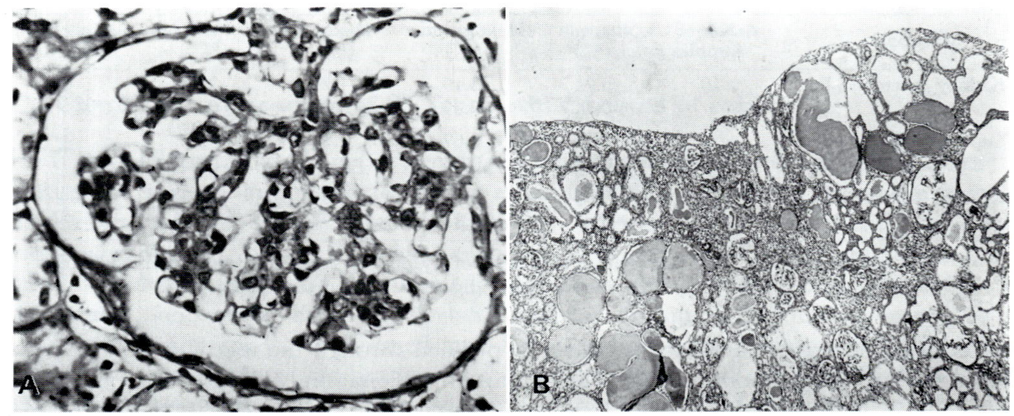

Fig. 2-2

A: Glomerular changes in a rat killed 12 days after injection of antiserum against fraction-3 of kidney (cortex)-ST. Morphologic changes of typical proliferative glomerulonephritis manifested by mesangial cell proliferation, lobulation and adhesion of glomerular tufts to Bowman's capsule.

B: Kidney section from a rat injected with rabbit antiserum against fraction-3 of kidney (cortex)-ST and killed 4 months later, showing typical chronic glomerulonephritis (so-called contracted kidney).

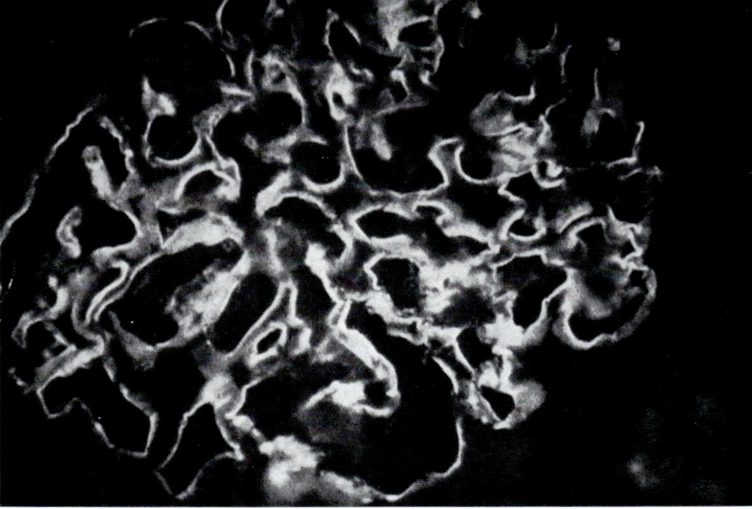

Fig. 2-3 Frozen section of kidney from a rat killed 14 days after the injection of non-labeled rabbit antiserum against fraction-3 of rat kidney (cortex)-ST. The section was treated with fluorescein isothiocyanate-labeled sheep antiserum against rabbit gamma-globulin. Note the fluorescence of the GBM.

III. Chemical Purification of the Soluble Antigen

1. Chemical purification of the antigen isolated from the anatomically pure GBM

Krakower and Greenspon studied the localization of the nephrotoxic antigen within the isolated renal glomerulus [13], and found in 1951 that the GBM was 20 times more active antigenically than the combined visceral epithelial and endothelial cells [20].   Moreover, in 1956, Ortega and Mellors [29] reported that the renal localization of nephrotoxic antibodies is primarily and exclusively in the membranes of the glomerular tufts.

Thus, it was important to determine whether purified material from the GBM was similar in its chemical composition to that of fraction-3 from kidney (cortex)-ST.

The antigen that produces nephrotoxic antiserum was isolated as GBM-ST from highly purified GBM, and then purified chemically as Fr-αS by starch block electrophoresis and molecular sieving through Sephadex G200 [38]:

A screening experiment was tried to ascertain the distribution in the starch block of the nephrotoxic serum antigen (Fig. 2-4).   The localization of antigenic material that induces nephrotoxic antiserum was limited to the following three fractions: α-fraction (-1 cm to -5 cm), β-fraction (-1 cm to $+1$ cm) and γ-fraction ($+1$ cm to $+5$ cm).

Immunization revealed that the antigenicity of the α-fraction was far greater than that of the other two fractions.   The α-fraction yielded only one peak in which the peaks of hexose and protein co-incided.

Reasonable purity of Fr-αS was revealed by immunoelectrophoretic and ultracentrifugal analysis:

The purified Fr-αS showed only a single sedimentation boundary with an $S_{20,w}$ of 1.02S

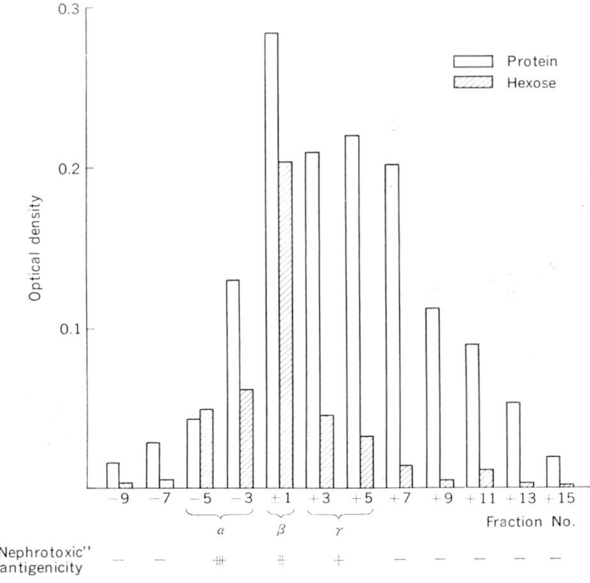

Fig. 2-4 Distribution of protein, hexose and antigenic substance following block electrophoresis of GBM-ST. (From Shibata, S. et al.: *J. Immunol. 102*: 593–601, 1969)

at 9.2 mg/ml by analysis in a Spinco Model E (Fig. 2-5). Due to the paucity of purified antigen [yielded only 5.5 mg (dry weight) from 390 mg (dry weight) of GBM-ST, starting from 3.0 kg (wet weight) of rat perfused renal cortex], further ultracentrifugal characterization was not feasible.

The chemical composition of Fr-αS was that of glycoprotein and the analytic data, including the results of amino acids analysis and studies on the monosaccharide composition, resembled those obtained with kidney (cortex)-ST as shown in Tables 2-4, 2-5, and 2-6. With the increase of purification, a remarkable decrease in the values of both glucosamine and phosphorus was noted.

In other words, it is possible to say that the more detailed structure of the active antigenic principle, which induces nephrotoxic antiserum, can be determined chemically, even when the starting material is a crude kidney (cortex)-ST, which contains tubular and vascular elements, as well as glomeruli or GBM.

In rats that received a single intravenous injection of antiserum against Fr-αS, acute proliferative glomerulonephritis was induced without a latent period and then progressed continuously [36]. The nephrotoxic potency of the antisera was so high that typical

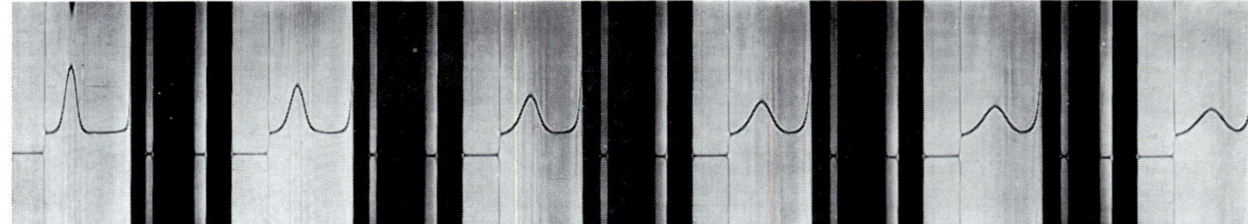

Fig. 2-5 Ultracentrifugal pattern of Fr-αS. Analysis was performed on a synthetic boundary cell at 55,430 rpm in 0.1 M NaCl. Phase angle, 65°. The pictures shown were taken at 1, 17, 33, 49, 65 and 81 min, respectively. The direction of the sedimentation is toward the right. (From Shibata, S. et al.: *J. Immunol. 102*: 593–601, 1969)

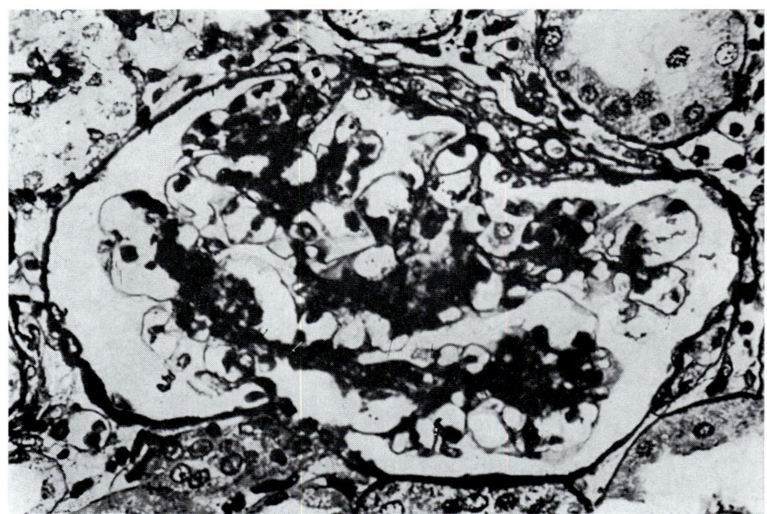

Fig. 2-6 Kidney section from a rat that was injected with rabbit antiserum against Fr-αS and killed 52 days later, demonstrating that glomerular scarring developed and progressed in the mesangium. PAM stain. (From Shibata, S. et al.: *J. Immunol. 102*: 593–601, 1969)

Table 2-4   Chemical properties of Fr-αS and fraction-3.

	Carbon	Hydrogen	Nitrogen	Hexose	Hexosamine	Phosphorus
Fr-αS	40.86*	6.90*	11.53*	11.06	0.28	0.12
Fraction-3			8.03**	12.45	0.43	0.11

    * Carbon, hydrogen and nitrogen were determined by elemental analysis.
    ** Nitrogen value was used in exchange for protein value.
(From Shibata, S. et al.: *J. Immunol. 102*: 593–601, 1969 [38])

Table 2-5   Amino acid composition of Fr-αS, fraction-3 and B-fraction of TR-Pron-GBM [38, 39].

Amino acid	Fr-αS Sample I (mol %)	Fr-αS Sample II (mol %)	Fraction-3 (mol %)	B-fraction of TR-Pron-GBM (mol %)
Glycine	37.78	34.25	37.76	39.69
Alanine	6.57	6.89	3.99	5.53
Valine	3.46	3.74	3.37	2.35
Leucine	5.54	6.18	6.44	5.50
Isoleucine	2.81	3.01	3.37	2.43
Proline	8.33	7.62	8.59	9.33
Phenylalanine	2.55	2.57	2.86	2.31
Tyrosine	0.84	1.07	Trace	0.80
Threonine	3.35	3.54	3.07	2.84
Serine	5.00	6.96	5.11	8.04
Cysteic acid	—*	—	4.50	—
Cystein	—	—	—	—
Methionine	1.09	1.15	—	0.68
Arginine	2.47	2.46	2.04	2.27
Histidine	1.09	0.98	0.51	1.44
Lysine	1.61	2.27	1.33	1.74
Aspartic acid	7.03	6.80	6.14	5.76
Glutamic acid	10.48	10.64	11.15	9.29
Hydroxyproline	—	—	Trace	—

    * Not detectable

Table 2-6   Monosaccharide composition of 90% phenol water layer,
Fr-αS, fraction-3 B-fraction of TR-Pron-GBM.

Material	Glucose	Galactose	Mannose
90% phenol water layer	1	0.14	0
Fr-αS	1	0.38	0.03
Fraction-3	1	0.65	0.06
B-fraction of TR-Pron-GBM	1	0.24	0

chronic glomerulonephritis with progressive scarring of glomeruli was observed even in rats which were killed 3 months after a single injection.

As shown in Fig. 2-6, glomerular scarring developed and progressed obviously in the mesangium as in human glomerulonephritis [14].

When glomerulonephritis induced by antisera against insoluble GBM (Masugi nephritis) was compared with that induced by antisera against soluble glycoprotein (fraction-3 or Fr-αS), the immunologic process of the latter cannot be explained by Kay's two step theory [15, 16] (combination of heterologous and autologous phases), but can be explained by a heterologous phase only (Fig. 2-7).

It is noteworthy that morphologic changes of the kidney produced by antiserum against

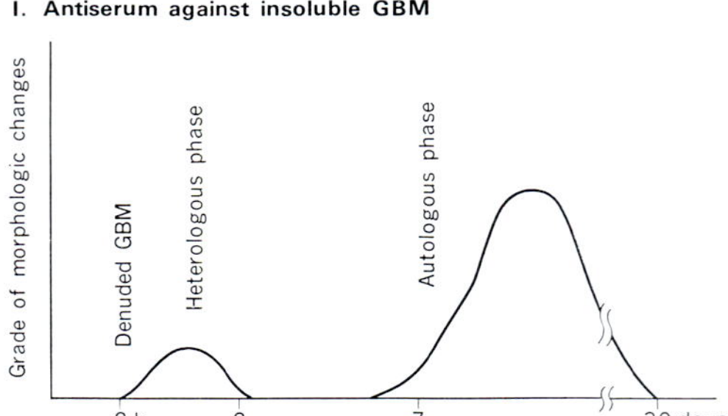

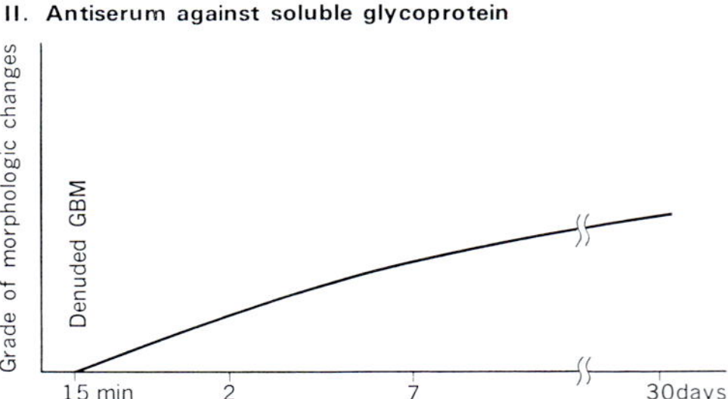

Fig. 2-7 Schematic demonstration of immunological events (glomerulonephritis) occurring in rats injected with antiserum against insoluble GBM (I) and in rats injected with antiserum against soluble glycoprotein from GBM (II). Note the presence of autologous phase only in (I). (From Shibata, S.: *In* Kefalides, N.A. (ed.) *Biology and Chemistry of Basement Membranes*, 535–559, Academic Press, New York, 1978)

Fr-αS also resembled those of experimental glomerulonephritis induced with antisera against fraction-3 from kidney (cortex)-ST [36, 37]. Immunofluorescence studies demonstrated that both of fraction-3 and Fr-αS are derived from the GBM (linear pattern).

Considering these results, it may be concluded that Fr-αS from GBM-ST and fraction-3 from kidney (cortex)-ST are very similar in both chemical composition and biologic activity.

2. Role of the protein and polysaccharide moieties in maintaining the antigenic properties

As the next step of the investigation, we attempted to determine the role of the protein and polysaccharide moieties in maintaining the antigenic properties of this glycoprotein, and these attempts resulted in further purification of this antigenic substance [39].

First, periodate oxidation which breaks carbon-carbon bonds — two adjacent unsubstituted hydroxyl groups or a hydroxyl group adjacent to primary or secondary amino group — was carried out to clarify the relationship between the polysaccharide moiety and antigenicity, and the results indicated that this procedure destroyed almost all of the antigenic property that induces nephrotoxic antibody.

In the next experiment, GBM-ST was digested with pronase-P for 3 hours, and zone electrophoresis was carried out for 10 hours for the purpose of removing the remaining pronase-P. These procedures resulted in a material (B-fraction of TR-Pron-GBM) that had a remarkably low protein content, without a decrease in antigenic activity. Amino acid composition of this material is shown in Table 5.

Although the monosaccharide composition of the glycoprotein obtained from GBM-ST was composed of glucose, galactose and a trace of mannose [38], the monosaccharide composition of the material obtained by pronase-digestion and zone electrophoresis of GBM-ST was found to be composed mainly of glucose, with a trace of galactose (see Table 2–6).

Therefore, the mannose component appears to be unnecessary for maintaining the antigenic property that induces nephrotoxic antibody. A very similar phenomenon was also observed by subfractionation of the β-fraction of GBM-ST: we have attempted to extract the polysaccharide fraction from the active glycoprotein without affecting the antigen that induces nephrotoxic antibody. For this purpose we used the 90% phenol extraction procedure [52]. Almost all of the antigenic property of active fraction, which had been shown to contain no nucleic acid after zone electrophoresis [38], shifted in the water-layer (Fig. 2–8). The monosaccharide composition of this fraction was revealed to be mainly glucose, with only a trace of galactose.

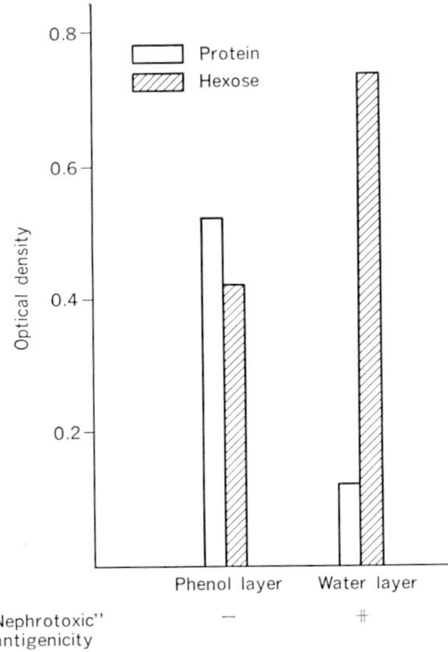

Fig. 2-8   Distribution of protein and antigen following 90% phenol fractionation. (From Shibata, S. et al.: *J. Immunol. 104*: 215–223, 1970)

Thus, our attempts to isolate and purify the antigenic substance that induces nephrotoxic antibody from the GBM yielded a glycoprotein that possessed mainly glucose and a trace of galactose as the polysaccharide moiety, and in which the protein content was remarkably low.

Recently, Klemer et al. [18, 19] isolated from normal and arteriosclerotic aorta a glycoprotein in which the polysaccharide moiety was shown to consist of glucose residues. However, they did not investigate the biologic activity of this glycoprotein.

Consequently, we have not seen any previous report of a soluble glycoprotein derived from normal GBM, in which the polysaccharide moiety was shown to consist mainly of glucose residues, and which has the biologically active antigenicity that induces nephrotoxic antibody.

IV. Specific Interaction of Nephrotoxic Serum Antigen and Concanavalin A

1. In vitro interaction of the antigen and concanavalin A

It has been reported from our laboratory that enzymatic digestion of the basement membrane yields a water-soluble glycoprotein, which contains as the carbohydrate composition glucose, galactose, a trace of mannose and glucosamine [37-39].   The glycoprotein has antigenic activity, which induces nephrotoxic antibody (nephrotoxic serum antigenicity) [37-39].

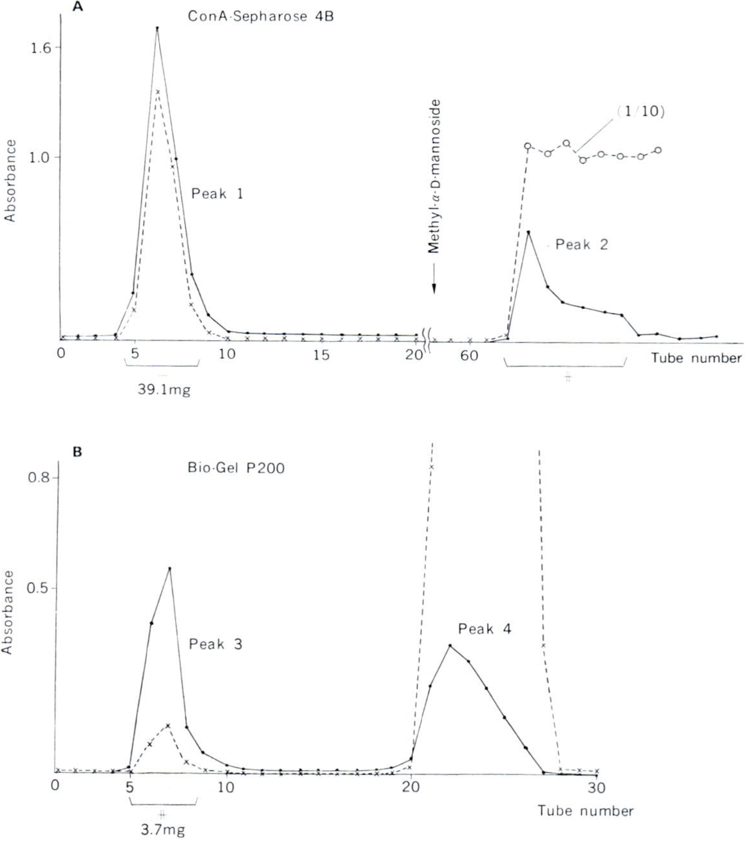

Fig. 2-9

A: Chromatography of the α-fraction of renal glycoprotein on Con A-Sepharose 4B. ●——●, Absorbance at 280 nm; ×······×, hexose content (anthrone method); ○——○, hexose content, scale compressed 10 times to show the mannoside front; +, −, antigenic activity, estimated by the Ouchterlony method using rabbit antiserum against the α-fraction of renal glycoprotein as testing antibody. 80 mg of the α-fraction of renal glycoprotein were applied.

B: Removal of methyl α-D-mannopyranoside from peak 2 of Fig. 9A by gel filtration on a column of Bio-Gel P200 equilibrated with 0.05 M pyridine acetate buffer, pH 5.5. The material (peak 3) retained by Con A and subsequently eluted with methyl α-D-mannopyranoside was revealed to be nephrotoxic antiserum producing antigen.

(From Shibata, S. et al.: *Biochim. Biophys. Acta 499*: 392–403, 1977)

The nephrotoxic serum antigenicity of the water-soluble glycoprotein was destroyed after periodate oxidation [38] and this evidence strongly suggests that nephrotoxic serum antigenicity relates more closely to the carbohydrate moiety. Furthermore, the trace of mannose was shown to be unnecessary for the production of nephrotoxic antiserum [38].

On the other hand, it is well known that concanavalin A (Con A), a lectin isolated from jack beans, binds specifically to α-D-glucopyranosyl, α-D-mannopyranosyl and β-D-fructo-furanosyl groups and forms precipitates with polysaccharides and glycoproteins containing these groups at the nonreducing terminus [4, 9-11, 47, 48].

Thus, active water-soluble glycoprotein was applied to a column of Con A affinity chromatography. As shown in the upper part of Fig. 2-9, the high and non-retarded peak was shown to contain no nephrotoxic serum antigenicity. However, in the material retained by Con A and subsequently eluted with α-D-methylmannoside, we found almost all of the principal nephrotoxic serum antigenicity. As shown in the lower part of this figure, the active water-soluble glycoprotein was sharply separated and purified from contaminated α-D-methylmannoside by gel filtration in a Bio-Gel P200 column. These results suggest that the active principle is a glycoprotein with a oligosaccharide having an α-D-glucopyranosyl or an α-D-mannopyranosyl unit at the non-reducing terminus.

A simple procedure, trichloroacetic acid treatment, was successfully introduced for removal of the mannose component. 0.25 vol. of 25% trichloroacetic acid was added to

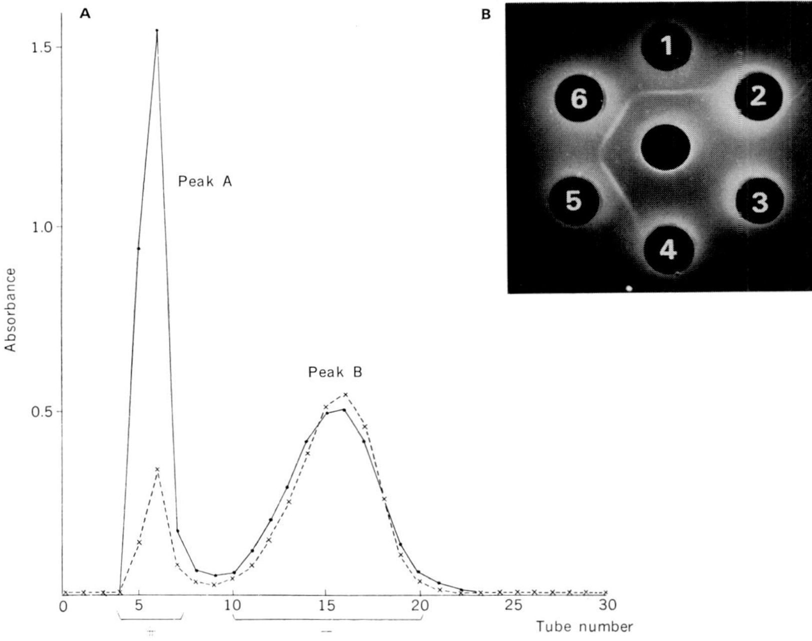

Fig. 2-10

A: The pattern of elution of the purified renal glycoprotein (fraction 1) from Bio-Gel P200. The active peak A (11.51 mg) was sharply separated from the inactive peak B (53.36 mg), starting from 100 mg of renal glycoprotein fraction 1.

B: Ouchterlony gel diffusion demonstrating the existence of a one common precipitin line between peak A, peak II and the α-fraction of renal glycoprotein and antiserum against peak 3. 1, peak A (Fig. 2-10A); 2, peak B (Fig. 2-10A); 3, peak II′ (Fig. 2-12); 4, peak I (Fig. 2-11); 5, peak II (Fig. 2-11); 6, the α-fraction of renal glycoprotein. Center well, anti-serum against peak 3.

(From Shibata, S. et al: *Biochim. Biophys. Acta 499*: 392–403, 1977)

the water-soluble renal glycoprotein and the mixture was centrifuged after overnight settling. Since nephrotoxic serum antigenicity was found mainly in the supernatant fluid, the precipitate was discarded.

The supernatant thus obtained was then applied to a column of Bio-Gel P200. Two hexose peaks (A and B) were obtained, and nephrotoxic activity was demonstrated only in the first peak A (Fig. 2-10). Monosaccharide composition of the active peak A was glucose and galactose in the ratio of 1 : 0.29 and mannose was not detected in this fraction.

Fig. 2-11 shows the representative elution patterns of peak A of Fig. 2-10 (the non-retarded and retarded fraction) in the column of Con A-Sepharose 4B.

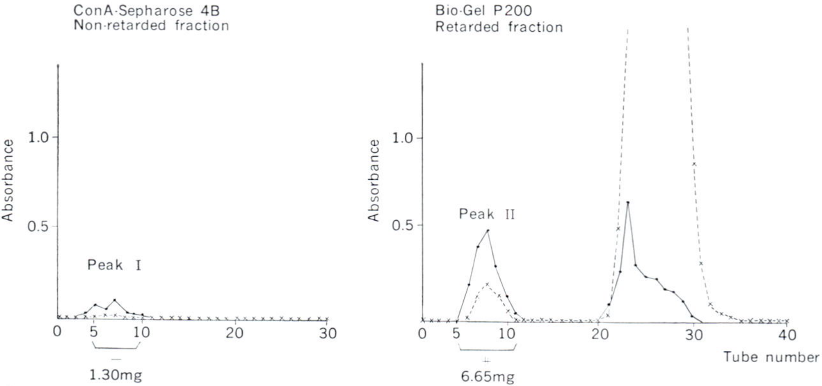

Fig. 2-11 Chromatography of active peak A of Fig. 10 on ConA-Sepharose 4B. ●——●, Absorbance at 280 nm; ×······×, hexose content (anthrone method); +, −, nephrotoxic activity (the antigenic activity that induces nephrotoxic antibody, estimated by Ouchterlony method using rabbit antiserum against peak 3 as testing antibody). Peak I : the non-retarded material, after removal of salt by gel filtration on a column of Bio-Gel P-6. Peak II : the retarded material, after removal of methyl α-D-mannopyranoside by gel filtration on a column of Bio-Gel P200. The presence of the significant hexose peak (glycoprotein) was found only in active fraction (peak II) with nephrotoxic activity. (From Shibata, S. et al.: *Biochim. Biophys. Acta 499*: 392–403, 1977)

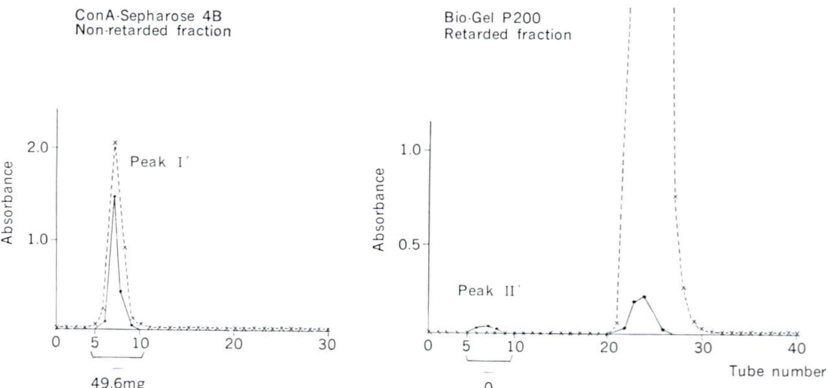

Fig. 2-12 Chromatography of inactive peak B of Fig. 2-10 on ConA-Sepharose 4B. ●——●, Absorbance at 280 nm; ×······×, hexose content (anthrone method); +, −, nephrotoxic activity (the antigenic activity that induces nephrotoxic antibody, estimated by Ouchterlony method using rabbit antiserum against peak 3 as testing antibody): Peak I′: the non-retarded material after removal of salt by gel filtration on a column of Bio-Gel P-6. Peak II′: the retarded material after removal of methyl α-D-manno-pyranoside by gel filtration on a column of Bio-Gel P200. Note the absence of the significant hexose peak in the active fraction (peak II′). (From Shibata, S. et al.: *Biochim. Biophys. Acta 499*: 392–403, 1977)

Table 2-7   Recovery of peak II (Con A) from 1 kg purified renal cortex.

Renal cortex	1 kg	(wet weight)
↓		
Basement membrane (insoluble)	2,141 mg	(dry weight)
↓		
Renal glycoprotein	700 mg	(dry weight)
↓		
Renal glycoprotein fraction 1 (supernatant)	305 mg	(dry weight)
↓		
Peak II (Con A)	10.14 mg	(dry weight)

(From Shibata, S. et al.: *Biochim. Biophys. Acta 499*: 392–403, 1977 [44])

There was no significant hexose content and no nephrotoxic activity in peak I (the non-retarded fraction), and a high glycoprotein component with nephrotoxic serum antigenicity was detected as peak II in the retarded fraction.   The yield of active glycoprotein was 10.14 mg (dry weight), starting from 1 kg (wet weight) of rat renal cortex or 700 mg of renal glycoprotein (Table 2-7).

When the second (inactive) peak B of Fig. 2-10 was applied to a column of Con A-Sepharose 4B, no significant glycoprotein component was detected in peak II′ (active fraction) of Fig. 2-12, and a high glycoprotein component was found only in peak I′ (inactive fraction).

It is noteworthy that in the non-retarded fraction we could not demonstrate nephrotoxic serum antigenicity.   If this activity was present in the non-retarded fraction, even to a very small extent, mild proliferative glomerulonephritis with moderate proteinuria might be induced in rats which received a single intravenous injection of antiserum against this fraction.

Thus, it can be concluded as follows: examination of the material retained by the un-solubilized Con A and subsequently eluted with methyl α-D-mannopyranoside reveals that the principal high affinity receptor for Con A is the water-soluble renal glycoprotein, having antigenic activity that induces nephrotoxic antibody.   Evidence was given to show that this finding is specific.   (This purified glycoprotein has also nephritogenicity; i.e. the activity capable of inducing glomerulonephritis in homologous animals by a single footpad injection with Freund's incomplete adjuvant [40–43].)

2. In vivo interaction of GBM and injected concanavalin A

The water-soluble renal glycoprotein, which interacts specifically with Con A, is shown to originate in the normal rat GBM.   Therefore, if the surface (the endothelial side) of normal rat basement membrane is composed of this renal glycoprotein, then the injected Con A should be found to bind to GBM.

To confirm this, the following in vivo experiments were carried out: 1) rats were injected with 1 ml of FITC-labeled Con A through the renal artery, and killed one hour after injection.   As shown in Fig. 2-13, the injected Con A interacted specifically with the capillary walls (and the mesangium) of the glomeruli, as well as with those of the peri-tubular capillaries.   The specificity was proved by the complete inhibition of this binding when rats were injected with both FITC-labeled Con A and methyl α-D-mannopyranoside (Fig. 2-14); and 2) rats were given intravenously 0.5, 1.0 or 2.0 mg non-labeled Con A/100g body weight and killed one hour after injection.   By the use of FITC-labeled antiserum against Con A (non-labeled Con A) in the kidney is exactly the same as that induced by the injection of FITC-labeled Con A.   Consequently, it appears likely that

On the other hand, a marked increase in the number of polymorphonuclear leukocytes in glomeruli appeared 2 hours after injection in animals given antiserum against soluble GBM-glycoprotein, as well as in those receiving antiserum against insoluble GBM.   Therefore, the exfoliation of endothelial cytoplasm denuding the GBM is difficult to explain with the aid of leukocytic mediator.

Furthermore, electron microscopic studies of the GBM itself in animals which were examined up to 4 hours after injection, failed to reveal any dramatic alteration in its structure.   The lamina densa remained intact as a continuous electron-dense band, and no differences could be distinguished between zones of the basement membrane in intimate contact with polymorphonuclear leukocytes and the basement membrane in capillary loops unaffected by polymorphonuclear leukocytes.

Table 2-8   Comparison of glomerulonephritis by anti-insoluble GBM serum and anti-soluble glycoprotein serum [46].

	Anti-insoluble GBM	Anti-soluble glycoprotein
Latent period	7–8 days	–
Its immunologic explanation	1. Heterologous phase	
	2. Autologous phase	Heterologous phase only
Early morphologic changes:		
1. Exfoliation of endothelial cytoplasm	2.5 hr	10–15 min
2. Polymorph infiltration	2.5 hr	2 hr
3. GBM only	24–48 hr	24–48 hr

The results are summarized in Table 2-8, and these seem to suggest strongly that the initial and significant morphologic changes induced in the glomeruli of rats by the intravenous injection of antiserum against soluble GBM-glycoprotein are not the GBM damage, but are the exfoliation of endothelial cytoplasm denuding the GBM, without endothelial cell necrosis and prior to infiltration of polymorphonuclear leukocytes.   In other words, it seems likely that nephrotoxic serum antigen is not the GBM as a whole, but only a structural component of the GBM or a coating material on the endothelial aspects of the GBM.

This view may be supported by the chemical findings in our laboratory [44] that nephrotoxic serum antigen, which is the water-soluble substance isolated from normal rat GBM, is chemically the receptor glycoprotein for Con A, having an α-D-glucopyranosyl unit at the non-reducing terminus facing the endothelial aspects of the glomerular capillary loop. The yield of the active glycoprotein was only 1/219 of insoluble GBM.

VI.   Conclusion

Although classical nephrotoxic serum nephritis is well known as a useful model for studying the mechanism of human glomerulonephritis, morphologic changes of this nephritis (especially of rats) are not so similar to those of human adult progressive glomerulonephritis (Ellis type II): namely, 1) the main histologic features of classical nephrotoxic serum nephritis in rats are not "glomerulitis", but "thickening of the GBM", and 2) rats receiving a single injection of nephrotoxic antisera show no morphologic changes of chronic glomerulonephritis with progressive scarring.

One of the reasons for this may be that nephrotoxic antisera has been prepared by immunizing animals with water-insoluble saline suspension of whole kidney homogenate, glomerulus, or GBM.

The nephritis induced in rats by a single intravenous injection of antiserum against water-soluble kidney (cortex)-ST was revealed to be similar to that of human adult progressive glomerulonephritis, and has the following features in contrast with nephrotoxic serum nephritis:

First, in rats that received a single injection of antisera against kidney (cortex)-ST (or GBM-ST) severe proteinuria and typical histologic changes of proliferative glomerulonephritis developed without a latent period and then progressed continuously and steadily.

Second, the immediate production and continuous progression of this experimental glomerulonephritis (regardless of species) strongly suggest that the direct interaction of circulating antibody with antigens contained in the GBM produces glomerular "injury", and that the latent period as the time required for the formation of antibodies against rabbit serum (i.e. the carrier-protein of anti-rat kidney serum) [15, 16] is not necessary for the development of morphologic changes of diffuse glomerulonephritis.

Thus, it seems reasonable to expect that the mechanism by which the injection of classical nephrotoxic antiserum results in the development of glomerulonephritis should be re-investigated, using antisera against purified antigens such as those we have demonstrated.

REFERENCES

1. Arakawa, M. and Kimmelstiel, P.: Circumferential mesangial interposition. *Lab. Invest. 21*: 276–284, 1969.
2. Baxter, J.H. and Goodman, H.C.: Nephrotoxic serum nephritis in rats. I. Distribution and specificity of the antigen responsible for the production of nephrotoxic antibodies. *J. Exp. Med. 104*: 467–486, 1956.
3. Churg, J., Grishman, E., Goldstein, M.H., Yunis, S.L., and Porush, J.G.: Idiopathic nephrotic syndrome in adults. *New Engl. J. Med. 272*: 165–174, 1965.
4. Clarke, A.E. and Denborough, M.A.: The interaction of concanavalin A with blood-group-substance glycoproteins from human secretions. *Biochem. J. 121*: 811–816, 1971.
5. Cochrane, C.G., Unanue, E.R., and Dixon, F.J.: A role of polymorphonuclear leukocytes and complement in nephrotoxic nephritis. *J. Exp. Med. 122*: 99–116, 1965.
6. Cole, L.R., Cromartie, W.J., and Watson, D.W.: A specific soluble substance involved in nephrotoxic nephritis. *Proc. Soc. Exp. Biol. Med. 77*: 498–501, 1951.
7. Faith, G.C. and Trump, B.F.: The glomerular capillary wall in human kidney disease: acute glomerulonephritis, systemic lupus erythematosus, and preeclampsia-eclampsia. Comparative electron microscopic observation and a review. *Lab. Invest. 15*: 1682–1719, 1966.
8. Glynn, L.E. and Holborow, E.J.: Conversion of tissue polysaccharides to autoantigens by group-A-hemolytic streptococci. *Lancet ii*: 449–451, 1952.
9. Goldstein, I.J., Hollerman, C.D., and Merrick, J.M.: Protein-carbohydrate interaction. I. The interaction of polysaccharides with concanavalin A. *Biochim. Biophys. Acta 97*: 68–76, 1965.
10. Goldstein, I.J., Hollander, C.E., and Smith, E.E.: Protein-carbohydrate interaction. II. Inhibition studies on the interaction of concanavalin A with polysaccharides. *Biochemistry 4*: 876–883, 1965.
11. Goldstein, I.J. and So, L.L.: Protein-carbohydrate interaction. III. Agar-gel-diffusion studies on the interaction of concanavalin A, a lectin isolation from jack bean, with polysaccharides. *Arch. Biochem. Biophys. 111*: 407–415, 1965.
12. Goodman, H. and Baxter, J.H.: Nephrotoxic serum nephritis in rats. II. Preparation and characterization of a soluble protective factor produced by trypsin digestion of rat tissue homogenate. *J. Exp. Med. 104*: 487–499, 1956.
13. Greenspon, S.A. and Krakower, C.A.: Direct evidence for the antigenicity of the glomeruli in the production of nephrotoxic serums. *Arch. Path. 49*: 291–297, 1950.
14. Jones, D.B.: Inflammation and repair of the glomerulus. *Amer. J. Path. 27*: 991–998, 1957.
15. Kay, C.F.: The mechanism by which experimental nephritis is produced in rabbits injected with nephrotoxic duck serum. *J. Exp. Med. 72*: 559–572, 1940,

16. Kay, C.F.: The mechanism of a form of glomerulonephritis, nephrotoxic nephritis in rabbits. *Amer. J. Med. Sci. 204*: 483–490, 1942.

17. Kimmelstiel, P., Osawa, G., and Beres, J.: Some glomerular changes by electron microscopy with predominant mesangial reaction. *Proceedings of the Third International Congress of Nephrology, Washington, 1966,* Vol. 2, pp. 17–32, Karger, New York, 1967.

18. Klemer, A. and Memple, D.: Chemische Untersuchungen an Chondroitinschwefelsäure-protein-komplexen normaler und sklerotischer Aorten. III. *Z. Naturforsch. 20b*: 553–559, 1965.

19. Klemer, A. and Nager, C.: Über Glykoproteide aus menschlichen Aorten. II. *Z. Naturforsch. 22b*: 456, 1967.

20. Krakower, C.A. and Greenspon, S.A.: Localization of the nephrotoxic antigen within the isolated renal glomerulus. *Arch. Path. 51*: 629–639, 1951.

21. Lerner, R.A. and Dixon, F.J.: Transfer of ovine experimental allergic glomerulonephritis (EAG) with serum. *J. Exp. Med. 124*: 431–442, 1966.

22. Lerner, R.A., Glassock, R.J., and Dixon, F.J.: The role of anti-glomerular basement membrane antibody in the pathogenesis of human glomerulonephritis. *J. Exp. Med. 126*: 989–1004, 1967.

23. Masugi, M.: Über die spezifisch zytotoxische Wirkung des Antinieren- und Leberserums sowie die sog. ungekehrte Anaphylaxie. *Tr. Jap. Path. Soc. 19*: 132–137, 1929.

24. Masugi, M.: Über das Wesen der spezifischen Veränderungen der Niere und der Leber durch das Nephrotoxin bzw. das Hepatotoxin. Zugleich ein Beitrag zur pathogenese der Glomerulonephritis und der eklamptischen Lebererkrankung. *Beitr. Path. Anat. 91*: 82–112, 1933.

25. Masugi, M.: Über die experimentelle Glomerulonephritis durch das spezifische Antinierenserum. Ein Beitrag zur Pathogenese der diffusen Glomerulonephritis. *Beitr. Path. Anat. 92*: 429–466, 1934.

26. Nagasawa, T. and Shibata, S.: Immunofluorescence studies on the anatomic distribution of the soluble antigen responsible for the production of nephrotoxic serum nephritis. *J. Immunol. 103*: 736–740, 1969.

27. Nagasawa, T. and Shibata, S.: Production of glomerulonephritis by antiserum against the soluble antigen (tryptic digested ultrasupernatant substance) from various rat organs. *Jap. J. Exp. Med. 39*: 143–151, 1969.

28. Naruse, T. and Shibata, S.: Mechanical extraction of the water-soluble antigen that induces nephrotoxic antiserum from rat glomerular basement membrane. *Immunology 22*: 925–932, 1972.

29. Ortega, L.G. and Mellors, R.C.: Analytical pathology. IV. The role of localized antibodies in the pathogenesis of nephrotoxic nephritis in the rat. *J. Exp. Med. 104*: 151–170, 1956.

30. Pressman, D., Eisem, E.N., and Fitzgerald, P.J.: The zone of localization of antibodies. VI. The rate of localization of anti-mouse-kidney serum. *J. Immunol. 64*: 281–287, 1950.

31. Raistrick, H. and Topley, W.W.C.: Immunizing fractions isolated from Bact. Aertrycke. *Brit. J. Exp. Path. 15*: 113–130, 1934.

32. Sarre, H. and Wirtz, H.: Geschwindigkeit und Ort der Nephrotoxic-bindung bei der experimentelle Glomerulonephritis. *Klin. Wochenschr. 18*: 1548–1550, 1939.

33. Shibata, S., Nagasawa, T., Takuma, T., Naruse, T., and Miyakawa, Y.: Isolation and properties of the soluble antigen specific for the production of nephrotoxic glomerulonephritis. I. Immunopathological demonstration of the complete antigenicity of the soluble antigen. *Jap. J. Exp. Med. 36*: 127–142, 1966.

34. Shibata, S., Nagasawa, T., Takuma, T., Naruse, T., and Miyakawa, Y.: Isolation and properties of the soluble antigen specific for the production of nephrotoxic glomerulonephritis. II. Purification of the active principle from the soluble antigen. *Jap. J. Exp. Med. 36*: 143–160, 1966.

35. Shibata, S. and Naruse, T.: Further purification of nephrotoxic serum antigen. *Jap. J. Exp. Med. 36*: 103–105, 1966.

36. Shibata, S., Nagasawa, T., Naruse, T., and Miyakawa, Y.: Glomerulonephritis induced in rats by antiserum against a glycoprotein from rat kidney. A new experimental model of glomerulonephritis. *Jap. J. Exp. Med. 37*: 337–353, 1967.

37. Shibata, S., Naruse, T., Nagasawa, T., Takuma, T., and Miyakawa, Y.: Purification by starch block electrophoresis of renal antigen that induces nephrotoxic antibody. *J. Immunol. 99*: 454–464, 1967.

38. Shibata, S., Miyakawa, Y., Naruse, T., Nagasawa, T., and Takuma, T.: A glycoprotein that induces nephrotoxic antibody: Its isolation and purification from rat glomerular basement membrane. *J. Immunol. 102*: 593–601, 1969.

39. Shibata, S., Naruse, T., Miyakawa, Y., and Nagasawa, T.: Further purification of the glycoprotein that induces nephrotoxic antibody: Isolation of the active polysaccharide fraction mainly composed of glucose. *J. Immunol. 104*: 215–223, 1970.

40. Shibata, S., Nagasawa, T., Miyakawa, Y., and Naruse, T.: Nephritogenic glycoprotein. I. Proliferative glomerulonephritis induced in rats by a single injection of the soluble glycoprotein isolated from homologous glomerular basement membrane. *J. Immunol. 106*: 1284–1294, 1971.

41. Shibata, S., Sakaguchi, H., Nagasawa, T., and Naruse, T.: Nephritogenic glycoprotein. II. Experimental production of membranous glomerulonephritis in rats by a single injection of homologous renal glycopeptide. *Lab. Invest. 27*: 457–465, 1972.

42. Shibata, S. and Nagasawa, T.: Nephritogenic glycoprotein. III. Immunochemical studies on nephritogenic activity of homologous water-soluble glycoprotein extracted from various rat organs. *Immunology 26*: 217–228, 1974.

43. Shibata, S., Sakaguchi, H., and Nagasawa, T.: Induction of chronic progressive glomerulonephritis with immunofluorescent "Mesangial pattern" in rats. *Nephron 16*: 241–255, 1976.

44. Shibata, S., Nagasawa, T., and Miura, K.: Nephritogenoside, the receptor glycoprotein for concanavalin A in rat glomerular basement membrane. Demonstration of α-D-glucopyranosyl unit at the non-reducing terminus. *Biochim. Biophys. Acta 499*: 392–403, 1977.

45. Shibata, S., Sakaguchi, H., and Nagasawa, T.: Exfoliation of endothelial cytoplasm in nephrotoxic serum nephritis. A study using antiserum against water-soluble glycoprotein isolated from the glomerular basement membrane. *Lab. Invest. 38*: 201–207, 1978.

46. Shibata, S.: Immunologic and non-immunologic aspects of experimental glomerulonephritis. *In* Kefalides, N.A. (ed.) *Biology and Chemistry of Basement Membranes*, 535–559, Academic Press, New York, 1978.

47. So, L.L. and Goldstein, I.J.: Protein-carbohydrate interaction. Application of the quantitative hapten inhibition technique to polysaccharide-concanavalin A interaction. Some comments on the forces involved in concanavalin A-polysaccharide interaction. *J. Immunol. 99*: 158–163, 1967.

48. So, L.L. and Goldstein, I.J.: Application of the quantitative precipitin method to polysaccharide-concanavalin A interaction. *J. Biol. Chem. 242*: 1617–1622, 1967.

49. Spühler, O., Zollinger, H.U., and Enderlin, M.: Zur Mechanismus der Masugi-nephritis. *Schweiz. Med. Wschr. 81*: 904–908, 1951.

50. Steblay, R.W.: Glomerulonephritis induced in sheep by injections of heterologous glomerular basement membrane and Freund's complete adjuvant. *J. Exp. Med. 116*: 253–272, 1962.

51. Unaue, E.R., Dixon, F.J., and Feldman, J.D.: Experimental allergic glomerulonephritis induced in the rabbit with homologous renal antigens. *J. Exp. Med. 125*: 163–176, 1967.

52. Westphal, O. and Lüderitz, O.: Chemische Erforshung von Lipopolysacchariden Gram-negative Bacterien. *Angewandte Chem. 66*: 407–414, 1954.

53. Winemiller, R., Steblay, R.W., and Spargo, B.: Electron microscopy of acute anti-basement membrane serum nephritis in rats. *Fed. Proc. 20*: 408–409, 1961.

Chapter **3**

Immunohistochemistry of Nephrotoxic Nephritis

Yozo MASUGI

I. Introduction

Nephrotoxic nephritis, also known as Masugi nephritis [50, 51] is a significant milestone for immunopathologic research not only of pathogenic mechanisms of glomerulonephritis per se, but also all antigen-antibody reaction mediated vascular injuries. Especially in the field of nephrology, this model has become the prototype of anti-glomerular basement membrane (GBM) antibody mediated glomerular damages.

The chronological review of nephrotoxic nephritis is given in a separate section, therefore in this chapter the author will describe mainly recent progress in the researches of nephrotoxic nephritis, related models of experimental glomerulonephritis and their human counterparts, in which immunohistochemical observations concerning immunopathologic points of view will be stressed.

II. General Remarks on Immunopathology of Nephrotoxic Nephritis

1. Heterologous phase

As is well known, nephrotoxic nephritis in experimental animals can be produced by passive administration of antikidney serum produced by another species of animal. This antiserum of heterologous origin has been known traditionally as nephrotoxic serum or nephrotoxin. When a proper amount of this potent antiserum is given to experimental animals, biphasic biological reactions usually ensue in the glomeruli [24, 33, 97].

After administration, some portion of the nephrotoxin immediately conjugates with the host GBM along its anatomical distribution, which can be easily observed by immuno-fluorescent technique. On the other hand, an appreciable amount of nephrotoxin, being heterologous protein in nature, is phagocytosed by the reticuloendothelial cells in various organs and serves as an antigenic stimulus to the host lymphatic apparatus. Such efficient conjugation of the nephrotoxin to the GBM might be explained from the following reasons [97]. The glomerulus is physiologically active in excreting intravascular contents through the GBM which is exposed to the capillary lumen by fenestrated pores of the endothelial layer. Furthermore, the circulatory blood volume of the kidney in unit time is measured to be much larger than that of other organs.

The conjugation of the administrated nephrotoxin in the circulatory blood to the GBM is observed to be terminated within almost 20 minutes after injection, measured by ^{131}I-labeled heterologous nephrotoxic globulin in mice [70], although some evidence suggests that antibody of low avidity lasts for a relatively longer time interval [95].

As already described, the results can be visualized by the immunofluorescent technique as a continuous uniform linear deposition of the heterologous nephrotoxic globulin along the host GBM (Fig. 3-1).   On this point, a very characteristic feature is that the positive antikidney antibody conjugation in the kidney is strictly confined to the GBM and rarely noted in the other components such as the tubular basement membrane (TBM).   This evidence is in sharp contrast to the observation that if the antikidney antibody is applied directly to the kidney section in vitro, it usually reacts not only to the GBM but also to the TBM and all other components for which antikidney antibody contains immunologic activities [28].

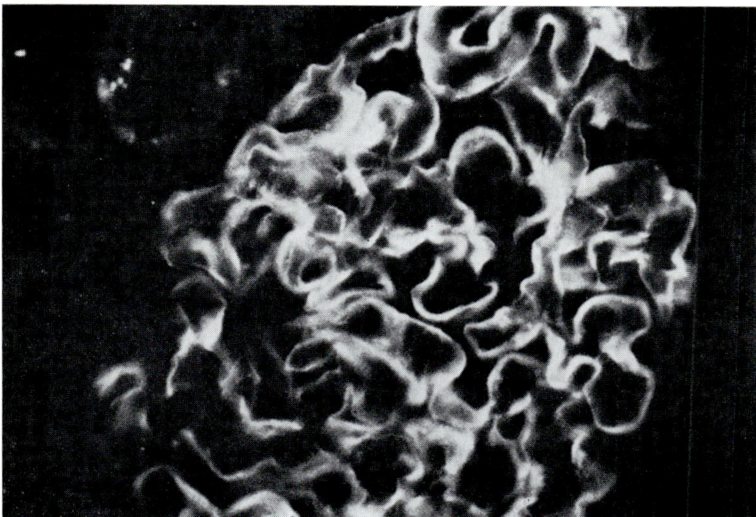

Fig. 3-1   A glomerulus of rat, 24 hours after receiving rabbit antirat GBM serum. The linear fluorescence of IgG (nephrotoxic globulin) along the GBM is shown. $\times 200$.

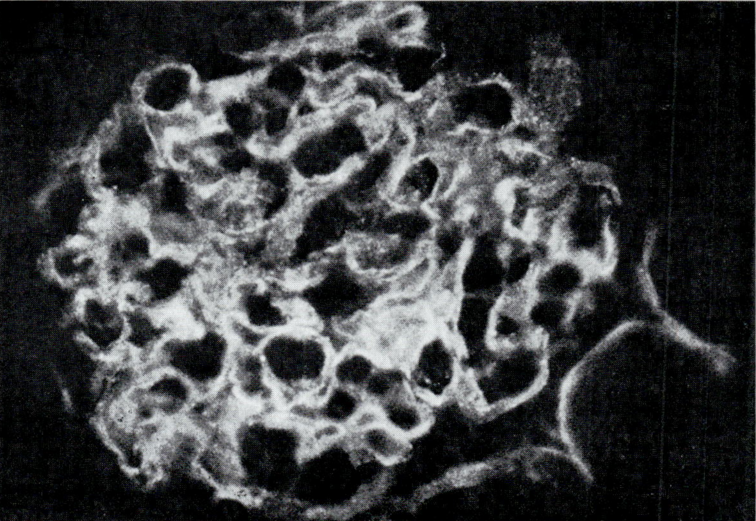

Fig. 3-2   A glomerulus of rat, 3 days after receiving rabbit antirat GBM serum. Mainly linear fluorescence of rat C_3 along the GBM is noted. $\times 200$.

Concomitant with conjugation of the nephrotoxin to the GBM, if the nephrotoxic antiserum is from a mammalian source, although some exceptions exist, the host complement system is usually activated and conjugated to the GBM together with the nephrotoxic globulin [24, 94, 97] (Fig. 3-2).

This initial occurrence is generally referred to the heterologous phase of nephrotoxic nephritis. Furthermore, the conjugation of the nephrotoxic antibody to the GBM may be followed immediately by proteinuria or by histological evidence of glomerulonephritis, although the glomerular alteration may depend much on the host species, the species origin of the nephrotoxin, amount of the nephrotoxic antibody used and the intensity of the host immune responses. For instance, avian nephrotoxin such as duck origin must be used in relatively large amounts to produce an immediate glomerular alteration in this heterologous phase [24, 25, 27, 74, 94]. However, in general, the glomerular alteration seen in this phase is usually not very conspicuous.

From the above results, the nephritogenic antigen(s) against the nephrotoxic antibody in the kidney should be localized in the GBM. The immunohistochemical studies of the precise localization and distribution of the nephritogenic antigen(s) in the GBM are the important theme of this article.

In this case, however, when a small amount of avian nephrotoxin is administered to mammals, although nephrotoxic globulin is localized along the GBM, the host complement system is not activated in this heterologous phase and morphological and functional glomerulonephritic changes are as a rule mild or not observed. However, the presence or abscence of the detectable complement components along the GBM in the heterologous phase in relation to the occurrence of glomerular alterations has also been debatable problem. This will be discussed again later.

2. Autologous phase

In the next step, the prolongation of the nephrotoxic nephritis process can be achieved by the following mechanisms. If the nephrotoxin treated animal has the capacity to make an immune response to the immunoglobulin(s) of the animal species used as the source of the nephrotoxin, prolonged and much more florid glomerulonephritic processes ensue after a certain latent period of usually six or more days.

This mechanism can be explained from the fact that fixation of the above newly formed antibody is superimposed upon the already attached heterologous nephrotoxic globulin along GBM [96]. By immunofluorescence, such host immunoglobulin(s) can be visualized also linearly along the GBM (Fig. 3-3). Concomitant with this event, further activation of the host complement system participates and this newly formed immune complex along the GBM can add further immunologic insult to the glomerular capillaries. This new event is referred to the autologous phase of the nephrotoxic nephritis. For this reason, it can be concluded that the severity of the glomerular lesion at this phase depends mainly on the amount of the initially attached heterologous nephrotoxic globulin to the GBM. If only a minute amount of antikidney antibody is administered originally to the experimental animals, unless active or passive immunization to the heterologous γ-globulin of the species supplying the nephrotoxic antibody is given at the same time, proteinuria or pathomorphologic alterations of glomeruli usually do not develop [96].

Because the nephrotoxic globulin, host antibody and complement system attached to the GBM usually is present as long as the original glomerular capillary architecture remains, the injurious effect of the immunologic reaction to glomeruli progresses. If a relatively small amount of the nephrotoxin of avian source is administered to mammals, the func-

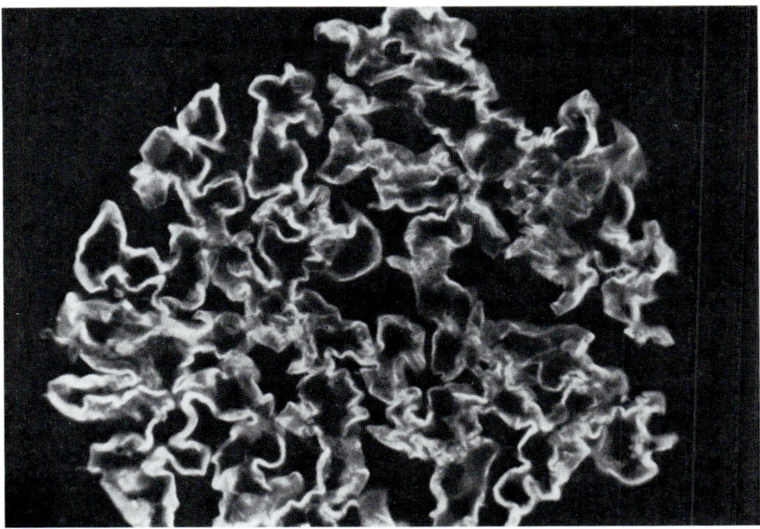

Fig. 3-3 A glomerulus of rabbit, 23 days after receiving guinea pig antirabbit GBM serum. The linear fluorescence of rabbit IgG along the GBM is obvious. ×200.

tional and morphological glomerulonephritic signs can be observed usually after the initiation of this autologous phase, because in this time the activation of the host antibody together with complement system can take place [94].

The fate of the pathomorphologic alterations of the kidney in the autologous phase depends not only upon the intensity of the host antibody response capable of fixing to the GBM-bound nephrotoxin, but also on the species difference of the experimental animals used. If potent nephrotoxin is administered, rats ordinarily follow a progressive disease course throughout the heterologous and autologous phases, terminating in chronic glomerulonephritis. On the other hand, rabbits usually show one of two distinct courses in the autologous phase. One is amelioration of the symptoms with morphologic cure, the other is a rapidly progressing subacute self-perpetuating course with predominant glomerular crescent formation which is eventually fatal.

In the nephrotoxic nephritis, as already stated, the initial event and the propagatory force of the entire disease process is the conjugation of the antikidney antibody to the GBM. If the antiGBM antibody, which is antibody to the mechanically isolated and purified GBM fragments, is used instead of the anti whole kidney antibody, the efficiency of conjugation of the antibody to the GBM and its phlogogenic effects are much more pronounced. In other words, the nephritogenic antigen(s) in the kidney as the target for the antikidney antibody should be localized in the GBM itself. However in this case too, if a kidney section is overlaid with the purified antiGBM antibody in vitro, the antibody conjugates not only to the GBM but also to the glomerular mesangial areas and total TBM.

From this reason, the investigation of precise in vivo localization of the antiGBM antibody in submolecular level may represent the structural localization of the nephritogenic antigen(s) in the GBM. For this purpose, the immunoelectron microscopic study rather than the light microscopic immunofluorescence should be used for detecting the distribution of the anti-GBM antibody along the GBM. In addition, the chemical nature of the nephritogenic antigen(s) is worthy of investigation. Before proceeding to these subjects, the results of the conventional transmission electron microscopic studies of the nephrotoxic nephritis will be surveyed.

III. Conventional Electron Microscopic Observation

The electron microscopic studies of the experimental animals in this nephrotoxic nephritis model have been reported many times, so that only the universal findings and their pathogenetic considerations will be summarized here.   In the heterologous phase, usually the displacement of glomerular endothelial cells by polymorphonuclear leukocytes (PMNs) or fibrin deposits or both [7, 26, 80], thickening and rarefaction of the lamina lucida int. [4, 6, 17, 21, 64] are the most consistent abnormalities that have been reported.   Edematous swelling or disarrangement of the mesangial matrices and accumulation of blood monocytes in the glomerular capillary lumina and further infiltration into the mesangial areas have also been considered [41, 80].   Besides, subendothelial deposits of wispy, poorly delineated substances are occasionally noted in this heterologous phase [6, 16, 17, 57, 64, 69].   However the GBM itself may fail to show alterative features of comparative severity, despite the considerable light microscopic and functional abnormalities in this heterologous phase of the complement-dependent antiGBM antibody mediated glomerular injury.

As an explanation for this discrepancy, the alteration of chemical constituents of the GBM, which was not evident by electron microscopy, was speculated.   For instance, reduction in sialoprotein was discussed by Chiu and Drummond [5] and Mohos and Skoza [63], explaining that sialic acid which was possibly partly responsible for maintaining the gel filtration property of the GBM and usually associated with the nephritogenic GBM antigen, would be reduced by the localization of nephrotoxic antibody to the GBM. Relationship between proteinuria and reduction in sialoprotein of the GBM especially at the level of epithelial cells and epithelial slits pores was also recently confirmed in autologous immune complex nephropathy of Heymann type [12].   On the other hand, Gang and Kalant [21] and Gang et al. [22] suggested that the loss of lipid phosphorous from the GBM at the molecular level caused by the initial attack of the heterologous nephrotoxic antibody, eventually led to proteinuria.   As far as the permeability of the GBM is concerned, the validity of these observations must be confirmed in the future.

In the following autologous phase, gradual deterioration of the GBM architecture, such as irregular thickening of the GBM with uneven distribution of electron density, proliferation of mesangial cells with widening of mesangial matrices and deposition of collagenous fibers in mesangial areas are usual findings in accord with the development of glomerulonephritic changes [6, 18, 91].   Furthermore, peripheral interposition of mesangial cells between endothelial cells and GBM [41, 91], separation of the capillary lumina by dendritic mesangial cell projections were reported [41].   The accumulation of PMNs in this phase is usually not conspicious compared to the heterologous phase.   Furthermore, electron dense deposits are reported to be found not only in the subendothelial but also in the subepithelial spaces along the GBM [4, 64, 81].   The biological nature of these deposits will be discussed again later.

From the above described conventional electron microscopic studies, detailed morphologic changes are known; however, the precise localization of the nephrotoxic antibody along the GBM or mode of submolecular interaction of antibody with the nephritogenic antigen(s) must be await the immunoelectron microscopic studies of the glomeruli.

IV. Immunoelectron Microscopic Observations

Immunohistocytological study on the electron microscopic level was started, using horse ferritin as a marker for the antibody globulin molecule by Singer [83] in 1959.   The excellence of this method was that iron micelle of the ferritin molecule gave a sharp contrast on the electron micrograph and that ferritin and antibody globulin could make an isomolecular compound [48, 86]. This method has been used widely in the biological field. However, because the large size of ferritin labeled antibody molecule has been main hindrance against the penetration of labeled antibody through the limiting membrane of tissue or cells, the alternative method such as enzyme labeled antibody technique especially using horseradish peroxidase as a marker was started by Nakane and Pierce [67] or Avrameas and Uriel [3] in 1966 and has been widely used. In this method, the localization of peroxidase as a marker of the antibody must be detected by a secondary histochemical method using a substrate such as diaminobenzidin which can give considerable density on the electron microscopic observation.

These two immunoelectron microscopic methods have also been used in the field of the kidney research including nephrotoxic nephritis.

1. In vitro incubation method by labeled "anti-nephrotoxic globulin" antibody

For the identification of intraglomerular localization of the nephrotoxic antibody or in other words the demonstration of distribution of the nephritogenic antigen(s) along the GBM at the submolecular level, the immunoelectron microscopic study by means of the in vitro ferritin labeled antibody technique on the rabbit nephrotoxic nephritis was originally performed by Andres et al. [1] in 1962, and was soon followed by Arhelger et al. [2]. These two articles showed that the entire width of the GBM is the target of the nephrotoxic antibody. The ferritin molecules labeled to the "anti-nephrotoxic globulin" antibody (antibody to the immunoglobulin(s) of the animal species from which the nephrotoxic serum originated) and served as the tracer of the nephrotoxic globulin, were found

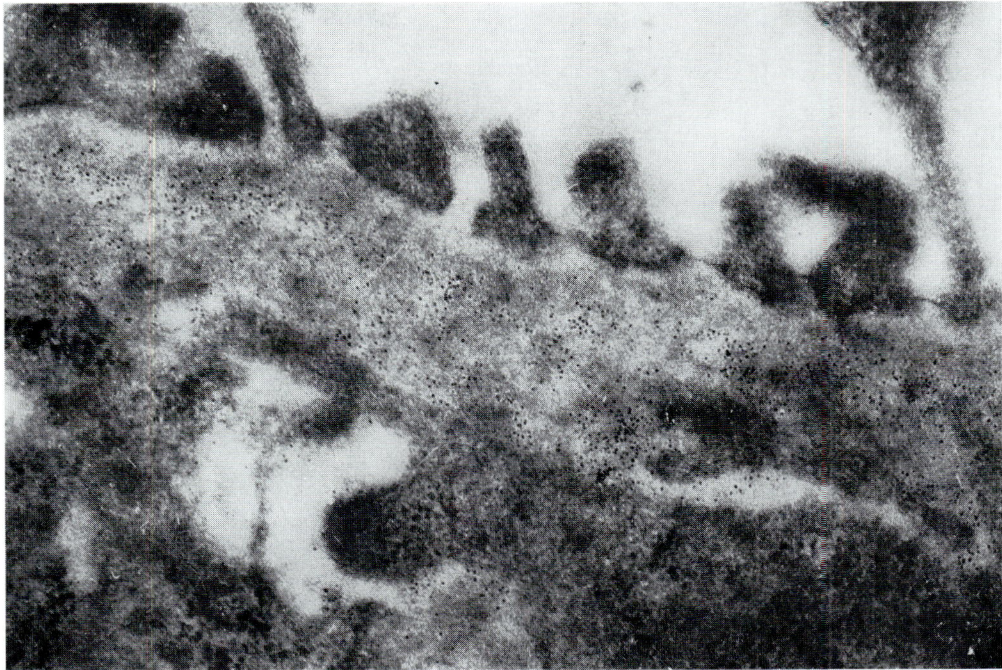

Fig. 3-4 A peripheral GBM of rat, 5 hours after receiving antiGBM antibody. Ferritin particles which represent localization of nephrotoxic antibody, disseminate throughout the GBM. The lamina densa and parts of lamina lucida int. apper to be more heavily infiltrated with ferritin particles. ×70,000.

either throughout the three layered GBM [1] or located to a greater extent in the inner and outer layers of the membrane [2].   Moreover, both groups reported further labeling of ferritin particles on the cytoplasm of the adjacent epithelial and endothelial cells in the glomeruli.   Especially, Andres et al. pointed out ferritin labeling of the amorphous material in cisternae of the endoplasmic reticulum of the epithelial cells.   Despite their belief that this finding might be specific and suggestive of either synthesis of new GBM material or just intracellular transport, its validity is not certain because of the technical instability of this method and the impurity of the antikidney antibody used by them at that time. These results were later confirmed by Masugi [52] who reported that the ferritin particles as tracers of nephrotoxic γ-globulin in the nephrotoxic nephritis model of rats, were observed to be located throughout the GBM especially the lamina densa and parts of lamina lucida int. (Fig. 3-4).   Furthermore, the ferritin particles were also found in lesser amounts in the mesangial matrices and intracytoplasmic vesicles of the mesangial cells (Fig. 3-5), although the immunofluorescent method done at the same time usually revealed no or just faintly detectable nephrotoxic γ-globulin in the mesangial areas.   The meaning of this finding in the mesangial areas will be mentioned later.

These immunoferritin findings were further confirmed by the in vitro technique with horseradish peroxidase labeled "anti-nephrotoxic globulin" antibody at the electron microscopic level by Hoedemaeker et al. [29] and Druet et al. [14] in 1972.   They also studied the mode of distribution of nephrotoxic globulin in glomeruli, in the heterologous phase of nephrotoxic nephritis.

Hoedemaeker et al. [29] used the multilayer peroxidase technique for detecting the distribution of the nephrotoxic antibody between 24 hours to 6 weeks after the admini-

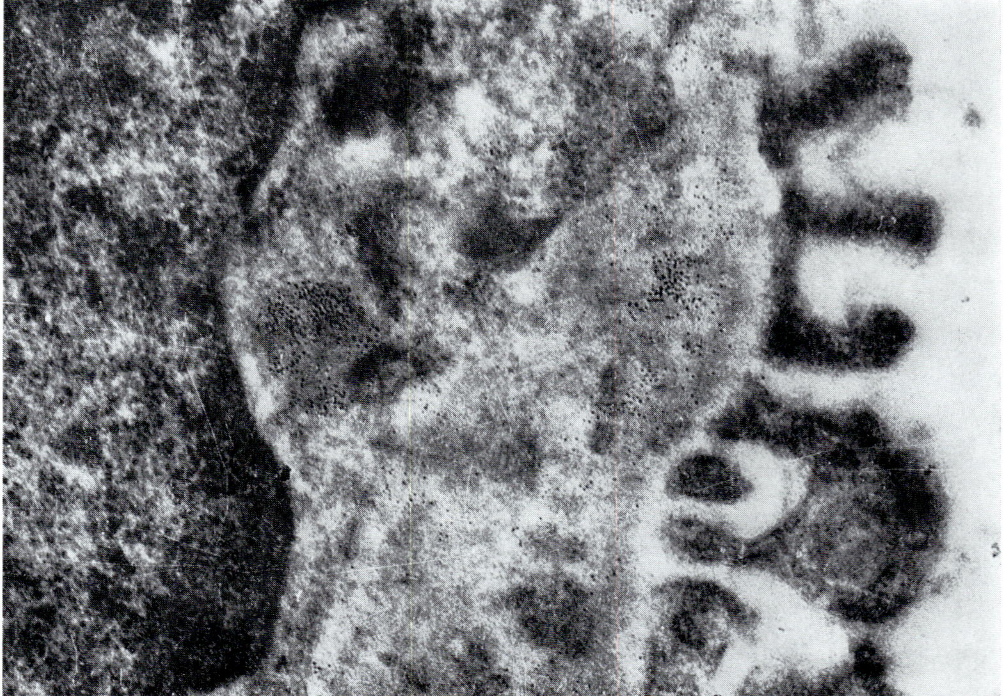

Fig. 3-5   A mesangial part of the glomerulus of same rat as in Fig. 4. Ferritin particles are also noted in the axillary region of the GBM, mesangial matrix and vesicle of mesangial cell. $\times 70,000$.

stration to rats.   They claimed that the reaction products of the peroxidase as the tracer of the nephrotoxic globulin were seen only in the peripheral BM of the glomerular capillaries, while the parts encircling the mesangial areas, also called axillary regions of the GBM, remained negative, as were the mesangial areas themselves (Fig. 3-6).   They explained that this localization could be due to the fact that only the peripheral parts of the GBM could be actively infiltrated by the injected nephrotoxic globulin and that during this filtration process the nephrotoxic globulin had the opportunity to bind the antigenic sites in the GBM.   The labeling along the peripheral GBM was observed throughout the entire width of the GBM, and the highest concentration of the labeling was occasionally found in the lamina densa, in accordance with the previous reports.   However, the findings at the axillary GBM and the mesangial areas were considerably different from the previous reports when the ferritin labeled antibody method was used.   They speculated that nephrotoxic globulin drained by the mesangial areas probably did not come in contact with the GBM or GBM-like substances in the mesangial matrices.   From this point of view, if availability or accessibility of the GBM antigen(s) to the in vivo administrated nephrotoxic antibody is taken into account, the precise anatomic distribution of the nephritogenic antigen(s) in the glomeruli may not be ascertainable.   However, this explanation may not have much experimental support, because the varied markers including macromolecules administrated to the experimental animals could easily pass into the mesangial areas of the glomeruli [15, 16, 42, 61, 62].   In case of the nephrotoxic nephritis in rats too, Mauer et al. [56] reported an increased radiolabeled aggregated human IgG uptake in the mesangium compared to the control animals.

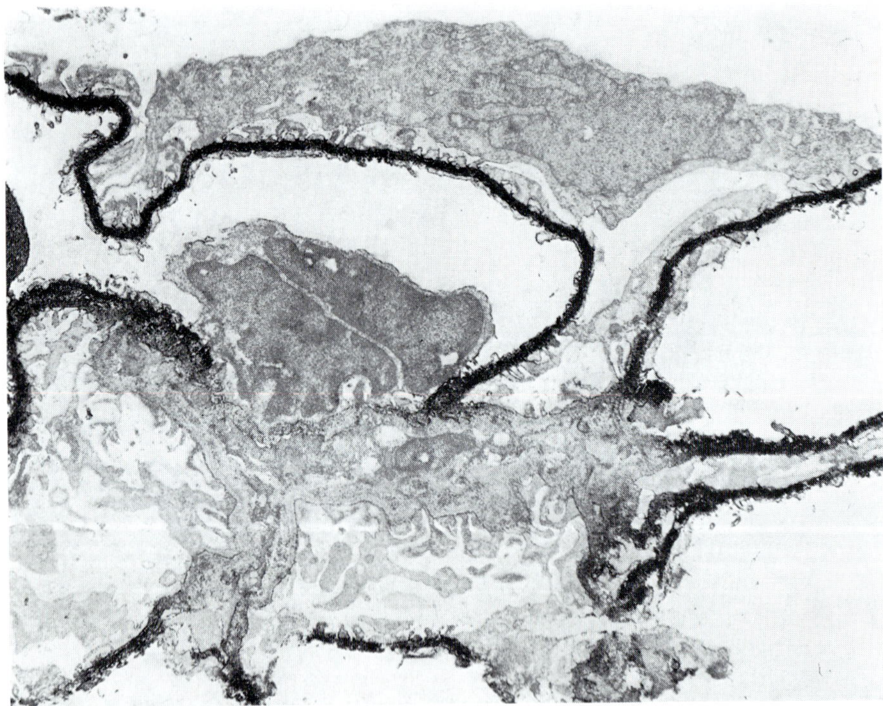

Fig. 3-6   Part of a glomerulus of a rat that received rabbit nephrotoxic globulin. The black enzymatic product indicating the presence of nephrotoxic globulin is observed in the peripheral GBM. The axillary portion of the GBM is negative.   ×6,5000. (From Hoedemaeker, P.J. et al.: *Lab. Invest. 26*: 610–613, 1972)

Druet et al. [14] used peroxidase labeled whole and Fab fragment of "anti-nephrotoxic globulin" antibody in the nephrotoxic nephritis rats. In addition to in vitro incubation method, they simultaneously performed an in vivo administration method with peroxidase labeled nephrotoxic antibody. In their study, both the in vitro and in vivo observations were reported to confirm each other showing that fixation of the heterologous nephrotoxic antibody was observed primarily in the GBM of the peripheral capillary loops mostly in its inner and outer aspects (Fig. 3-7). They also found that enzymatic reaction products were noted in the mesangial matrices and the GBM adjacent to the mesangial areas, although they were less intense than in the GBM of the peripheral capillary loops. Furthermore, the membranoid material between endothelial and mesangial areas was also positive. They postulated that nephrotoxic antibody might penetrate more readily into the peripheral glomerular capillary loops than inside the mesangial material. In other words, the nephrotoxic antibody might be largely consumed at the peripheral GBM and only a minor portion of the antibody might enter the mesangial areas or axillary portions of the GBM. Recently, McCauseland et al. [57] did a similar in vitro study using pero-

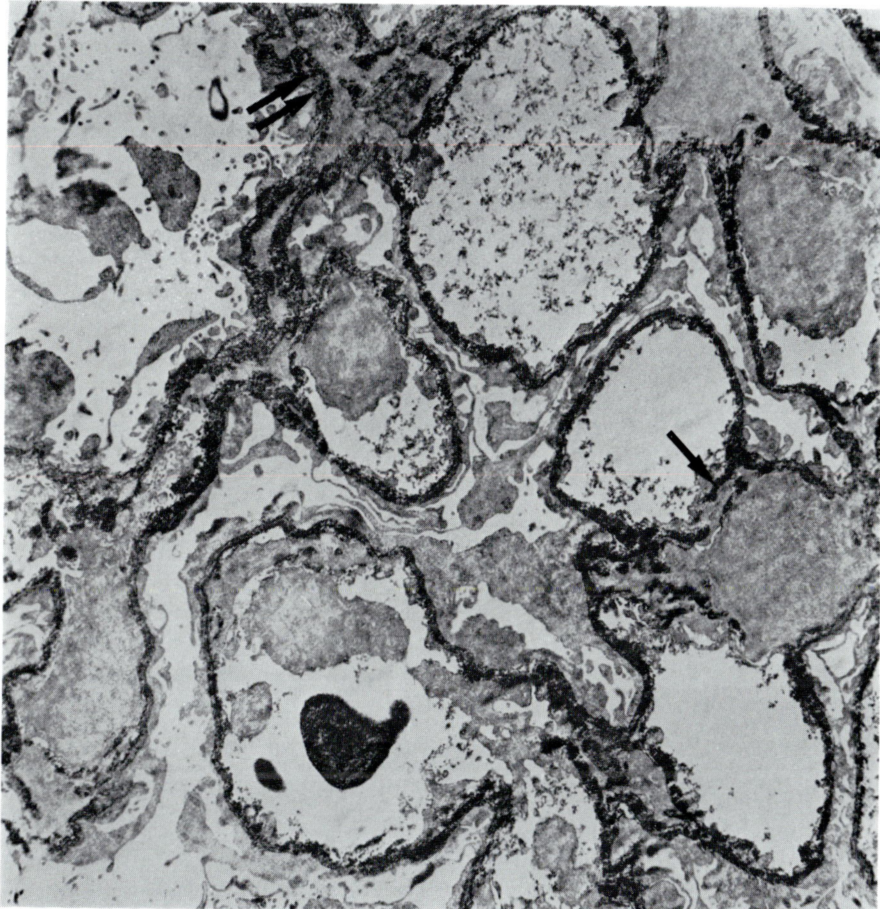

Fig. 3-7 Part of a glomerulus of a rat, 2 days after receiving the last injection of rabbit nephrotoxic serum. In vitro incubation with peroxidase-labeled goat Fab anti-rabbit IgG. The black enzymatic reaction product is observed on all of the GBM. The BM over the mesangial area and the mesangial matrix are less intensely labeled (double arrow) but the mesangial material between the endothelial cell and the mesangial area is strongly labeled (single arrow). ×5,8000. (From Druet, P. et al.: *Lab. Invest. 27*: 157–164, 1972)

xidase labeled antirabbit IgG (anti-nephrotoxic antibody) applied directly to mechanically isolated renal glomeruli from the nephrotoxic nephritis rats. They found that the enzymatic reaction products distributed throughout the peripheral GBM. Especially the lamina lucida int. and ext. usually exhibited a stronger enzymatic reaction than the lamina densa. In the mesangial areas, on the other hand, the concentration of enzymatic reaction products was found to be appreciably lower. It may be a logical conclusion that this apparent discrepancy between immunofluorescent and immunoelectron microscopic studies concerning the attitude of the axillary portions of the GBM and the mesangial areas to the nephrotoxic antibody, is a consequence of the thickness of the section used for each study, as Druet et al. [14] believed. McCauseland et al. [57] further observed high concentration of the antiGBM antibody in the subendothelial deposits, noted in the initial stage of the nephrotoxic nephritis. This evidence will be mentioned later again.

2. In vivo administration method of labeled nephrotoxic antibody

As far as the in vivo administration method of the labeled nephrotoxic globulin is concerned, the original experimental procedure of this type appears to have been started by Shibata et al. at the fluorescent microscopic level [75], although considerable loss of antibody activity could not be avoided by fluorescent dye labeling. Nevertheless, they disclosed continuous linear distribution of the labeled nephrotoxic γ-globulin strictly confined to the GBM. The similar idea was soon applied to the electron microscopic level. For instance, Vogt et al. [99] injected the ferritin labeled nephrotoxic γ-globulin to rats, and noted a heavy accumulation of the ferritin particles on the GBM almost exclusively at its endothelial side. Although higher concentration of the ferritin particles was demonstrated

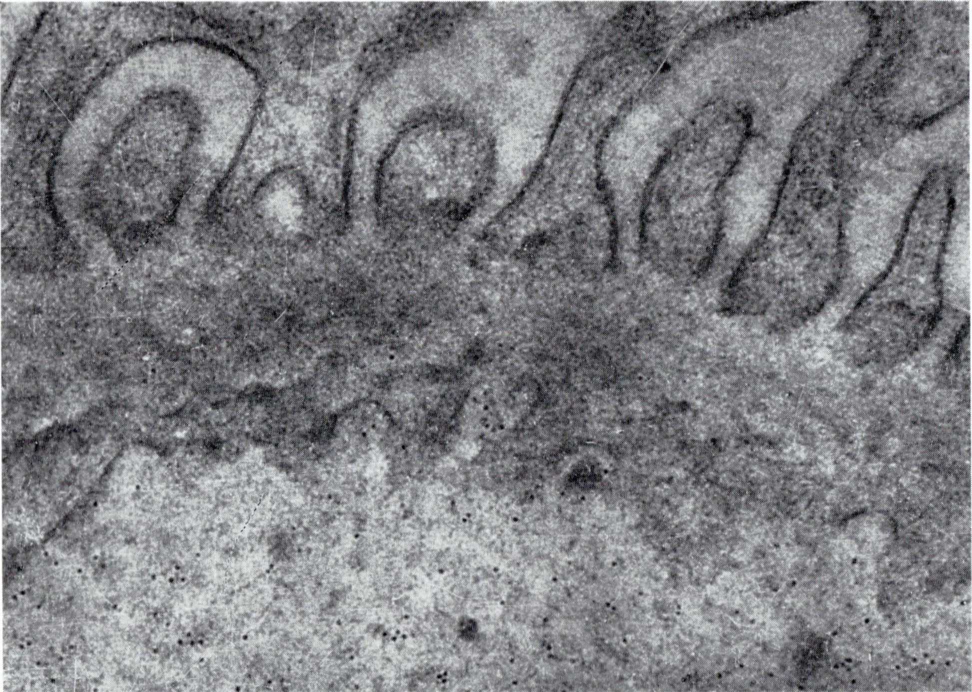

Fig. 3-8   A peripheral part of the glomerular capillary wall of a rat, directly after receiving ferritin labeled nephrotoxic globulin. Ferritin particles are seen to reach the BM from the capillary lumen through endothelial pores and possibly transendothelial pathway. $\times 80,000$.

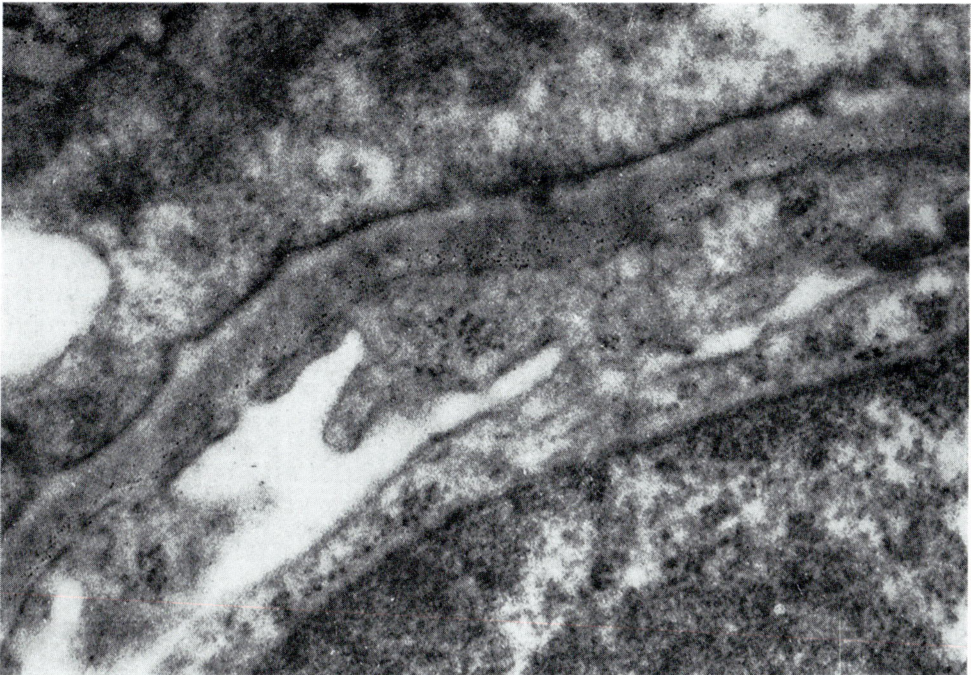

Fig. 3-9 A peripheral part of a glomerular capillary wall of a rat, 5 hours after receiving ferritin labeled nephrotoxic globulin. Ferritin particles are seen to be distributed fairly even along the subendothelial side of the GBM. $\times 68,000$.

on the peripheral GBM, they noted ferritin particles also in the axillary regions of the GBM, mesangial matrices and in membrane limited vacuoles, vesicles and also in dense bodies of the mesangial cells.   They suspected that these mesangial accumulations of ferritin particles might be non specific, because similar finding was also noted in the control cases. Successively Masugi [52] also reported the results of the in vivo administration method of the ferritin labeled nephrotoxic γ-globulin to rats.   Ferritin particles were observed to react with the GBM through the endothelial pores and even across the endothelial cell cytoplasms, immediately after the injection of the labeled nephrotoxic γ-globulin (Fig. 3-8), and later they were found to be distributed fairly evenly along the subendothelial side of the peripheral GBM (Fig. 3-9) in accordance with the observation of Vogt et al. [102]. Furthermore, although less densely, ferritin particles were found also in the axillary GBM, mesangial matrices and vesicles of the mesangial cells from the initial stage of the heterologous phase (Fig. 3-10).   At the same time, the mesangial cells were observed to be degenerated.   The control rats that received ferritin alone or normal rabbit γ-globulin conjugated ferritin, revealed very irregular and focal random absorption of ferritin particles in the GBM and in the mesangial matrices.   Though ferritin particles were also taken into the cytoplasmic vesicles of the mesangial cells, they usually disappeared within 1 to 2 weeks after the administration, leaving no alteration of the glomeruli.

On the other hand, as already described, the reaction product of the peroxidase labeled nephrotoxic antibody administered in vivo to the experimental animals by Druet et al. [14], was found to be localized on the entire width of the peripheral GBM, especially concentrated on its inner and outer sides, and less intensely in the mesangial areas.   This result might be due to easier penetrability of the peroxidase labeled nephrotoxic antibody than ferritin conjugated, possibly because of the smaller molecular size of peroxidase than

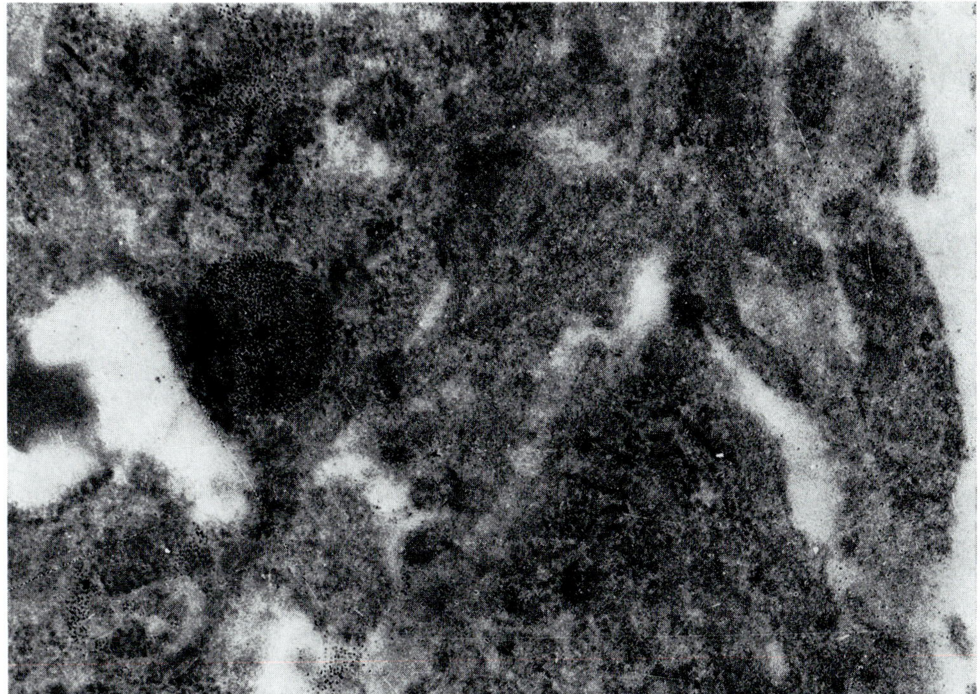

Fig. 3-10 A mesangial part of the glomerulus of same rat as in Fig. 9. Ferritin particles are also noted in the mesangial matrix and vesicle of mesangial cell. The mesangial cell is seen to be considerably degenerated after incorporation of aggregated and disperssed ferritin particles. ×60,000.

ferritin. Druet, using Fab fragment instead of whole IgG molecule of the nephrotoxic antibody for the peroxidase labeling, disclosed a more even distribution of the reaction products throughout the GBM. In addition to the peripheral GBM localization of the peroxidase labeled nephrotoxic antibody, Fresen and Vogt [19] who also administered the peroxidase labeled antibody to rats, observed enzymatic reaction products being further located in the spongy material between mesangial and endothelial cells, in accordance with Druet et al. [14]. Although the axillary regions of the GBM showed no enzymatic activity, it was found in a few mesangial cytoplasmic vesicles.

3. Immunopathologic considerations

By referring to the results of the immunoelectron microscopic studies, done by both ferritin and peroxidase labeled antibody techniques including in vitro and in vivo methods, one obvious point is that at least the BM of the peripheral glomerular capillaries possibly its entire width must be the principal site of localization of the administered nephrotoxic antibody. In other words, the nephritogenic antigen(s) should be distributed at least in the peripheral GBM itself. However, concerning the relationship of the axillary GBM and the mesangial regions against the nephrotoxic antibody, the reported results showed considerable differences from one article to the another.

The explanation for this discrepancy is not certain, but the differences of the amount and avidity of the original or labeled nephrotoxic antibodies used and the differences of the preparatory methods might be responsible. Furthermore, as already described, the lack of availability of the nephritogenic antigen(s) in the axillary GBM and the mesangial areas to the injected nephrotoxic globulin was discussed by Hoedemaeker et al. [29]. However, this may not be of much concern, for the reason already pointed out.

As previously stated, in the author's immunoelectron microscopic observation of nephrotoxic nephritis [52] performed by the in vitro incubation method of the ferritin labeled antibody, the localization of the nephrotoxic antibody was seen to be fairly evenly distributed throughout the GBM of the peripheral and even axillary regions of the capillaries, although in general the lamina densa was comparably heavily involved than the laminae lucidae. Besides, some of nephrotoxic antibody was constantly found in the mesangial matrices and vesicles of the mesangial cells. The author feels that this latter finding is specific for the previously described reasons, although control cases showed similar findings but to a lesser extent.

In general, from a pure morphologic standpoint, the mesangial area is the first recognized site for the widening of its matrix and degeneration or proliferation of regional mesangial cells, in case of both human and experimental glomerulonephritis. At this time, the mesangial matrix would play a role on the one hand as the supporting component of a BM like substance sharing the same antigenicity with the original GBM, and on the other hand as a reserved space for transportation and deposition of trapped macromolecules in the glomeruli [15, 42, 62]. The mesangial cells also show phagocytic activity [16, 42] and may manufacture a new BM like matrix. From the evidence of the localization of the nephrotoxic antibody itself in the mesangial matrix and cytoplasmic vesicles, the author introduces the possibility of an active transport mechanism of the GBM antigen(s)-antibody complex from the original combining sites along the GBM and possibly in the mesangial matrix to the mesangial cell cytoplasm. This may happen slowly, bacause the immunofluorescent studies usually do not show a clear cut distribution of immunoreactants in the mesangial areas. Finally, it is speculated that such a transported intracytoplasmic immune complex may exert phlogogenic effects on the regional mesangial cells for the initiation of glomerulonephritis when their physiological protective capacities are overcome. The morphologic evidence indicated that such noxious macromolecules in the cytoplasmic vesicles led to degeneration of the mesangial cells, as already described. Hoyer et al. [30] recently observed increased colloidal carbon uptake in the mesangium of the nephrotoxic nephritis of rats compared to the control animals, and also speculated that the presence of increased quantities of macromolecules such as an immune complex within the mesangial cells over prolonged periods, similar to the persistence of increased carbon in this model, may lead to inflammatory change of the glomerular mesangial areas. Mauer et al. [55, 56] also discussed the possibility of mesangial damage after uptake and processing of the potentially noxious macrolecules such as an immune complex of any kind.

The possible transportation mechanism of the GBM antigen(s)-antibody complex from the original combining sites is also speculated even in the GBM itself, where the initial linear appearance of the immunoreactants became granular later on [52, 81]. This will be discussed later.

V. Chemical Nature of the Nephritogenic Antigen(s)

As already described, from pathogenetic point of view, one of the important points concerning the occurrence of the nephrotoxic nephritis would be the identification of the antigenically active nephritogenic component(s) in the GBM as the main target of anti-GBM antibody. Besides morphological studies described above, the chemical analysis of the GBM, especially of its nephritogenic property is to be described.

For this purpose of investigation, first of all the GBM must be collected as pure as possible and second it must be solubilized by suitable means such as by proteolytic enzymes or by pure chemicals.   Finally, if some component is thought to be responsible for the antigenic activity, its nephritogenic property must be confirmed by bioassay using nephrotoxic nephritis series.   Generally speaking, the chemical studies of the intact GBM have revealed the presence of at least two carbohydrate rich proteins, one is collagen and the other is non collagenous glycoprotein [34, 35, 84, 85].   The antigenic element(s) may reside in these components.

Shibata et al. [76, 77] from their long continuing studies of the chemical analysis and biological assays of trypsin digested rat GBM, concluded that nephritogenic potentiality laid principally in the polysaccharide moiety of the water soluble GBM glycoproteins. Furthermore, they claimed that a single injection of the glycopeptide which was pronase digested and trichloracetic acid treated above described nephritogenic glycoprotein with Freund's incomplete adjuvant to rats could produce proliferative glomerulonephritis [78], and very recently they stated that the most active nephritogenic property was observed to be localized in the glucose dominant glycogenic fraction having concanavalin A combining capacity [79].   The precise results are being given in Chapter 2 by Shibata.

On the other hand, Huang and Kalant [31] suspected that the essential antigenic structure in the GBM for eliciting potent nephrotoxic antibody was more closely related to the peptide portion than to the carbohydrate moiety of the non collagenous glycoprotein, based on the fact that proteolytic digestion of collagenase treated rat GBM destroyed its nephrotoxic antigenicity, although destruction of much of the carbohydrate composition by exposure to mild alkali did not affect its nephrotoxigenicity.   Rothbard and Watson [71] pointed out that by in vitro and in vivo immunofluorescent methods, antibodies to rat collagen and to rat kidney showed the regular linear fluorescence along the glomerular capillaries.   Absorption of each antiserum with its homologous antigen completely removed the antibody by immunofluorescence.   However, nephrotoxicity in the antikidney antibody could persist even after absorption by collagen.   The anticollagen antibody itself seemed not to have any nephrotoxic capacity.   From the above observations, non collagenous glycoprotein in the GBM seemed to be responsible for the nephritogenic antigen(s).

In human cases also, Marquardt et al. [49] found at least seven distinct GBM antigens in collagenase solubilized human GBM by an immunoadsorbent method, and suspected that this antigenic heterogeneity was due to the heterogenous carbohydrate composition in structural non collagenous glycoprotein of the GBM.   They finally concluded that the nephritogenic antigen(s) to which patients with antiGBM glomerulonephritis such as Goodpasture's syndrome produced antibody, should be localized in this non collagenous portion of the GBM, judged from inhibition assay.

Similarly, it was reported that human circulating or eluted antiGBM antibodies could react to collagenase solubilized GBM in radioimmunoassay, which has not been blocked by absorption with isolated di- or heteropolysaccharide moieties of GBM [106].

On the other hand, McPhaul and Mullins [60] disclosed that the sera or the renal eluates from the antiGBM antibody mediated glomerulonephritis cases showed antibody activities to one of each or both of collagenase digested and trypsin digested human GBM antigens, based on the surveys of passive hemagglutination or radioimmunoassay.   The author's own observation [53] of human cases also disclosed that eluted IgG of kidneys from 5 of 7 fatal chronic glomerulonephritis cases obtained by autopsy, showed positive antiGBM activity to the trypsin or collagenase digested and solubilized human GBM on passive hemagglutination by Boyden's method, but negative by Middlebrook's method.   Furthermore, if such solubilized GBM antigens were deproteinized by trichloracetic acid, their antigenicities were completely lost even by Boyden's method. This evidence suggests that trypsin or collagenase digestion resistant and trichloracetic acid inactivated protein or polypeptide moiety of the GBM constituents might play a major antigenic role against the antiGBM antibody rather than the polysaccharide moiety. In addition, there is another much conflicting report which disclosed inhibitory activity of disaccharide containing glycopeptide of GBM to human antiGBM antibody in Goodpasture's disease against sodium dodecylsulfatesolubilized human GBM antigen in radioimmunoassay [47].

In this chapter, the author will not go into further detail about the chemical composition of nephritogenic antigen(s). Nevertheless, it must be noticed that the simple linear fluorescence of the nephrotoxic antibody along the GBM in the experimental nephrotoxic nephritis so far has raised an important information concerning the identification of the nephritogenic antigen(s) both at morphological and chemical levels. These two approaches of investigation must be combined for further clarification of this subject.

VI. Analysis of Deposition along the Glomerular Basement Membrane

As stated already, in the heterologous phase of nephrotoxic nephritis, by electron microscopic studies of the glomeruli, deposits of varied sizes and densities are noted on the subendothelial spaces of the GBM [6, 17, 18, 57, 64, 69], although fluorescent microscopic study ordinarily discloses only a thin linear appearance of immunoreactants along the GBM. Furthermore, these subendothelial deposits at the electron microscopic level do not always show a fibrillar appearance of polymerized fibrin, and such deposits can be seen even after administration of the antibody against the purified GBM fragments. The latter evidence may be against the idea that these subendothelial deposits are due to incorporation of non GBM antigen(s)-antibody complex.

The origin of these subendothelial deposits has not been known. Although the possibility of nonspecific infusion by plasma protein can not be excluded, they might in some way be related to an immune complex, because of their location and electron density. For convincing this fact, McCausland et al. [57] did find heavy concentration of antiGBM antibody in those subendothelial deposits by immunoenzymatic electron microscopic study, as already described. Therefore, the possible pathways for this GBM antigen-antibody complex must be sought.

First of all, subendothelial concentration of the host GBM antigen(s) against the nephrotoxic antibody may be considered together with the secondary incorporation of plasma proteins at the site of antigen(s)-antibody reaction [73]. However, the previous immunoelectron microscopic observations, especially immunoperoxidase studies of the nephrotoxic nephritis did not totally support this explanation. Alternatively another source of the GBM antigen(s)-antibody complex must be considered. Certain evidence exists that normal animals continuously release the GBM like antigen(s) into plasma [59]. It could be speculated that this circulating GBM like antigen(s) may be caught by the administrated heterologous nephrotoxin, forming an immune complex in the circulation and then be trapped in the subendothelial spaces of the GBM at the initial stage of the heterologous phase.

In the following autologous phase of the nephrotoxic nephritis, besides subendothelial deposits [18], the electron microscopic subepithelial deposits along the GBM [4, 64, 81] are more prone to be produced. The immunofluorescent studies also disclosed a fairly granular pattern of the immunoreactants including nephrotoxic globulin along the GBM in the advances autologous phase [52, 81]. If these subepithelial deposits represent GBM antigen(s)-antibody complex or nephrotoxic globulin-antibody complex, they might be in some way catabolized at the original combining sites along the GBM and thereafter transported to the subepithelial spaces, as mentioned in the previous section. The author feels that this is the most likely explanation. Alternatively, in the autologous phase of nephrotoxic nephritis, autoantibody might be formed against the altered GBM substance because of injury from the heterologous antibody. Thereafter, this autoantibody cross reacted with the circulating GBM like antigen(s), and this autologous immune complex might be later trapped in the subepithelial spaces of the GBM, just as in the heterologous immune complex type glomerulonephritis. However until now, this autoimmune thesis has not been proved.

The real nature of these subendothelial and subepithelial deposits in the heterologous and the autologous phases of nephrotoxic nephritis must be analyzed by a more precise and specific immunoelectron microscopic method, for detecting not only serum globulin but also antigenic element(s) in question.

VII. Necessity of Complement Activation

The roles of complement activation and intraglomerular aggregated PMNs in mediating the heterologous nephrotoxic nephritis have been well documented [7, 9, 26, 94, 103]. Especially, as already described, the role of complement which is usually noted linearly along the GBM with other immunoreactants by immunofluorescence in nephrotoxic nephritis has been thought to be principal element for the occurrence of glomerular injury together with its chemotactic activity to PMNs. However, the precise role of complement in this system has not been clarified. Whether complement can exert a direct deleterious effect on the GBM similar to its effect on erythrocytes, cellular membranes or bacterial cell walls is not known at present.

It has also been recognized that glomerular injury could be induced by some nephrotoxic antibodies which apparently neither fixed complement nor needed the presence of PMNs [24, 25, 27, 74, 93], including nephrotoxin of avian source as already described. Furthermore, apparently complement-independent glomerulonephritis could be produced by nephrotoxic antiserum, selectively depleted of, or congenitally deficient in complement components [7, 8, 26, 45]. Recently, the same observation was also noted in even the autologous phase of nephrotoxic nephritis in decomplemented rabbit [93].

Generally, the glomerular lesions induced by a complement-independent pathway usually require more bound antibody globulin, because they usually represent only minor fractions of the nephrotoxic properties of the antiGBM antibody. For instance, sheep γ_2 and avian nephrotoxic antisera which do not fix complement must be administered in relatively large doses for the induction of glomerular injury [24, 27]. Furthermore, it has been said that complement-independent nephrotoxic glomerulonephritis usually lacked humoral and cellular exudative components in glomeruli, characteristics of complement mediated glomerular injuries [8, 24, 27].

Recent detailed studies of nephrotoxic nephritis induced by injection of purified γ_1 and γ_2 nephrotoxic guinea pig antibodies to rats [38, 39, 68] disclosed that a marked proteinuria could be induced in animals without complement fixation by γ_1 antibody or its $F(ab)_2$ fragment. On the other hand, guinea pig γ_2 antiGBM antibody which can activate complement also induced a transient proteinuria similar to that produced by complement-independent γ_1 antibody [68]. Furthermore, it was reported that proteinuria induced by γ_2 antibody was significantly increased by prior deposition of γ_1 nephrotoxic antibody to the GBM [68].

Simpson et al. [82] recently reported the occurrence of the nephrotoxic nephritis in guinea pigs both conventional and C_4-deficient strains by using each one of sheep non complement fixing γ_2 and complement fixing γ_2 subclasses of antiGBM antibody or $F(ab')_2$ fragment of γ_1. In addition, complement depletion by cobra venom factor in this system also failed to reduce the glomerular injuries. This glomerulonephritis seemed to be largely independent of the complement system both in the classical and alternative complement activation pathways, and to be due to the fixation of the $F(ab')_2$ of the antibody molecules to the GBM. They suspected that antibody itself might be capable of destroying the functional integrity of the permeability barrier of the GBM by combination with the corresponding GBM antigen(s). However, $F(ab')$ or $F(ab)$ monomeric fragments of the anti-GBM antibody, though fixing on the GBM, did not cause proteinuria. The guinea pig appeared to be more sensitive to the nephrotoxic antibody than the rat or rabbit. Simpson et al. calculated that only 7 to 10 microgram antibody to 1.0 gram kidney were requirement to initiate proteinuria in this species. Recently, Couser et al. [13] further confirmed the evidence of considerable alteration of GBM permeability in not only heterologous but also autologous phases of nephrotoxic nephritis in guinea pig induced by sheep γ_1 and γ_2 nephrotoxic serum, which did not involve complement and PMN dependent mechanisms.

In another system of experimental glomerulonephritis, Couser et al. [10, 11] also reported that an autologous antiGBM antibody mediated glomerulonephritis in guinea pig actively immunized with human GBM incorporated with Freund's complete adjuvant, might have occurred through an undefined mechanism that apparently did not involve activation of the complement system or participation of PMNs. Furthermore, Rudofsky et al. [72] found that C_4-deficient guinea pigs were not protected from the experimental autoimmune tubulo-interstitial disease produced by the injection of rabbit TBM with Freund's complete adjuvant, although in this case a possible activation of an alternative complement pathway could not be disregarded.

In human glomerulonephritis cases too, IgG deposits without detectable incorporation of any complement component in glomeruli occur rarely in the immune complex type glomerulonephritis but occur possibly in 25 per cent of antiGBM antibody induced glomerulonephritis [105]. Verroust et al. [101]. thought glomerular injuries observed in these instances might be mediated by complement-independent pathways similar to those utilized by avian and some mammalian antiGBM antibodies.

Finally, it must be further clarified whether complement-independent glomerular injury of nephrotoxic nephritis can be produced from only GBM antigen(s)-antibody conjugation per se or requires incorporation of another mediating system other than complement activation.

VIII. Coagulation System

One can not underestimate the pathogenetic role of the coagulation process in the occurrence of nephrotoxic nephritis [100]. The linear deposition of fibrin or fibrinogen along the glomerular capillaries early in the production of experimental nephrotoxic nephritis is usually noted by the immunofluorescent method.

When a state of intravascular clotting was induced in rabbits by intravenous injection of thrombin or thromboplastin [99], a number of histologic lesions were observed in glomeruli, such as swelling and proliferation of the endothelial and mesangial cells, PMN infiltration, clumping of platelets and deposition of fibrin and fibrinoid material along the GBM. Furthermore, variable features in the development of progressive glomerular obliteration were seen.

Thus in the particular case, the characteristic lesions of glomerulonephritis can be produced in a situation in which an immunological mechanism does not participate. However, in the case of nephrotoxic nephritis, the deposition of fibrin or fibrinoid material along the GBM must be one of the sequential events, triggered by the nephritogenic antigen(s) and nephrotoxic antibody interaction. In support of this fact, it was said that treatment with anticoagulants resulted not only in the prevention of fibrin and fibrinoid deposits along the GBM but also in a marked diminution or suppression of mesangial cell swelling and proliferation, and further prevention of epithelial crescent formation in Bowman's space [23, 37, 100, 104]. Watanabe and Tanaka [104] further described that inhibition of fibrinolysis with trans-aminomethylcyclohexane carboxylic acid increased intraglomerular fibrin deposition and accelerated morphological glomerular injuries. In any case, nephrotoxic antibody and host immunoglobulin(s) were detected continuously along the GBM and proteinuria was said to be not diminished.

Thomson et al. [92] again recently investigated the protective effect of anticoagulant such as heparin or of defibrination with ancrod in nephrotoxic nephritis in rabbits and found that these treatments did not reduce intrarenal fixation of nephrotoxic antibody, complement activation or host antibody response, although massive doses of heparin or ancrod prevented intraglomerular fibrin deposits. These and other observations [65, 66] suggested that fibrin deposition plays no initiating role in the primary allergic events causing capillary damage.

IX. Anti-Tubular Basement Membrane Antibody

In nephrotoxic nephritis, as already described, nephrotoxic antibody conjugation is confined only to the GBM and rarely found along the TBM. However, recently the pathogenicity of the antiTBM antibody has gradually gained attention among other experimental models.

In 1971, Steblay and Rudofsky [88] reported that guinea pigs immunized by purified rabbit TBM with Freund's complete adjuvant, developed autoantibody against their own TBM, which was recognized by extensive linear deposition of IgG along the cortical TBM in immunofluorescence. The tubulo-interstitial nephritis with destruction of urinary tubules and variable amounts of interstitial mononuclear cell infiltration developed with symptoms of proteinuria, glucosuria and azotemia. Furthermore, passive transfer of serum from such diseased animals to normal recipient guinea pigs induced an identical or even more fatal kidney disease [89]. The necessity of complement activation through the classical pathway was questioned in this experimental model as previously described [72]. Recently Lehman et al. [44] produced similar interstitial nephritis with minimal glomerular abnormalities in guinea pigs, immunized with bovine renal BM, and concluded that the TBM apparently contained antigens both different from and common to the GBM. Furthermore, a study of Hyman et al. [32] disclosed the importance of the genetic factor for the production of antiTBM antibody and the occurrence of tubulo-interstitial nephritis among different inbred strains of guinea pigs immunized by rabbit TBM in Freund's complete adjuvant.

A similar pathologic observation was again noted in rabbits [36] immunized with the homologous rabbit kidney incorporated in Freund's complete adjuvant, and in rats [90] especially Brown Norway (BN) and Lewis-BN (L/BN) F_1 hybrid rats immunized with homologous Sprague-Dawley rat kidney together with pertussis vaccine. This latter evidence was further confirmed by a cross transplantation study by Lehman et al. [43] in 1974. They confirmed that BN and L/BN rats possess a specific TBM antigen which is not present in the TBM of L rats. Transplantation of L/BN rat kidneys into L rats induced antiTBM antibody which bound to the TBM of donor (L/BN) but not recipient (L) kidneys. In contrast, transplantation of L/BN kidneys into BN rats failed to induce such an antibody, although severe rejection phenomena occurred.

The human counterparts of antiTBM antibody activities in variable kidney diseases including antiGBM antibody mediated glomerulonephritis were well documented by Lehman et al. [45] in 1975. They however decided that in such human cases, the pathogenetic contribution of the antiTBM antibody to tubular damage was difficult to assess, in contrast to the above described well documented animal experiments. The linear fluorescence of the host immunoglobulin(s) along the TBM observed in the human cases were thought to be a secondary phenomenon.

Nevertheless, it would be an important problem to clarify the pathway through which the antiTBM antibody can react on the final target. The antibody globulin may react to the TBM by diffusion through peritubular capillary walls or a transtubular epithelial pathway by reabsorption of intraluminally filtered antibody from the glomeruli. However, the effectiveness of either route is difficult to confirm. In any case, because the TBM is not the capillary wall, the pathogenetic mechanism of antiTBM antibody mediated local tissue lesion must be differently analyzed from the antiGBM antibody mediated glomerular capillary damage.

In the fully developed autoimmune tubulo-interstitial disease of the kidney, besides antiTBM antibody activity, lymphocytes and other monocytic cells are found to migrate from peritubular vessels into the interstitium where they are often found in direct contact with the TBM. These lymphocytes were reported to show some features of activated motile lymphocytes [90]. The author's provisional study [54] revealed their T-cell characteristic from the specific surface marker stained by fluorescent labeled anti-T cell antibody. This evidence would suggest the possibility of the participation of cellular hypersensitivity for the occurrence of this type of TBM injury other than antiTBM serum antibody activity. On the other hand, Van Zwieten et al. [98] recently produced anti-TBM antibody mediated renal disease in guinea pigs by Lehman's method [44] and further demonstrated the occurrence of the identical renal lesions in the healthy guinea pigs by transfer of the serum, but failed by transfer of the lymphnode cells from diseased animals. Furthermore, they obtained the evidence that infiltrated mononuclear cells in the interstitium around the damaged urinary tubules of these animals revealed mostly the characteristics of monocyte or macrophage and not of B-lymphocyte, judged from the sheep red cell (EA and EAC), rosetting technique performed on the frozen kidney sections. However, unfortunately, they did not examine T-cell population among these infiltrating cells in the renal interstitium.

Nevertheless, in the case of nephrotoxic nephritis mediated by the circulating antiGBM antibody, even in its fully developed autologous phase, the participation of sensitized lymphocytes for alteration of the GBM has so far not been convincingly reported.

X. Final Remarks

The fundamental contribution of nephrotoxic nephritis to the medical and biological fields would be the establishment of the pathogenetic pathway of the antiGBM antibody to kidney, based upon functional, immunologic and morphologic aspects. Although, in the case of nephrotoxic nephritis, its antibody is heterologous in nature, the GBM antigen(s)-antibody conjugation per se initiates the successive glomerular injuries. The complement activation is thought to be not always an essential factor.

This experimental model further opened the possibility of the selfperpetuating autoimmune pathogenetic pathway of the autologous antiGBM antibody mediated experimental glomerulonephritis [87]. In the antiGBM antibody mediated glomerulonephritis cases, the GBM antigen(s) and autologous antibody conjugation is also capable of inducing the injurious effects upon the glomerular structure, just as the heterologous antiGBM antibody insult in nephrotoxic nephritis.

However, the identification and distribution of the antigenic determinant(s) on the GBM as the target of the antiGBM antibody have still not been completely settled among the investigators concerned both with the immunoelectron microscopic and chemical approaches. Furthermore, the mode of in vivo availability of the nephritogenic antigen(s) on the GBM and the manner of its turnover after combination with the antiGBM antibody should also be clarified in near future.

The human counterparts of the antiGBM antibody mediated glomerulonephritis were thoroughly studied by Wilson and Dixon [105], and by McPhaul and Mullins [60]. The overall rate of occurrence in all glomerulonephritis cases was calculated to be 5 per cent by the former and 11 to 16 per cent by the latter authors. Except for well documented Goodpasture's syndrome cases with lung involvement and rapidly progressive glomerulonephritis, both groups included a considerable number of cases with mild morphologic renal change. Especially, McPhaul and Mullins [60] reported cases consisting of a wide variety of morphologic features ranging from normal or minor glomerular abnormalities to an end stage proliferative glomerulonephritis. These varieties must be due to the different biological status of the immunologic reactions and different individual susceptibilities to them. The author's own observations as already described [53], also revealed the renal eluates from occasional fatal chronic glomerulonephritis cases showed in vitro antiGBM activity.

However, in certain human renal disease cases, the linear fluorescence of immunoglobulins especially IgG along the GBM has been noted in some nephrotic glomerulonephritis cases with satisfactory steroid therapy response, in the early stage of systemic lupus erythematosus (SLE) kidneys without functional abnormalities [40] or in some diabetic glomerulosclerosis kidneys [20, 58]. In such cases the complement system has usually not been found in glomeruli and the staining intensity of IgG along the GBM as usually not as bright as in the typical heterologous phase of nephrotoxic nephritis. Furthermore, the eluted immunoglobulin(s) from such SLE and diabetic kidneys were reported not to have shown any antiGBM antibody activity [20, 40]. The glomeruli-bound immunoglobulin(s) of such cases might be either an antibody reaction to a non-nephritogenic antigen such as collagen, as Koffler et al. stated [40] or only a non immunologic phenomenon possibly secondary to the elevated permeability of the GBM. The real nature of this phenomenon has not as yet been established. Nevertheless, one thing to be careful of is that the immunohistologic linear fluorescence of immunoglobulin(s) along the GBM in the human cases does not always denote nephrotoxic antiGBM antibody activity. The same thing may also be true about the linear distribution of immunoglobulin(s) along the TBM of some cases of human renal disease.

Finally, it must be stressed that the efficiency of the occurrence of nephrotoxic nephritis is excellent, because as already stated the antigen is GBM-bound and the high accessibility of the glomerulus to the circulating antiGBM antibody due to possible organ specificity. This experimental model can be remain as a prototype of structural antigen antibody reaction mediated vascular damage, not only of the renal glomeruli but also of all vital organs throughout the body.

REFERENCES

1. Andres, G.A., Morgan, C., Hsu, K.C., Rifkind, R.A., and Seegal, B.C.: Electron microscopic studies of experimental nephritis with ferritin-conjugated antibody. The basement membrane and cisternae of visceral epithelial cells in nephritic rat glomeruli. *J. Exp. Med. 115*: 929–936, 1962.

2. Arhelger, R.B., Gronvall, J.A., Carr, O.B., and Brunson, J.G.: Electron microscopic localization of nephrotoxic serum in rabbit glomeruli with ferritin conjugated antibody. *Lab. Invest. 12*: 33–37, 1963.

3. Avrameas, S. et Uriel, J.: Méthod de marquage dántigenes et dáticorps avec des enzymes et son application en immunodiffusion. *Compt. Rend. Acad. Sci. 262*: 2543–2545, 1966.

4. Battifora, H.A. and Markowitz, A.S.: Nephrotoxic nephritis in monkeys. Sequential light, immunofluorescence and electron microscopic studies. *Amer. J. Path. 55*: 267–281, 1969.

5. Chiu, J. and Drummond, K.N.: Chemical and histochemical studies of glomerular sialoprotein in nephrotoxic nephritis in rats. *Amer. J. Path. 68*: 391–406, 1972.

6. Churg, J., Grishman, E., and Mautner, W.: Nephrotoxic serum nephritis in the rat. Electron and light microscopic studies. *Amer. J. Path. 37*: 729–749, 1960.

7. Cochrane, C.G., Unanue, E.R., and Dixon, F.J.: A role of polymorphonuclear leucocytes and complement in nephrotoxic nephritis. *J. Exp. Med. 122*: 99–116, 1965.

8. Cochrane, C.G.: Mediation of immunologic glomerular injury. *Transplant. Proc. 1*: 949–958, 1969.

9. Cochrane, C.G., Müller-Eberhardt, H.J., and Aikin, B.S.: Depletion of plasma complement in vivo by a protein of cobra venom: Its effect on various immunological reactions. *J. Immunol. 105*: 55–69, 1970.

10. Couser, W.G., Stilmant, M., and Lewis, E.J.: Experimental glomerulonephritis in the guinea pig. I. Glomerular lesion associated with antiglomerular basement membrane antibody deposits. *Lab. Invest. 29*: 236–243, 1973.

11. Couser, W.G., Spargo, B.H., Stilmant, M.M., and Lewis, E.J.: Experimental glomerulonephritis in the guinea pig. II. Ultrastructural lesions of the basement membrane associated with proteinuria. *Lab. Invest. 32*: 46–55, 1975.

12. Couser, W.G., Stilmant, M.M., and Darby, C.: Autologous immune complex nephropathy. I. Sequential study of immune complex deposition, ultrastructural changes, proteinuria, and alteration in glomerular sialoprotein. *Lab. Invest. 34*: 23–30, 1976.

13. Couser, W.G., Stilmant, M.M., and Jermanovich, N.B.: Complement-independent nephrotoxic nephritis in the guinea pig. *Kidney Internat. 11*: 170–180, 1977.

14. Druet, P.J., Bariety, J., Bellon, B., and Laliberte, F.: Ultrastructural localization of nephrotoxic rabbit antibodies using peroxidase-labeled conjugates. *Lab. Invest. 27*: 157–164, 1972.

15. Farquhar, M.G., Wissing, S.L., and Palade, G.E.: Glomerular permeability. I. Ferritin transfer across the normal glomerular capillary wall. *J. Exp. Med. 113*: 47–66, 1961.

16. Farquhar, M.G. and Palade, G.E.: Functional evidence for the existence of a third cell type in the renal glomerulus. Phagocytosis of filtration residues by a distinct "third" cell. *J. Cell Biol. 13*: 55–87, 1962.

17. Feldman, J.D., Hammer, D., and Dixon, F.J.: Experimental glomerulonephritis. III. Pathogenesis of glomerular ultrastructural lesions in nephrotoxic serum nephritis. *Lab. Invest. 12*: 748–763, 1963.

18. Feldman, J.D.: Pathogenesis of ultrastructural glomerular changes induced by immunological means. *In* Graber, P. and Miescher, P.A. (eds.): *Immunopathology IIIrd International Symposium*, 263–281, Schwabe, Basel/Stuttgart, 1963.

19. Fresen, K.O. and Vogt, A.: Ultrastructural localization of peroxidase-labelled nephrotoxic antibodies after intravenous application. *Exp. Path. 8*: 276–282, 1973.

20. Gallo, G.: Elution studies in kidneys with linear deposition of immunoglobulin in glomeruli. *Amer. J. Path. 61*: 377–386, 1970.

21. Gang, N.F. and Kalant, N.: Nephrotoxic serum nephritis. I. Chemical, morphologic and functional changes in the glomerular basement membrane during the evolution of nephritis. *Lab. Invest. 22*: 531–540, 1970.

22. Gang, N.F., Mautner, W., and Kalant, N.: Nephrotoxic serum nephritis. II. Chemical, morphologic and functional correlates of glomerular basement membrane during the evolution of nephritis. *Lab. Invest. 23*: 150–157, 1970.

23. Halpern, B., Milliez, P., Lagrue, G., Fray, A., and Morard, J.C.: Protective action of heparin in experimental immune nephritis. *Nature 205*: 257–259, 1965.

24. Hammer, D.K. and Dixon, F.J.: Experimental glomerulonephritis. III. Immunologic events in the pathogenesis of nephrotoxic serum nephritis in the rats. *J. Exp. Med. 117*: 1019–1034, 1963.

25. Hasson, M.W., Bevans, M., and Seegal, B.G.: Immediate or delayed nephritis in rats produced by duck anti-rat-kidney sera. *Arch. Path. 64*: 192–204, 1957.

26. Hawkins, D. and Cochrane, C.G.: Glomerular basement membrane damage in immunological glomerulonephritis. *Immunology 14*: 665–681, 1968.

27. Henson, P.M.: Release of biologically active components from blood cells and its role in antibody-mediated tissue injury. *In* Amos, B. (ed.): *Progress in Immunology I*, Academic Press, New York/London, 1971.

28. Hill, A.G.S., Cruickshank, B., and Crossland, A.: A study of antigenic component of kindey tissue. *Brit. J. Exp. Path. 34*: 27–34, 1953.

29. Hoedemaeker, P.J., Feenstra, K., Nijkeuter, A., and Arends, A.: Ultrastructural localization of heterologous nephrotoxic antibody in the glomerular basement membrane of the rat. *Lab. Invest. 26*: 610–613, 1972.

30. Hoyer, J.R., Elema, J.D., and Vernier, R.L.: Unilateral renal disease in the rat. II. Glomerular mesangial uptake of colloidal carbon in unilateral aminonucleoside nephrosis and nephrotoxic serum nephritis. *Lab. Invest. 34*: 250–255, 1976.

31. Huang, F. and Kalant, N.: Isolation and characterization of antigenic components of rat glomerular basement membrane. *Canad. J. Biochem. 46*: 1523–1532, 1968.

32. Hyman, L.R., Colvin, R.B., and Steinberg, A.D.: Immunopathogenesis of autoimmune tubulointerstitial nephritis. I. Demonstration of differential susceptibility in strain II and strain XIII guinea pigs. *Lab. Invest. 116*: 327–335, 1976.

33. Kay, C.F.: The mechanism by which experimental nephritis is produced in rabbits injected with nephrotoxic duck serum. *J. Exp. Med. 72*: 559–572, 1940.

34. Kefalides, N.A. and Winzler, R.J.: The chemistry of glomerular basement membrane and its relation to collagen. *Biochem. 5*: 702–713, 1966.

35. Kefalides, N.A.: Isolation and characterization of the collagen from glomerular basement membrane. *Biochemistry 7*: 3103–3112, 1968.

36. Klassen, J., McCluskey, T., and Milgrom, F.: Nonglomerular renal disease produced in rabbits by immunization with homologous kidney. *Amer. J. Path. 63*: 333–350, 1971.

37. Kleinerman, J.: Effects of heparin on experimental nephritis in rabbits. *Lab. Invest. 3*: 495–508, 1954.

38. Kobayashi, Y., Shigematsu, H., and Tada, T.: Nephritogenic properties of nephrotoxic guinea pig antibodies. I. Glomerulonephritis induced by guinea pig IgG_1 antibody in rats. *Virchows Arch. Abt. B Zellpath. 14*: 259–271, 1973.

39. Kobayashi, Y., Shigematsu, H., and Tada, T.: Nephritogenic properties of nephrotoxic guinea pig antibodies. II. Glomerular lesions induced by $F(ab)_2$ fragments of nephrotoxic IgG_1 antibody in rats. *Virchows Arch. Abt. B Zellpath. 15*: 35–44, 1973.

40. Koffler, D., Agnello, V., Carr, R.I., and Kunkel, H.G.: Variable patterns of immunoglobulin and complement deposition in the kidneys of patients with systemic lupus erythematosus. *Amer. J. Path. 56*: 305–316, 1969.

41. Kondo, Y., Shigematsu, H., and Okabayashi, A.: Cellular aspects of rabbit Masugi nephritis. III. Mesangial changes. *Lab. Invest. 34*: 363–371, 1976.

42. Latta, H. and Maunsbach, A.B.: Relationship of the centrolobular region of the glomerulus to the juxterglomerular apparatus. *J. Ultrastruct. Res. 6*: 562–578, 1962.

43. Lehman, D.H., Lee, S., Wilson, C.B., and Dixon, F.J.: Induction of antitubular basement membrane antibodies in rat by renal transplantation. *Transplant. 17*: 429–431, 1974.

44. Lehman, D.H., Marquardt, H., Wilson, C.B., and Dixon, F.J.: Specificity of autoantibodies to tubular and glomerular basement membranes induced in guinea pigs. *J. Immunol. 112*: 241–248, 1974.

45. Lehman, D.H., Wilson, C.B., and Dixon, F.J.: Extraglomerular immunoglobulin deposits in human nephritis. *Amer. J. Med. 58*: 765–786, 1975.

46. Lindberg, L.H. and Rosenberg, L.T.: Nephrotoxic serum nephritis in mice with a genetic deficiency in complement. *J. Immunol. 100*: 34–38, 1968.

47. Mahieu, P., Lambert, P.H., and Miescher, P.A.: Detection of antiglomerular basement membrane antibodies by a radioimmunological technique; Clinical application in human nephropathies. *J. Clin. Invest. 54*: 128–137, 1974.

48. Marinis, S., Vogt, A., and Brandner, G.: Isolation and characterization of immunoferritin conjugates. I. The molecular ratio. *Immunology. 17*: 77–83, 1969.

49. Marquardt, H., Wilson, C.B., and Dixon, F.J.: Isolation and immunological characterization of human glomerular basement membrane antigens. *Kidney Internat. 3*: 57–65, 1973.

50. Masugi, M.: Über das Wesen der spezifischen Veränderungen der Niere und der Leber durch das Nephrotoxin bzw. das Hepatotoxin. Zugleich ein Beitrag zur Pathogenese der Glomerulonephritis und der eklamptischen Lebererkrankung. *Beitr. path. Anat. 91*: 82–112, 1933.

51. Masugi, M.: Über die experimentelle Glomerulonephritis durch das spezifische Antinierenserum. Ein Beitrag zur Pathogenese der diffusen Glomerulonephritis. *Beitr. path. Anat. 92*: 429–466, 1934.

52. Masugi, Y.: Immunoelectron microscopic studies on local vascular changes after immunological tissue injuries; especially on the mechanism of nephrotoxic nephritis. *Acta Path. Jap. 19*: 265–281, 1969.

53. Masugi, Y., Sugisaki, Y., and Ishizaki, M.: The significance of the glomeruli-bound anti renal basement membrane active antibody as the pathogenetic factor of human chronic glomerulonephritis. *Acta Path. Jap. 24*: 633–650, 1974.

54. Masugi, Y., Ishizaki, M., and Sugisaki, Y.: Study on the anti-GBM antibody mediated glomerulonephritis in rats. (Abst. in Japanese). *Jap. J. Nephrol. 17*: 510–511, 1975.

55. Mauer, S.M., Fish, A.J., Blau, E.B., and Michael, A.F.: The glomerular mesangium. I. Kinetic studies of macromolecular uptake in normal and nephrotic rats. *J. Clin. Invest. 51*: 1092–1101, 1972.

56. Mauer, S.M., Fish, A.J., Day, N.K., and Michael, A.F.: The glomerular mesangium. II. Studies of macromolecular uptake in nephrotoxic nephritis in rats. *J. Clin. Invest. 53*: 431–439, 1974.

57. McCausland, I.P., Seelye, R.N., Gavin, J.B., and Herdson, P.B.: The electron microscopic localization of nephrotoxic antibodies in isolated glomeruli. *Pathol. 8*: 73–80, 1976.

58. McClusky, R.T.: The value of immunofluorescence in the study of human renal disease. *J. Exp. Med. 134*: 242s-255s, 1971.

59. McPhaul, J.J. and Dixon, F.J.: Immunoreactive basement membrane antigens in normal human urine and serum. *J. Exp. Med. 130*: 1395–1409, 1969.

60. McPhaul, J.J. and Mullins, J.D.: Glomerulonephritis mediated by antibody to glomerular basement membrane. Immunological, clinical and histopathological characteristics. *J. Clin. Invest. 57*: 351–361, 1976.

61. Menefee, M.G., Mueller, C.B., Bell, A.L., and Meyer, J.K.: Transport of globin by the renal glomerulus. *J. Exp. Med. 120*: 1129–1138, 1964.

62. Michael, A.F., Fish, A.J., and Good, R.A.: Glomerular localization and transport of aggregated proteins in mice. *Lab. Invest. 17*: 14–29, 1967.

63. Mohos, S.C. and Skoza, L.: Glomerular sialoprotein. *Science 164*: 1519–1521, 1969.

64. Movat, H.Z., McGregor, D.D., and Steiner, J.W.: Studies of nephrotoxic nephritis. II. The fine structure of the glomerulus in acute nephrotoxic enphritis of dogs. *Amer. J. Clin. Path. 36*: 306–321, 1961.

65. Naish, P., Penn, G.B., Evans, D.J., and Peters, D.K.: The effect of defibrination on nephrotoxic serum nephritis in rabbits. *Clin. Sci. 42*: 643–646, 1972.

66. Naish, P.F., Evans, D.J., and Peters, D.K.: The effects of defibrination with ancrod in experimental allergic glomerular injury. *Clin. Exp. Immunol. 20*: 303–309, 1975.

67. Nakane, P.K. and Pierce, G.B.: Enzyme-labeled antibodies: Preparation and application for the localization of antigens. *J. Histochem. Cytochem. 14*: 929–931, 1966.

68. Passos, H.C., Siqueira, M., Martinez, O.C., and Bier, O.G.: Studies on the nephrotoxic activity of guinea-pig gamma 1 and gamma 2 antibodies. *Immunology 26*: 407–416, 1974.

69. Piel, C.F., Dong, L., Modern, F.W.S., Goodman, J.R., and Moore, R.: The glomerulus in experimental renal disease in rats as observed by light and electron microscopy. *J. Exp. Med.* *102*: 573–580, 1955.

70. Pressman, D., Eisen, N.H., and Fitzgerald, P.J.: The zone of localization of antibodies. VI. The rate of localization of anti-mouse-kidney serum. *J. Immunol. 64*: 281–287, 1950.

71. Rothbard, S. and Watson, R.F.: Comparison of reaction of antibodies to rat collagen and to rat kidney in the basement membranes of rat renal glomeruli. *J. Exp. Med. 129*: 1145–1161, 1969.

72. Rudofsky, U.H., McMaster, P.R.B., Wai-Sai, M.A., Steblay, R.W., and Pollora, B: Experimental autoimmune renal cortical tubulointerstitial disease in guinea pigs lacking the fourth component of complement. *J. Immunol. 112*: 1387–1393, 1974.

73. Sakuma, S. und Vogt, A.: Electronenmikroskopische Untersuchungen während der akuten Phase der durch Kaninchenantirattennierenserum erzeugten Masugi-Nephritis der Ratte. *Hiroshima J. Med. Sci.*: *24*: 153–173, 1975.

74. Seegal, B.C., Hsu, K.C., and Andres, G.A.: Specific nephrotoxic nephritis: old facts and present concepts. *In* Graber, P. and Miescher, P.A. (eds.): *Immunopathology IIIrd International Symposium*, 208–219, Schwabe, Basel/Stuttgart, 1963.

75. Shibata, S., Nagasawa, T., Takuma, T., Naruse, T., and Miyakawa, Y.: Isolation and properties of the soluble antigen specific for the production of nephrotoxic glomerulonephritis. I. Immunopathological demonstration of the complete antigenicity of the soluble antigen. *Jap. J. Exp. Med. 36*: 127–142, 1966.

76. Shibata, S., Miyakawa, Y., Naruse, T., Nagasawa, T., and Takuma, T.: A glycoprotein that induced nephrotoxic antibody: its isolation and purification from rat glomerular basement membrane. *J. Immunol. 102*: 593–601, 1969.

77. Shibata, S., Naruse, T., and Nagasawa, T.: Further purification of the glycoprotein that induces nephrotoxic antibody: isolation of the active polysaccharide fraction mainly composed of glucose. *J. Immunol. 104*: 215–223, 1970.

78. Shibata, S., Sakaguchi, H., Nagasawa, T., and Naruse, T.: Nephritogenic glycoprotein. II. Experimental production of membranous glomerulonephritis in rats by a single injection of homologous renal glycopeptide. *Lab. Invest. 27*: 457–465, 1972.

79. Shibata, S., Miyakawa, Y., and Nagasawa, T.: Studies on the developing mechanism of glycoprotein nephritis: its immunological and pathomorphological aspects (Abst. in Japanese). *Jap. J. Nephrol. 18*: 117–118, 1976.

80. Shigematsu, H.: Glomerular events during the initial phase of rat Masugi nephritis. *Virchows Arch. Abt. B Zellpath. 5*: 187–200, 1970.

81. Shigematsu, H. and Kobayashi, Y.: The development and fate of the immune deposits in the glomerulus during the secondary phase of rat Masugi nephritis. *Virchows Arch. Abt. B Zellpath. 8*: 83–95, 1971.

82. Simpson, I.J., Amos, N., Evans, D.J., Thomson, N.M., and Peters, D.K.: Guinea-pig nephrotoxic nephritis. 1. The role of complement and polymorphonuclear leucocytes and the effect of antibody subclass and fragments in the heterologous phase. *Clin. Exp. Immunol. 19*: 499–511, 1975.

83. Singer, S.J.: Preparation of an electron-dense antibody conjugate. *Nature 183*: 1523–1524, 1959.

84. Spiro, R.G.: Studies on the renal glomerular basement membrane. Preparation and chemical composition. *J. Biol. Chem. 242*: 1915–1922, 1967.

85. Spiro, R.G.: Studies on the renal glomerular basement membrane. Nature of the carbohydrate units and their attachment to the peptide portion. *J. Biol. Chem. 242*: 1923–1932, 1967.

86. Sri Ram, J., Tawde, S.S., Pierce, G.B., and Midgley, A.R.: Preparation of antibody-ferritin conjugates for immune-electron microscopy. *J. Cell Biol. 17*: 673–675, 1963.

87. Steblay, R.W.: Glomerulonephritis induced in sheep by injection of heterologous glomerular basement membrane and Freund's complete adjuvant. *J. Exp. Med. 116*: 253–272, 1962.

88. Steblay, R.W. and Rudofsky, U.: Renal tubular disease and autoantibodies against tubular basement membrane in guinea pigs. *J. Immunol. 107*: 589–594, 1971.

89. Steblay, R.W. and Rudofsky, U.: Transfer of experimental autoimmune renal cortical tubular and interstitial disease in guinea pigs by serum. *Science 180*: 966–968, 1973.

90. Sugisaki, T., Klassen, J., Milgrom, F., Andres, G.A., and McCluskey, R.T.: Immunopathologic study of an autoimmune tubular and interstitial renal disease in Brown Norway rats. *Lab. Invest. 28*: 658–671, 1973.

91. Suzuki, Y., Churg, J., Grishman, E., Mautner, W., and Dach, S.: The mesangium of the renal glomerulus. Electron microscopic studies of pathologic alterations. *Amer. J. Path. 43*: 555–578, 1963.

92. Thomson, N.M., Simpson, I.J., and Peters, D.K.: A quantitative evaluation of anticoagulants in experimental nephrotoxic nephritis. *Clin. Exp. Immunol. 19*: 301–308, 1975.

93. Thomson, N.M., Naish, P.F., Simpson, I.J., and Peter, D.K.: The role of C_3 in the autologous phase of nephrotoxic nephritis. *Clin. Exp. Immunol. 24*: 464–473, 1976.

94. Unanue, E.R. and Dixon, F.J.: Experimental glomerulonephritis. IV. Participation of complement in nephrotoxic nephritis. *J. Exp. Med. 119*: 965–982, 1965.

95. Unanue, E.R. and Dixon, F.J.: Experimental glomerulonephritis. V. Studies on the interaction of nephrotoxic antibodies with tissues of the rats. *J. Exp. Med. 121*: 697–714, 1965.

96. Unanue, E.R. and Dixon, F.J.: Experimental glomerulonephritis. VI. The autologous phase of nephrotoxic serum nephritis. *J. Exp. Med. 121*: 715–725, 1965.

97. Unanue, E.R. and Dixon, F.J.: Experimental glomerulonephritis: Immunological events and pathogenetic mechanisms. *Adv. Immunol. 6*: 1–90, 1967.

98. Van Zwieten, M.J., Bhan, A.K., McCluskey, R.T., and Collins, A.B.: Studies on the pathogenesis of experimental anti-tubular basement membrane nephritis in the guinea pig. *Amer. J. Path. 83*: 531–546, 1976.

99. Vassali, P., Simon, G., and Rouiller, C.: Electron microscopic study of glomerular lesions resulting from intravascular fibrin formation. *Amer. J. Path. 43*: 579–617, 1963.

100. Vassali, P. and McCluskey, R.T.: The pathogenic role of the coagulation process in rabbit Masugi nephritis. *Amer. J. Path. 45*: 653–677, 1964.

101. Verroust, P.J., Wilson, C.B., Cooper, N.R., Edgington, T.S., and Dixon, F.J.: Glomerular complement components in human glomerulonephritis. *J. Clin. Invest. 53*: 77–84, 1974.

102. Vogt, A., Bockhorn, H., Kozima, K., and Sasaki, H.: Electron microscopic localization of the nephrotoxic antibody in the glomeruli of the rat after intravenous application of purified nephritogenic antibody-ferritin conjugates. *J. Exp. Med. 127*: 867–878, 1968.

103. Ward, P.A., Cochrane, C.G., and Müller-Eberhard, H.: The role of serum complement in chemotaxis of leucocytes in vitro. *J. Exp. Med. 122*: 327–346, 1965.

104. Watanabe, T. and Tanaka, K.: The role of coagulation and fibrinolysis in the development of rabbit Masugi nephritis. *Acta Path. Jap. 26*: 147–165, 1976.

105. Wilson, C.B. and Dixon, F.J.: Anti-glomerular basement membrane antibody induced glomerulonephritis. *Kidney Internat. 3*: 74–89, 1973.

106. Wilson, C.B. and Dixon, F.J.: The renal response to immunological injury. *In* Brenner, B.M. and Rector, F.C. (eds.): *The Kidney*, 838–940, W.B. Saunders, Philadelphia, 1976.

Chapter **4**

Scanning Electron Microscopy of the Glomerulus in Masugi Nephritis of Rabbits

Masaaki ARAKAWA, Masanobu EDANAGA, and Junichi TOKUNAGA

I. Introduction

Scanning electron microscopy, which is suited for the study of the stereoscopic surface ultrastructure of tissues and cells, has been introduced in the histopathological study of the kidney since Buss and Krönert [9] first studied normal rat glomeruli by this new methodology in 1969. Since then several research groups including the authors' have clarified some problems concerning the ultrastructure of the glomeruli, which have remained unknown until now in transmission electron microscope studies. One of the authors, Arakawa, has concentrated his efforts mainly to scanning electron microscopy of mammalian glomeruli in experimental nephropathies as well as of the human glomeruli in normal and pathologic situations [2–8]. He reported in 1974 on the scanning electron microscopy of Masugi nephritis in rabbits [6], which was produced by a single intravenous injection of nephrotoxic immune serum of heterogeneous origin (anti-rabbit kidney duck serum) according to Masugi's original method [12, 13].

In addition to previous observations, an attempt has been made in this investigation to observe an isolated single glomerulus in Masugi nephritis of rabbits, that is obviously a satisfactory method for an effective and extensive evaluation of glomerular lesions. The surface ultrastructure of normal rabbit glomeruli was also demonstrated in order to understand the pathological lesions more clearly.

II. Materials and Methods

Adult white rabbits weighing approximately 2 kg were used in this study. Glomerulonephritis was produced in ten rabbits by a single intravenous injection of anti-rabbit kidney duck serum at a dose level of 1 ml per kg of body weight. After a latent period of a few days all rabbits showed proteinuria and microscopic hematuria. Urine protein increased gradually up to the maximum level of 1.1 gm for 24 hours. Ten to 14 days after the injection they were sacrificed under general anesthesia for the examination. Two rabbits, which were not injected and showed no proteinuria, were examined as normal controls.

One kidney extirpated from either side after ligating the renal artery was used for light microscopy. The other kidney was perfused immediately from the abdominal aorta with approximately 500 ml of 2.5% phosphate-buffered glutaraldehyde (pH 7.4, 0.1M). Following perfusion fixation, it was separated into two or three blocks and immersed for several days in the fixative similar to that used for perfusion. It was then cut into small blocks suitable for scanning electron microscopic observation with a clean razor blade. The blocks were dehydrated in a series of graded acetone and dried in air.

On the other hand, glomeruli in a small cube were gently squeezed out into a buffered solution by gentle teasing with two forceps under a binocular microscope [14].　A single glomerulus could be readily isolated without noticeable damage to the glomerular surface under the scanning electron microscope.　One or a few isolated glomeruli were sucked up through a polyethylene capillary tube and blown out onto the back side of a copper grid (250-400 mesh), which had been previously immersed in acetone, hydrophylized with a sputter coating of gold and palladium, and placed in a Petri-dish.　Fifty percent ethanol was gently poured with a small pipette from the edge of the dish, and this was replaced succesively by a series of graded ethanols.　Absolute alcohol was finally replaced by amyl acetate.　The mesh was then dried by the critical point drying method using CO_2.　After drying, the surface of the specimen was coated by a sputter coating of gold and palladium.

The scanning electron microscopes, Hitachi HSM-2 and JEOL JSM-2, were used for observation.

III.　Results

1.　Scanning electron microscopy of the glomerulus in normal rabbits

Fig. 4-1 illustrates a general view of a glomerulus from a normal rabbit.　Bowman's capsule has been cut open.　Fig. 4-2 shows a portion of a glomerulus with well expanded, winding capillary loops.　They are covered by podocytes.　The cell body or nuclear portion of the podocyte containing its nucleus is noticed to be a round thickened mass and to be located in the curve of the loops.　The broad flat cytoplasmic layer frequently extends from the cell body towards the periphery and is very irregular in shape.　The surface of the cell body is rather smooth or slightly uneven.

Several cytoplasmic processes, primary processes, arise directly from the cell bodies and wind transversely or longitudinally around the capillary loops.　The width of these processes is very variable.　Occasionally they are larger at the periphery and ended into wide cytoplasmic area.　Some of the primary processes issue thinner secondary processes, which extend in the same manner as the primary ones and occasionally give rise to tertiary processes.　These cytoplasmic processes issue in turn into thin clubbed terminal processes.　They come out at right angle or radially like fern leaves.　The terminal processes are attached to the outer surface of the basement membrane, and correspond to the triangular profiles of "foot processes" seen by transmission electron microscopy.　They are relatively uniform in width, approximately 200 to 300 millimicrons, however, very variable in length, 500 to 3,500 millimicrons.　Thin string-like microprojections and lumpy cytoplasmic protrusions are occasionally noticed to be scattered on the surface not only of the cell bodies but also of the cytoplasmic processes.

2.　Light microscopy of the glomerulus in Masugi-nephritic rabbits

All rabbits show rather similar histologic alterations in the glomerulus.　They reveal a diffuse increase in mesangial nuclei and matrix, moderate to severe in most glomeruli.　Some of the glomeruli presents a PAS-positive, rather homogeneous, hyaline substance in Bowman's space, containing occasionally nuclear debri or fibrinous material.　Cellular proliferation of Bowman's epithelium, so-called crescent formation, is seen in some glomeruli, which is occasionally replaced by fibrinous tissue.　There are focal thickening and splitting of the peripheral basement membrane.　Neither complete hyalinization nor marked swelling of glomeruli is observed at this acute stage.

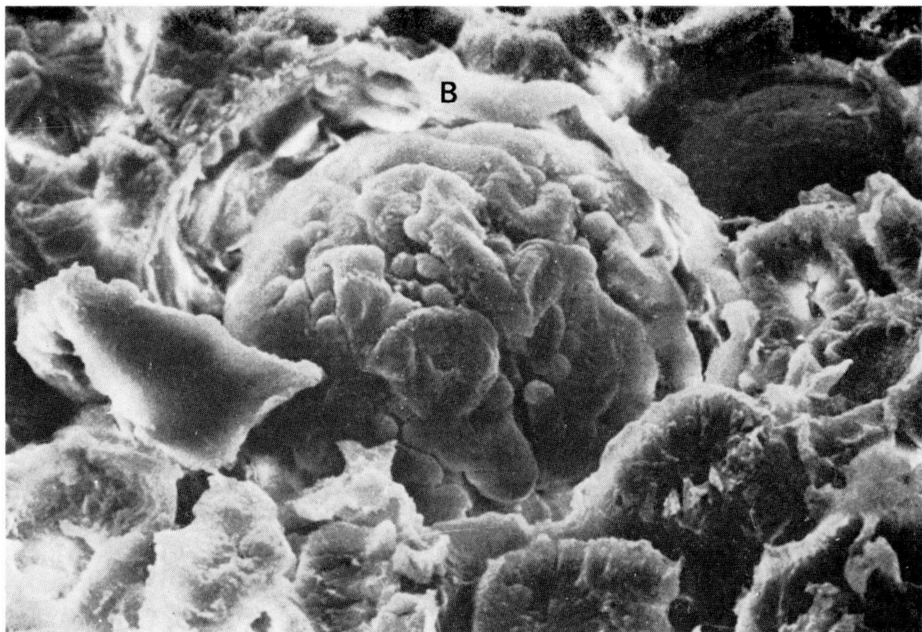

Fig. 4-1 A low power scanning electron micrograph of a normal rabbit glomerulus. Approximately one-half of the entire surface could be observed through the opened Bowman's capsule (B). The winding capillary loops are covered by podocytes. ×700.

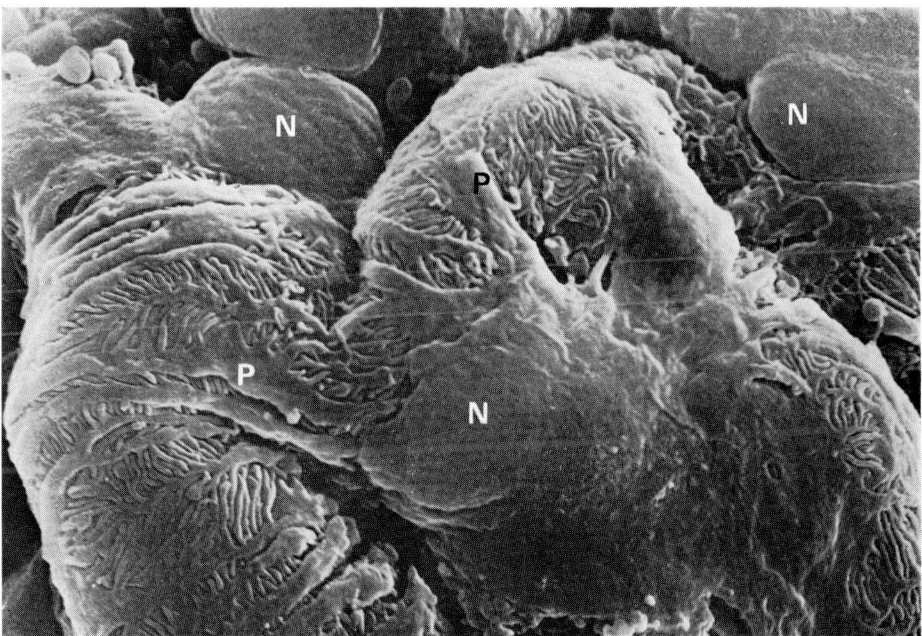

Fig. 4-2 A portion of the capillary loops of a normal rabbit glomerulus. The nuclear portion (N) of a podocyte, which extends as a broad flat cytoplasmic sheet, issues several cytoplasmic processes (P). Thin clubbed terminal processes branch out from the cytoplasmic processes, primary, secondary, or tertiary at a right angle or radially, and are regularly interdigitated with those of the different cells. ×4,900.

3. Scanning electron microscopy of the glomerulus in Masugi-nephritic rabbits

Figs. 4-3 to 4-7 represent the total view of an isolated single glomerulus observed from various directions. Fig. 4-3 shows the specimen placed perpendicular to the beam. Fig. 4-4 shows the same specimen tilted at 30°, the specimen was then rotated to an angle of 90° to the right as shown in Fig. 4-5. In Fig. 4-6 it was further rotated 90°, and in Fig. 4-7 a further 90°. Concerning the overall appearance of the glomerulus, it seems to be slightly enlarged with a rather prominent lobular appearance of the capillary loops. The capillary loops are swollen or expanded slightly as seen in these figures, while some are atrophied or collapsed in varying degrees.

The podocytes overlying the capillary loops increase in number in many glomeruli (Fig. 4-8). The cell body of a podocyte either becomes more round and smaller, protruding as a polyp, or represents a rather flat expansion (Figs. 4-8–4-10). The cytoplasmic processes, primary, secondary, and tertiary, are more or less shrunken. The terminal processes branching from these processes are markedly and irregularly atrophied or swollen. The loss of terminal processes is observed only in small parts of the glomeruli. There are occasionally many lumpy cytoplasmic projections, which are aggregated on the surface of some podocytes (Fig. 4-11). Numerous thin, tiny, string-like microprojections are also seen occasionally at the margin of nuclear portions as well as on the cytoplasmic processes (Fig. 4-12).

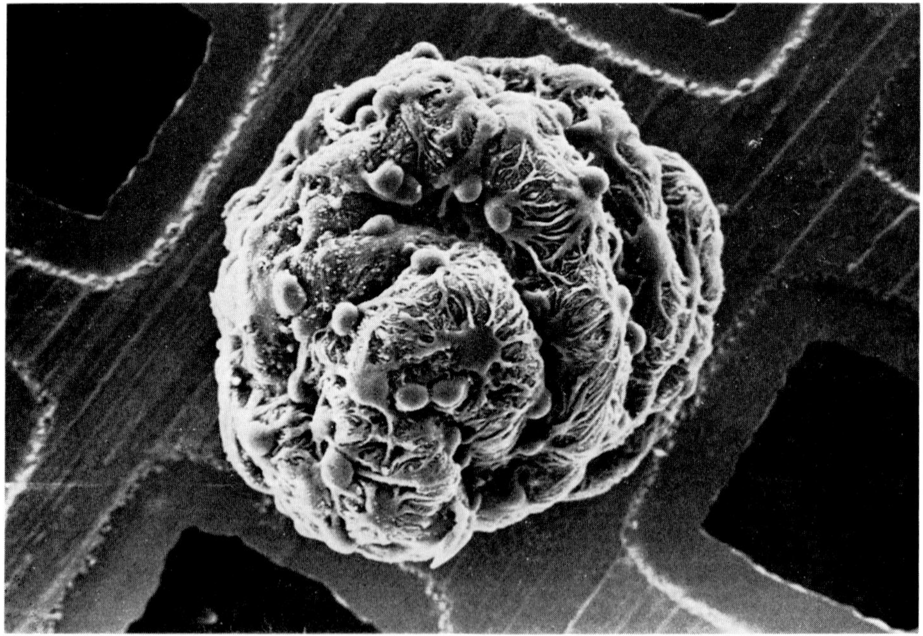

Fig. 4-3

Figs. 4-3 – 4-7 The scanning electron micrographs of an isolated single glomerulus of a Masugi-nephritic rabbit. ×680. Fig. 4-3 is the view of the entire glomerulus placed perpendicular to the beam. Fig. 4-4 shows the same specimen tilted at 30° to the beam. In Fig. 4-5 it was rotated to an angle of 90° to the right. In Fig. 4-6 it was further rotated 90°, and in Fig. 4-7 a further 90°.

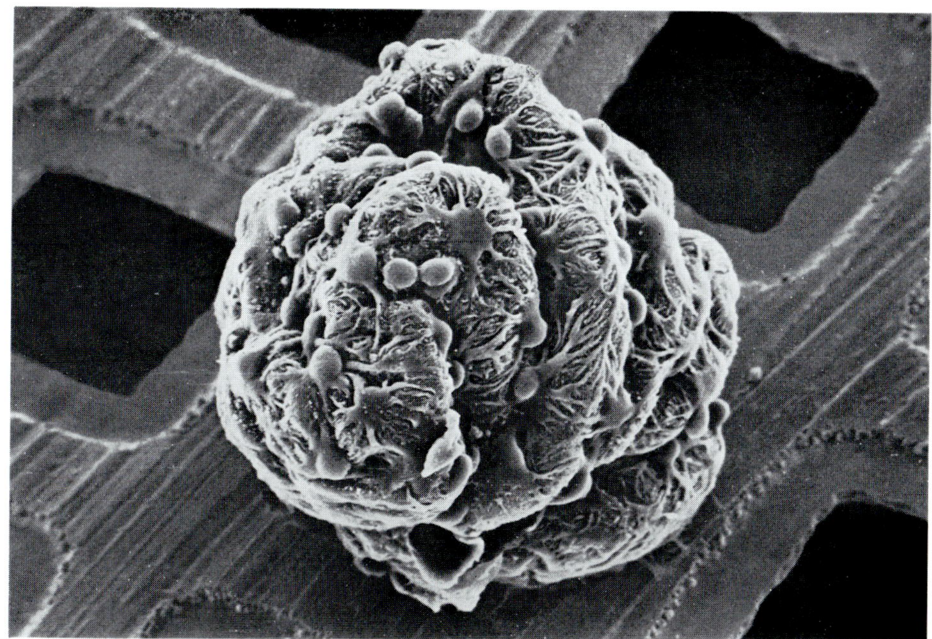

Fig. 4-4

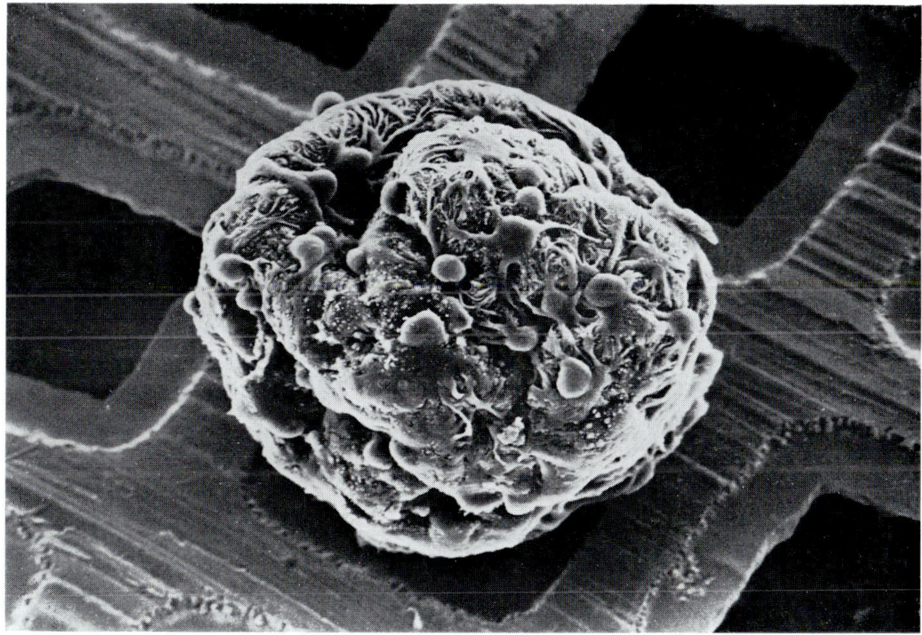

Fig. 4-5

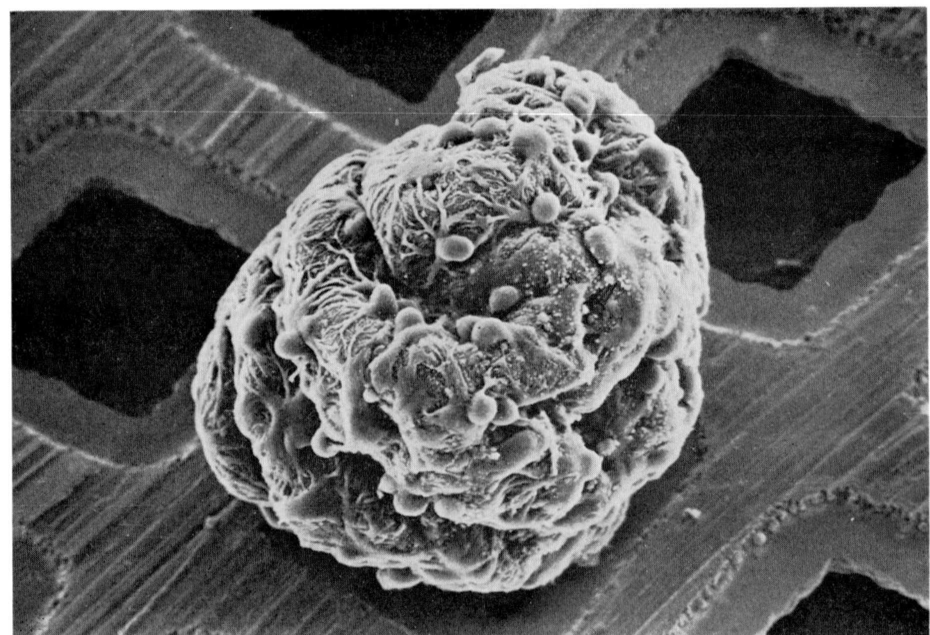

Fig. 4-6

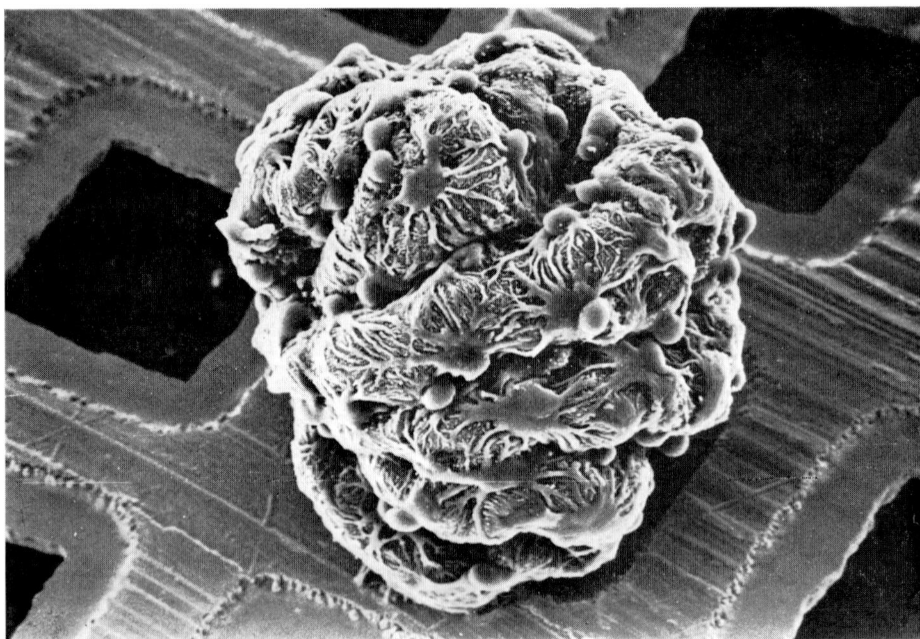

Fig. 4-7

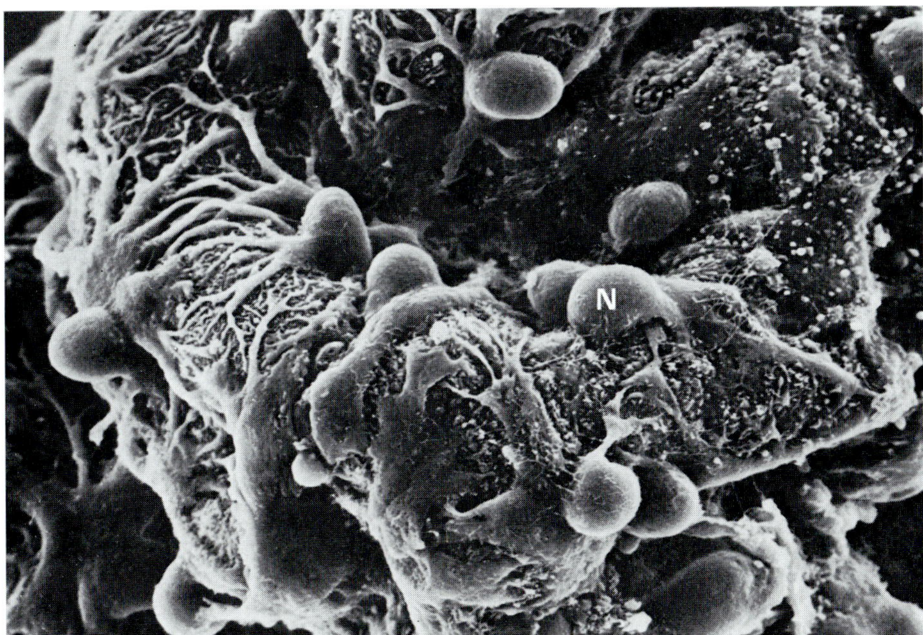

Fig. 4-8　A portion of a capillary loop of the glomerulus of a Masugi-nephritic rabbit. The cell bodies or nuclear portions (N) of the podocytes increase in number and become more round and smaller, presenting a polyp-like appearance. The cytoplasmic processes are irregularly atrophied.　×1,850.

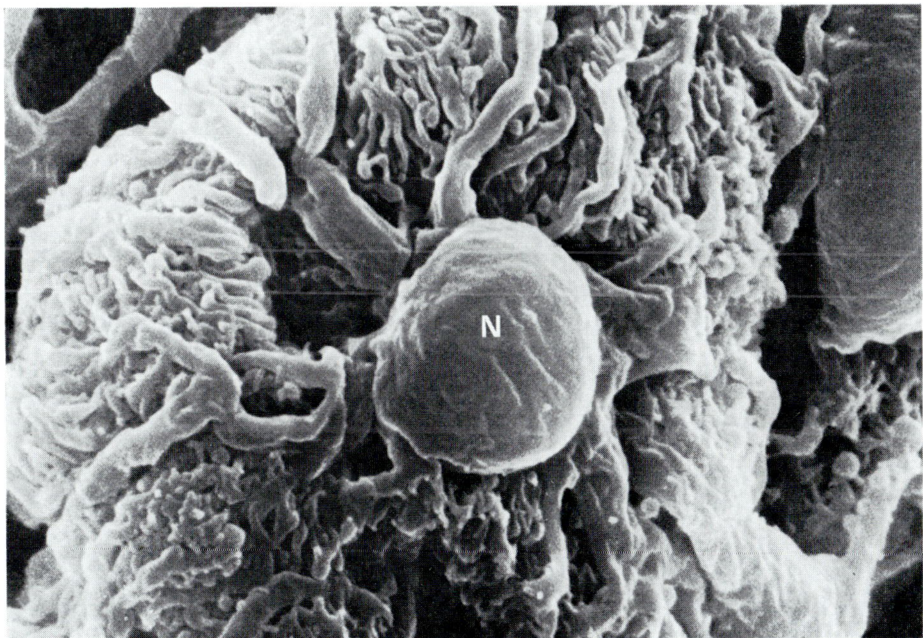

Fig. 4-9　Higher magnification of part of a podocyte. A polyp-like nuclear portion (N) and atrophied cytoplasmic processes are clearly shown. The terminal processes are well preserved, although they are irregularly arranged.　×6,620.

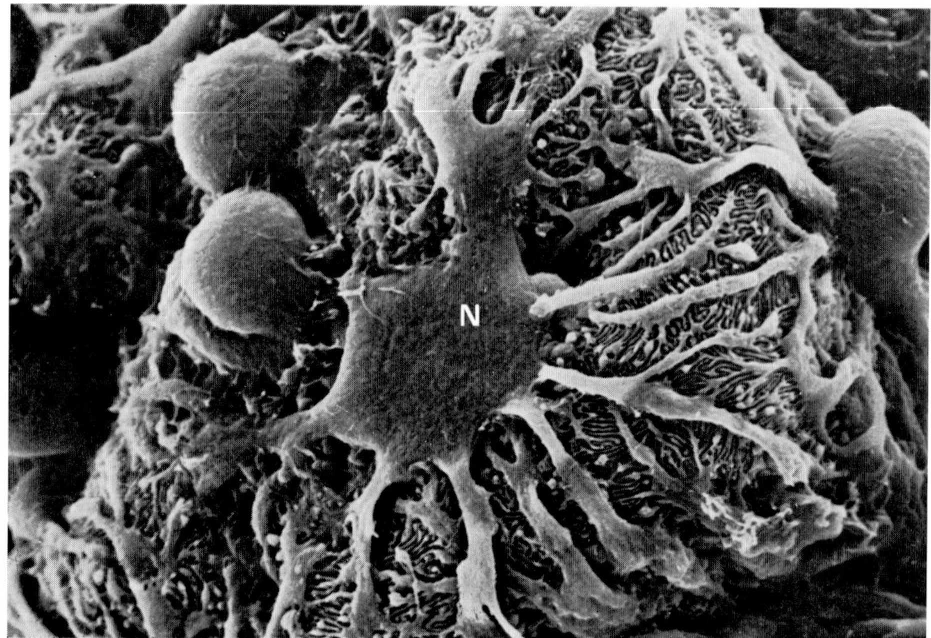

Fig. 4-10 Higher magnification of a nuclear portion (N) of a podocyte, which is spread out. Irregularly atrophied cytoplasmic processes are also observed. ×3,750.

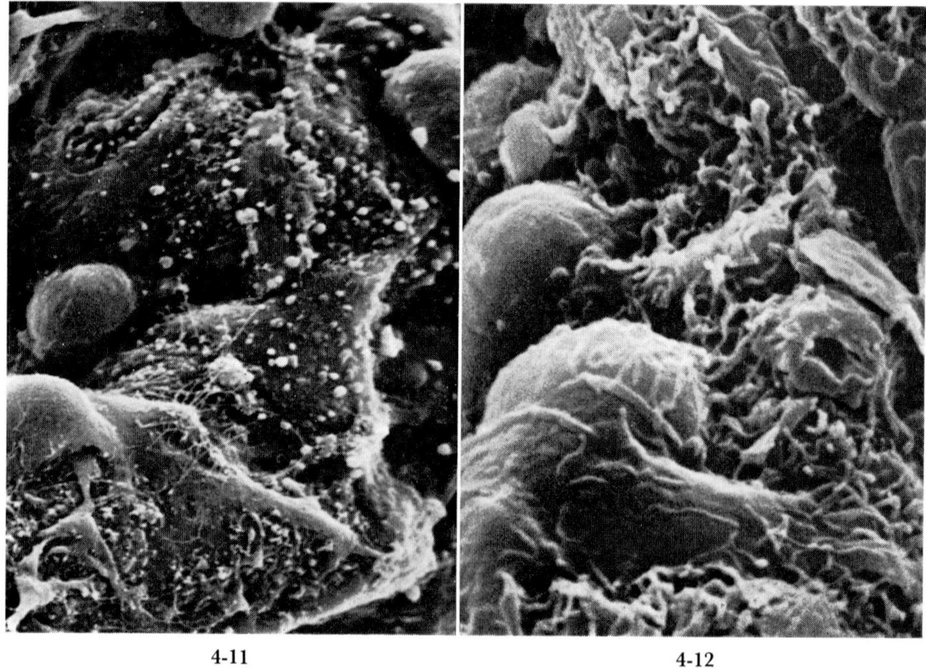

Fig. 4-11 Higher magnification of a portion of Fig. 4-8. Many small cytoplasmic protrusions are present on the surface of cell bodies and cytoplasmic processes. ×2,800.
Fig. 4-12 Higher magnification of parts of the podocytes. Numerous string-like microprojections branch directly from the nuclear portions or from the cytoplasmic processes. ×6,000.

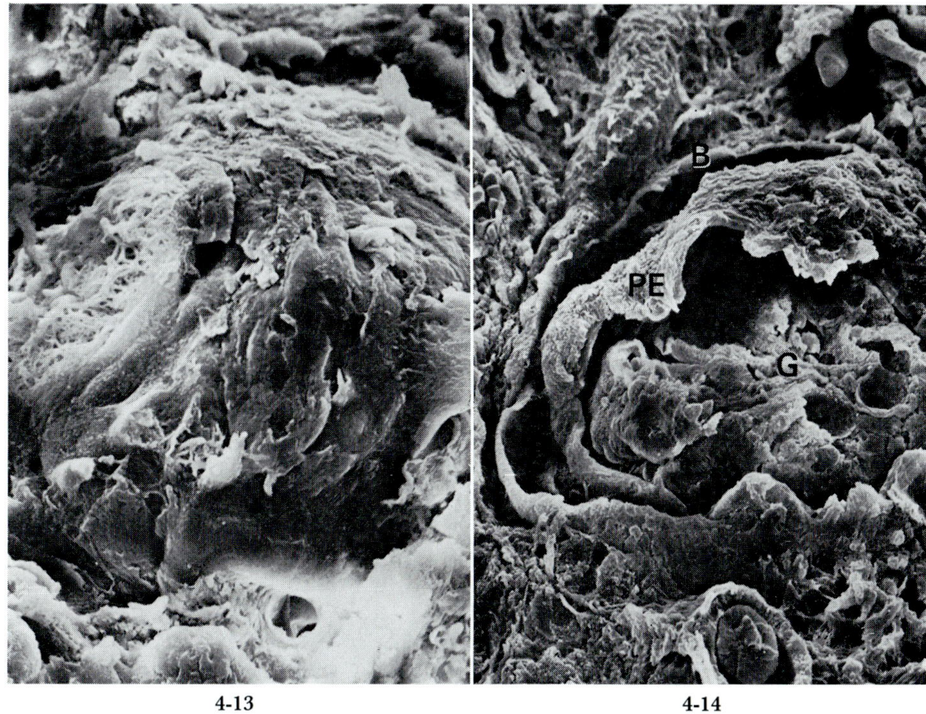

4-13 **4-14**

Fig. 4-13 A low power scanning electron micrograph of a glomerulus of a Masugi-nephritic rabbit, covered with homogenous, partly granular, or partly fibrinous substance. ×740.

Fig. 4-14 A cross section view of a glomerulus showing the same change as seen in Fig. 4-13. Granular or fibrinous solid substance (PE), assumed to be protein or fibrinous exudate, is seen between capillary loops (G) and Bowman's capsule (B). ×600.

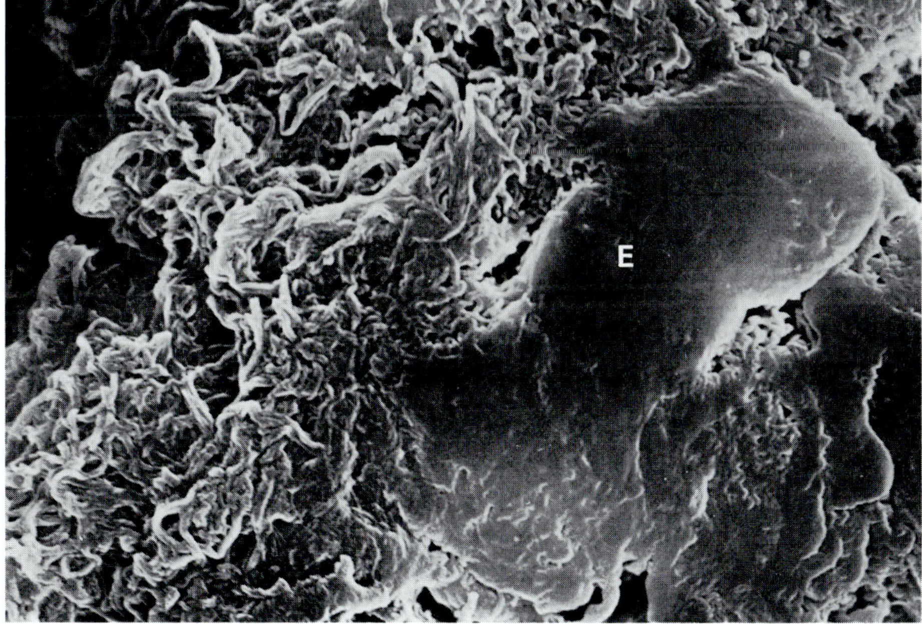

Fig. 4-15 At the border between a podocyte (E) and protein or fibrinous substance there are numerous fine fibrils represented as irregular wrinkling. ×5,600.

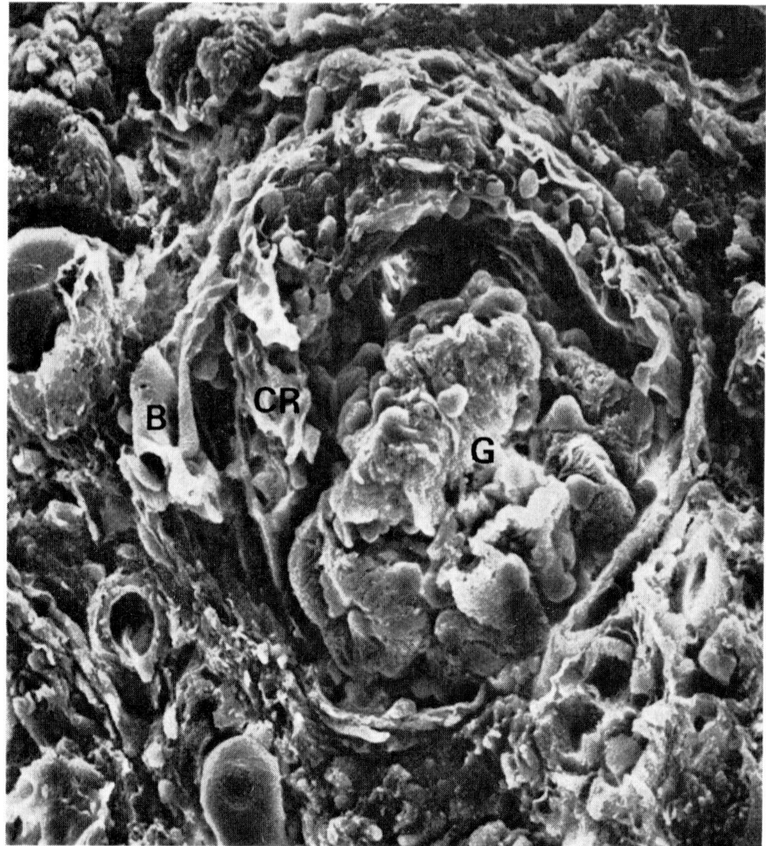

Fig. 4-16   A cross section of a glomerulus of a Masugi-nephritic rabbit. Increased small round cells have aggregated in semilunar form (CR) along the inner surface of Bowman's capsule (B). Glomerular capillary loops (G) have no direct connection with proliferating cells.   ×640.

Some glomeruli are covered with rather homogenous, partly granular, or partly fibrinous substance, which might correspond to protein or fibrinous exudate in Bowman's space seen in light microscopy (Fig. 4-13).   This irregularly shaped, board-like substance covered most parts of the glomerular surface, so that only small portions could be identified with a scanning electron microscope.   Fig. 4-14 reveals a cross section view of the glomerulus with this substance.   At the junction between podocytes and this substance fine fibrillar materials are seen to be wrinkled in various directions (Fig. 4-15).

The proliferation of Bowman's epithelium, so-called crescent formation, is occasionally observed in some glomeruli (Fig. 4-16).   Many small round cell bodies are aggregated together in a semilunar form along the inner surface of Bowman's capsule.   Fig. 4-16 clearly illustrates that the visceral epithelial cells have no direct relation to the crescent.

IV. Discussion

The principal renal lesion of Masugi nephritis in rabbits is diffuse proliferative glomerulonephritis.   The main reaction site in the glomerulus is the mesangium, which cannot be observed under a scanning electron microscope by the conventional specimen preparation.   However, the podocyte, which is a proper subject for scanning electron microscopy, is known to reveal extensive multiplication and syncytial cell formation by light microscopy (Germuth, 1973) [11].   This study represents some interesting findings in the podocytes such as increase in number, atrophy with polyp-like protrusion or flat expansion of the cell body, irregular atrophy and arrangement of the large cytoplasmic and small terminal processes and focal increase in lumpy protrusions or string-like microprojections of the cytoplasm.   Syncytial formation of neighboring cells could not be confirmed.   Similar alterations are also seen in proliferative glomerulonephritis of different pathogenesis, namely immune complex nephritis, such as acute serum sickness nephritis in rabbits and human acute poststreptococcal glomerulonephritis.   This means that the reaction of podocytes seems to be a secondary reaction to mesangial or endothelial cell proliferation in various conditions.

Buss and Lamberts [10] reported on the scanning electron microscopy of Masugi nephritis in rats, in which pronounced furrowing of the podocyte surface has been stressed as a special reactive form in this type of nephritis.   Furrowed podocytes were not observed in Masugi nephritis of rabbits as far as the authors observed.   There is some difference in the nature of Masugi nephritis between rats and rabbits.   In Masugi nephritis of rats, the first phase of nephritis is not a true proliferative glomerulonephritis, but a degenerative one, followed by mild proliferative glomerulonephritis with a marked nephrotic syndrome in the second phase.   They reported that the glomerulonephritis was mild and focal, and that proteinuria was also very mild [10].   On the other hand, Masugi nephritis of rabbits generally reveals a diffuse proliferative glomerulonephritis as seen in this study.   It is assumed that furrowing of the podocytes is a reaction only to a degenerative glomerulitis, and not to a proliferative one.   The furrowing of the podocyte surface was also seen in the course of aminonucleoside nephrosis in rats, although it was noticed occasionally in normal glomeruli [4].

In the early stage of acute poststreptococcal glomerulonephritis in man, 3 to 6 weeks after onset, the glomerulus represents a Rugby ball-like oval, but not globular swelling of the whole glomerulus, associated with prominent lobular appearance of the capillary loops [8].   It became less and less prominent in parallel with the course of nephritis.   It is also noticed in the severe stage of the nephrotic syndrome.   The reason that it was not seen in this experimental nephritis might be due to the stage or severity of the proliferative glomerulonephritis.

Many lumpy cytoplasmic protrusions on the podocyte surface are also seen in patients with a severe nephrotic syndrome or in the early and elapsed stage of acute glomerulonephritis [8].   They are seen in the experimental nephrotic syndrome such as aminonucleoside nephrosis [4] and daunomycin nephrosis [10] in rats.

Buss and Lamberts [10] thought that the lumpy protrusions, which were designated as "buds", contained excreted protein or coagulated protein of the glycocalyx.   Andrews [1] suggested that they corresponded to the presence of intracellular vacuoles containing protein, which were excreted partially into the urinary space.   The occurence of these protrusions seems to be related to marked proteinuria, because they were very evident in the nephrotic syndrome.   However, they were also seen in acute glomerulonephritis without proteinuria or even in normal glomeruli [8].

The loss of the terminal processes is seen in only small areas of all glomeruli, which is compatible with a mild degree of proteinuria in nephritic rabbits.   It is a nonspecific reaction to increased permeability of the basement membrane to serum protein.   The extent of disappearance is well correlated only with the grade of proteinuria, but not with the nature of glomerular damage as confirmed before [3, 4].   The mechanism of the loss of the terminal processes was clarified first by one of the authors, Arakawa [2–4].   He clearly demonstrated the disappearance and recovery process of the terminal processes in amino-nucleoside-nephrotic rats and also confirmed it in the renal biopsy specimens from humans with a nephrotic syndrome [3]. With the development of proteinuria, the terminal processes are irregularly swollen and retracted toward the nuclear portion of the cell, so that they became less and less interdigitated. Finally no interdigitation of the processes remained and the cells faced adjacent cells with straight cell borders. In the stage of recovery the reverse process is noticed in parallel with the decrease of proteinuria. According to the results, the loss of the terminal processes is not due to syncytial formation but to swelling and retraction of the processes. Because no syncytial formation takes place in this process, the term "fusion" of the terminal processes seems to be inappropriate. It may be preferable to use "loss" or "disappearance" of the processes.

The surface of the podocyte was veiled frequently with a rather homogeneous, partially granular, or partially fibrinous board-like substance, which corresponded to a protein and fibrinous exudate in Bowman's space seen in light microscopy (Figs. 4-13, 4-14). Fig. 4-15 showed clearly close relationship between aggregated, wrinkled fibrils and homogeneous substance covering the podocyte surface.

The cellular proliferation of Bowman's epithelium, which is known as extracapilary proliferation or crescent formation, was observed first in this study as seen in Fig. 4-16. Although the origin of proliferating cells could be either visceral epithelial cells, podocytes, or parietal epithelial cells, Bowman's epithelium, they came clearly from the latter in this figure. Further study will be expected in rapidly progressive glomerulonephritis showing marked crescent formation.

Concerning the scanning electron microscopic observation of the mesangium or basement membrane, which are the main reaction sites in proliferative glomerulonephritis as Masugi nephritis, the freeze cracking method should be applied, although there are still some problems in resolving power. Further studies will be needed in the near future.

V. Summary

The three-dimensional ultrastructural alterations of the glomerular surface, particularly of the podocytes, in Masugi nephritis were studied by scanning electron microscopy. The podocytes revealed increase in number, polyp-like protrusion or flat expansion of the cell body, irregular arrangement and atrophy of the cytoplasmic processes, and increase in lumpy cytoplasmic protrusions and string-like microprojections, which were assumed to be secondary reactions to proliferative glomerulonephritis showing primarily mesangial cell proliferation. The terminal processes remained intact in most parts of the glomeruli, although they were irregularly either atrophied or swollen. The three-dimensional view of protein or fibrinous substance in Bowman's space and crescents were clearly demonstrated first by the authors.

REFERENCES

1. Andrews, P.M.: Scanning electron microscopy of the nephrotic kidney. *Virchows Arch. B Cell Path. 17*: 195–211, 1975.
2. Arakawa, M.: A scanning electron microscopy of the glomerulus of normal and nephrotic rats. *Lab. Invest. 23*: 489–496, 1970.
3. Arakawa, M.: A scanning electron microscope study of the human glomerulus. *Amer. J. Path. 64*: 475–462, 1971.
4. Arakawa, M. and Tokunaga, J.: A scanning electron microscope study of the glomerulus. Further consideration of the mechanism of the fusion of podocyte terminal processes in nephrotic rats. *Lab. Invest. 27*: 366–371, 1972.

5. Arakawa, M. and Tokunaga, J.: Further scanning electron microscope studies of the human glomerulus. *Lab. Invest. 31*: 436–440, 1974.

6. Arakawa, M., Tokunaga, J., Shimotori, T., and Kinoshita, Y.: A scanning electron microscope study of the glomerulus of normal and nephritic rabbits. *Virchows Arch. B Cell Path. 17*: 185–194, 1974.

7. Arakawa, M., Edanaga, M., and Tokunaga, J.: Scanning electron microscopy of the isolated human glomerulus in normal, nephritic, and nephrotic situations. *In* Kluthe, R., Vogt, A., and Batsford, R. (ed.): *Glomerulonephritis,* 96–108, Georg Thieme, Stuttgart, 1976.

8. Arakawa, M. and Tokunaga, J.: A scanning electron microscope study of the human Bowman's epithelium. *In* Kobayashi, K. (ed.): *Contribution to Nephrology,* Vol. 6 Renal Research, 73–78, Karger, Basel, 1977.

9. Buss, H. and Krönert, W.: Zur Struktur des Nierenglomerulum der Ratte: rasterelektronenmikroskopischer Untersuchungen. *Virchows Arch. B Cell Path. 4*: 79–92, 1969.

10. Buss, H. and Lamberts, B.H.: Orthology and pathology of the renal podocytes. *In* Johari, O. and Corvin, I. (ed.): *Scanning Electron Microscopy* 1972, 574–580, I.I.T. Research Institute, Chicago, 1972.

11. Germuth, F.G. and Rodriguez, E.: *Immunopathology of the Renal Glomerulus: Immune Complex Deposit and Antibasement Membrane Disease.* Little, Brown, Boston, 1973.

12. Masugi, M.: Über das Wesen der spezifischen Veränderungen der Niere und der Leber durch das Nephrotoxin bzw. das Hepatotoxin. Zugleich ein Beitrag zur Pathogenese der Glomerulonephritis und der eklamptischen Lebererkrankung. *Beitr. path. Anat. 91*: 82–112, 1933.

13. Masugi, M.: Über die experimentelle Glomerulonephritis durch das spezifische Antinierenserum. Ein Beitrag zur Pathogenese der diffusen Glomerulonephritis. *Beitr. path. Anat. 92*: 429–466, 1934.

14. Tokunaga, J., Edanaga, M., Masu, Y., and Fujita, T.: Isolated renal glomeruli for scanning electron microscopy. *J. Electron Microscopy 24*: 109–114, 1975.

Chapter **5**

Fine Structure of Masugi Nephritis and Immune Complex Nephritis

Yoichiro KONDO and Hidekazu SHIGEMATSU

I. Introduction

The assumption that many human glomerular diseases might develop on the basis of immunologic mechanisms had been a matter of controversy until several decades ago. In fact a number of experimental attempts failed to prove beyond dispute an immune etiology for glomerulonephritis. This frustrating controversy was settled in two different ways. The first convincing evidence was presented by Masugi and associates [108–110]. By using a heterologous nephrotoxic serum, they produced a variety of glomerular diseases in rats or rabbits compatible with acute, subacute, and chronic glomerulonephritis in humans. Thus nephrotoxic serum nephritis (Masugi nephritis) became the first representative model of glomerulonephritis induced by immunologic means. It is now realized that heterologous nephrotoxic antibodies (NTAbs) are directed against a number of antigens situated in the glomerular basement membrane (GBM). On the other hand, the search for the pathogenesis of serum sickness led to an attempt to reproduce various serum sickness diseases experimentally in animals. Rich and Gregory clearly showed that hypersensitivity diseases including acute proliferative glomerulonephritis developed in rabbits that received large dose injection(s) of horse serum [154]. Subsequently it was revealed that the glomerulonephritis and other tissue lesions in acute serum sickness in animals are mediated by local deposition of antigen-antibody complexes (immune complexes) circulating in the blood. The pathogenesis of naturally occurring glomerular diseases in experimental animals, notably those observed in New Zealand strain mice and mink with Aleutian disease, have been interpreted in terms of an immune complex etiology [25]. Obviously the establishment of these two experimental models has greatly contributed to the search for the pathogenesis of human glomerular diseases. At present, on the basis of the underlying immunologic mechanisms, experimental as well as human glomerulonephritis can be separated into two major categories, consisting of antiGBM nephritis and immune complex nephritis [33]. The establishment of our concept of the pathogenesis of glomerulonephritis is undoubtedly indebted to ingenious immunologic methods currently introduced for investigations. The glomerular pathology has also been stimulated by the introduction of electron microscopy which has confirmed previous conflicting issues in light microscopy and has made it possible to provide a large number of new findings of interest. In this chapter, ultrastructural features of several representative models of immunologically induced experimental glomerulonephritis will be described with some pathogenetic considerations.

II. Ultrastructural Pathology

1. Masugi nephritis in rats

Since the original reports of Masugi and associates [108–110], many investigators have employed two kinds of NTAbs, namely duck NTAb and rabbit NTAb to induce nephrotoxic nephritis in the rabbit and rat respectively. It is well recognized that Masugi nephritis is devided into two phases, consisting of the first or heterologous phase and the second or autologous phase. The first phase, which is the result of a prompt fixation of NTAbs to the glomerulus, is best seen in rat Masugi nephritis induced by using rabbit NTAb. The glomerular alterations can be recognized immediately after the injection and persist for several days, and are then exacerbated following the initiation of the second phase whereby host antibody reacts with the antigen (rabbit NTAb) having been localized in the glomerulus.

a. The first phase

When compared to other experimental systems, there is a considerable advantage in examining rat Masugi nephritis caused by rabbit NTAb in that follow-up studies of a definite glomerulonephritis are possible from the very early stage. Piel et al. were pioneers who almost two decades ago examined rat Masugi nephritis with the aid of electron microscopy [149]. Because of technical difficulties in the preparation of specimens, they only clarified the presence of platelets in the glomerular capillaries and GBM thickening, which had been presumed to be present but not clearly recognized by light microscopy. The GBM alteration became apparent at 6 hours. Subsequently Miller and Bohle observed deposition of granular substances at the subendothelial aspect of the GBM [125]. Churg et al. clarified the disease process in some detail [18]. After 2 hours there was noticeable swelling of the endothelium, particularly of the attenuated layer, with partial disappearance of the endothelial pores. The capillary lumens contained many polymorphonuclear leukocytes (PMNs) which were often adherent to the capillary walls. At 24 hours migrant cells decreased in number and the capillary lumens were obliterated by swollen endothelial cytoplasm. The GBM irregularity was prominent. From 24 hours to 3 days the lumens were progressively filled with "hyaline" thrombi showing a fibrillar structure in electron microscopy with a predominant periodicity of 230Å. Feldman et al. noted wispy, poorly delineated deposits localized within or on the luminal side of the GBM as the earliest glomerular abnormality [45]. During the next 3 to 4 days swelling of the endothelium followed. The mesangial zone was dilated and contained an increased number of cells and increasing masses of basement membrane material. The exudative or degenerative nature of rat Masugi nephritis was emphasized by Fujimoto et al. [48]. Within several hours the GBM showed a wave-like distortion and the lumens were occluded with fibrin or fibrinoid thrombi, thereby providing a feature of fibrinoid degeneration of the capillary loops that resembled wire-loop lesions in human lupus nephritis. There was no definite proliferation of glomerular cells, though endothelial swelling was intense. Although intraluminal accumulation of PMNs was already described by the previous inverstigators, Cochrane and associates for the first time disclosed their pathogenetic role for the development of glomerular lesions [26]. With injections of an amount of rabbit NTAb known to yield considerable proteinuria in animals, an elevation in the numbers of PMNs in glomeruli was observed between 20 minutes to 12 hours, a peak accumulation being 2.5 hours. The PMNs infiltrated the endothelial pores gaining intimate contact with the GBM. Ultrastructural alterations of the PMNs, however, were not apparent; their

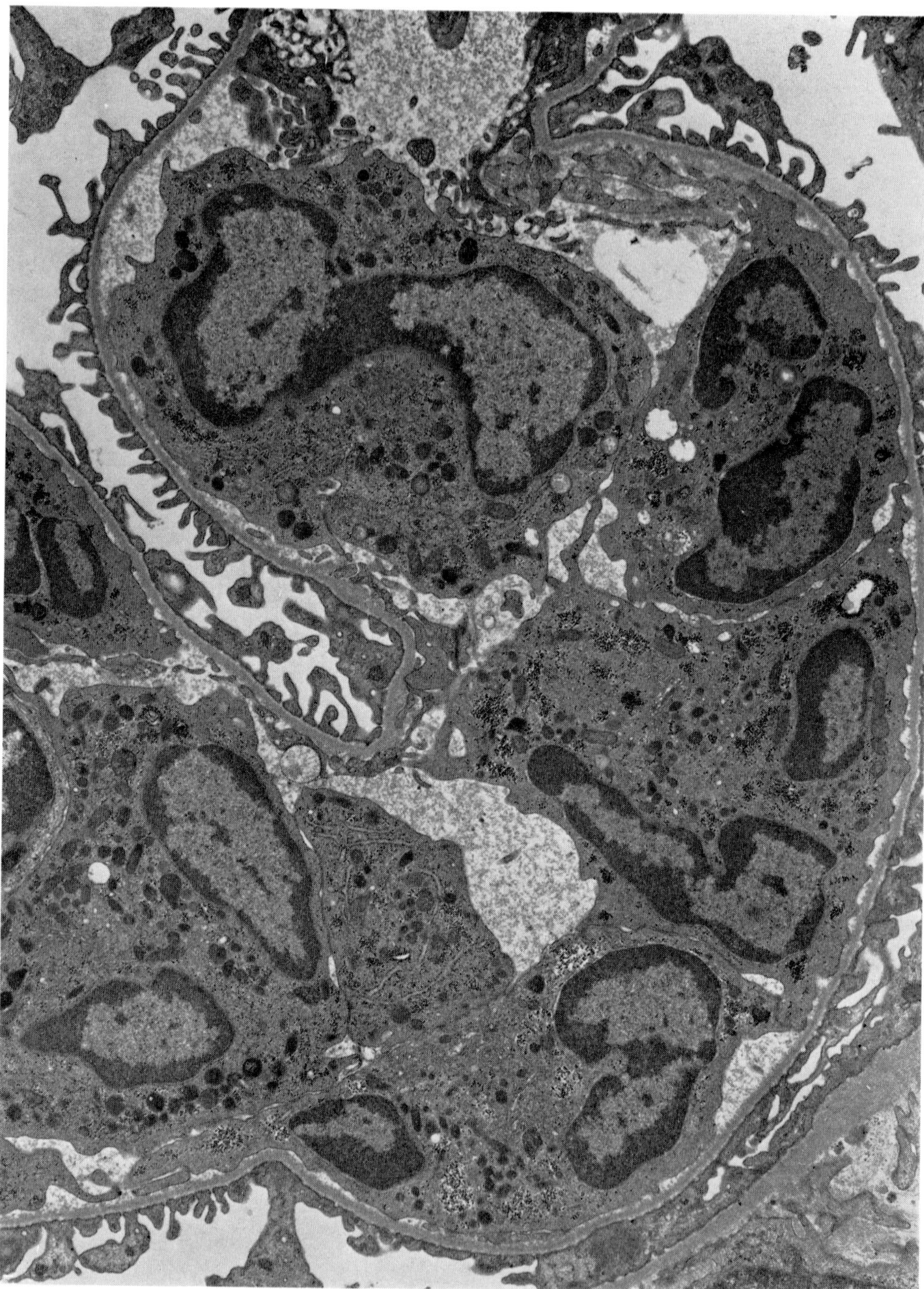

Fig. 5-1 First phase of rat Masugi nephritis (3 hours after injection of rabbit NTAb). Massive accumulation of PMNs and their attachment to the GBM associated with broad desquamation of endothelial layers. ×8,000.

phagocytosis and discharge of lysosomes could not be demonstrated.   The GBM showed no dramatic alterations.   Nonetheless it was found that proteinuria was entirely PMN-dependent.

The sequence of glomerular events has been extensively studied by Shigematsu [165]. There appeared massive accumulations of PMNs within 2 hours which often attached directly to the GBM.   It was found that the PMNs lost granules associated with the occurrence of a variety of phagocytic vacuoles.   Membrane-limited dense granules, possibly of PMN origin, were found to be intermixed with clotting material.   The intraluminal presence of PMNs and thrombotic material was much less prominent at 12 hours.   The latter seemed to be removed in part by mononuclear phagocytes (monocytes) which had now accumulated.   The monocytes or macrophages contained numerous phagosomes and were often located on the denuded GBM where PMNs had been attached.   Considerable accumulation of monocytic cells often provided a feature of proliferative glomerulonephritis.   After 3 days the monocytic cells decreased in number and the intraluminal changes were no longer remarkable.   At this stage the denuded GBM was almost entirely covered by regenerating endothelium, except for occasional cases undergoing a progressive luminal occlusion due to massive thrombosis.   No obvious GBM distortion was observed. More recently, using ultrastructural histochemistry, Morita et al. reconfirmed that the increase in number of mononuclear cells was the result of migration of blood monocytes but not of proliferation of glomerular cells [127].   In addition to these changes fusion of epithelial foot processes may be observed.   The podocytes sometimes showed long thin interlacing projections [18].   Various vacuoles with heterogeneous contents could also be found in the epithelial cytoplasm.

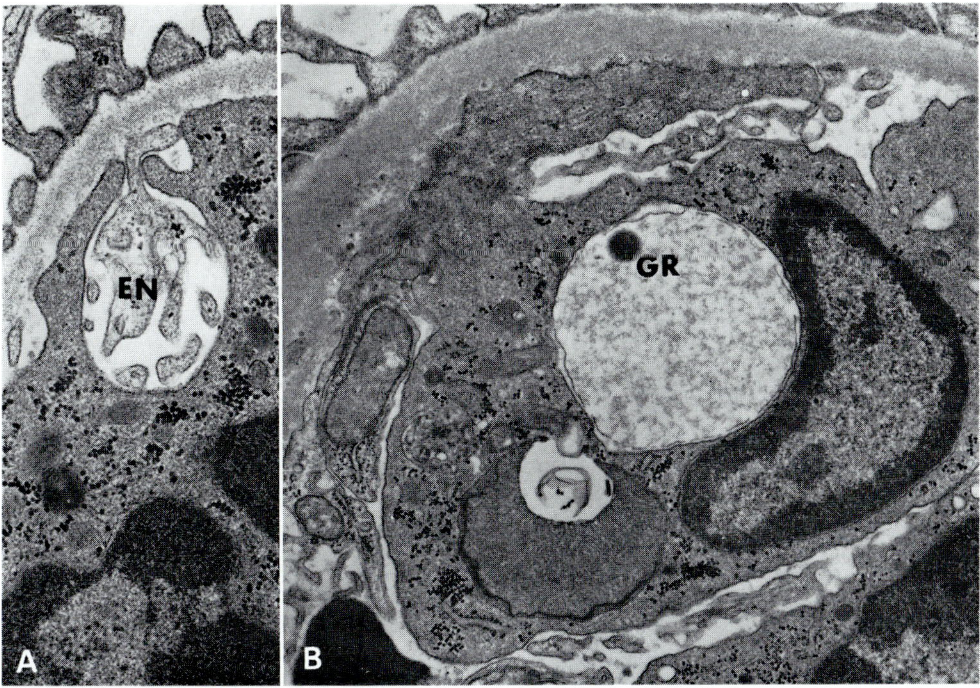

Fig. 5-2   First phase of rat Masugi nephritis (6 hours after injection of rabbit NTAb). *A*: A portion of a PMN showing endocytosis of endothelial fragments (EN).   ×29,000.   *B*: A PMN granule (GR) is released into a large vacuole.   ×14,000.

These observations have confirmed that the first phase indeed develops immediately after the injection of rabbit NTAb.   Obviously the amount of the NTAb capable of fixing to glomeruli is crucial in determining the intensity of glomerular injury.   Lesser amounts of NTAb may induce only mild immediate glomerulonephritis or no detectable glomerular abnormality at all even by electron microscopy [166].   The amount of NTAb to induce an immediate glomerulonephritis has been calculated [188].   The mildest form of glomerular lesion may be localized desquamation of the capillary endothelium which is rarely accompanied by other alterations.   Such a minimal injury can be readily repaired.   The injection of appropriate amounts of NTAbs causes a prominent exudative change characterized by a massive influx of PMNs but this does not always imply a poor prognostic course unless there is concurrent participation of the clotting process.

It seems reasonable to divide the first phase into two stages, consisting of acute exudative inflammation and subsequent repair [165].   The following description is a summary of the glomerular changes taking place during the first phase of rat Masugi nephritis. Because it has been revealed that rabbit NTAb and complement (C3) are specifically localized on the GBM entirely along the capillary loops [13, 145, 163, 187, 198], one might assume that the GBM is the initial site of injury.   A number of GBM abnormalities can be observed at the very early stage.   However, these are neither diffuse nor uniform and are sometimes hardly distinct from the normal range of GBM variations.   The most consistent alteration is localized mottling or deposits observed predominantly at the subendothelial aspect of the GBM as reported by Feldman et al. [45] The deposits may in part be derived from the damaged GBM and from insudation of proteinaceous material from the blood. Local or wide spread exfoliation of the endothelium is then observed.   Considerable portions of the deposits may disappear with the endothelial exfoliation but the denuded GBM still shows a fluffy profile at its subendothelial aspect.   Migrated PMNs often insert their cytoplasmic processes into mottled areas of the GBM or into the subendothelial space replacing the endothelial layer [26].   The PMNs do phagocytose endothelial fragments, platelets, and other substances of unknown origin.   The PMN granules are decreased in number while an aggregate of glycogen granules accumulates in the cytoplasm.   Presumably the granules are released into the phagocytic vacuoles and are in part discharged into the extracellular space, though the release process could rarely be observed in situ. The granules are also discharged externally following cell lysis.   Simultaneously abundant deposition of fibrin strands is seen mixed with intact as well as disintegrated platelets and cell debris.   Segmental areas of a glomerulus are occluded by these platelet-fibrin thrombi. Whenever the glomeruli are diffusely involved in the clotting process, total necrosis of glomerular cells inevitably ensues resulting in diffuse cortical necrosis similar to that observed in the generalized Shwartzman reaction.   Diffuse occlusion of tubules by hyaline casts (massive cylinduria) within a few hours suggests the prospect of such a severe outcome. The endothelial cell body is generally preserved despite remarkable loss of the peripheral attenuated portions.   There is no proliferation of the endothelial cells during the acute stage.   The mesangium shows edematous swelling of the matrix and cellular hypertrophy. The duration of the acute, exudative stage is usually selflimiting and a reparatory process may appear as early as 24 hours [165].   PMNs, platelets, and cellular debris had mostly disappeared from the glomeruli at 24 hours leaving a patent capillary lumen.   The denuded GBM is gradually covered by cytoplasmic extension of the endothelium.   Such a regenerating layer is swollen with decreased numbers of pores as compared to the normal layer.   The new endothelial covering is not always intimately applied to the GBM and sometimes there remains a broad subendothelial space which is often filled with proteinaceous material.   Mitotic proliferation of the endothelial cells may occasionally be

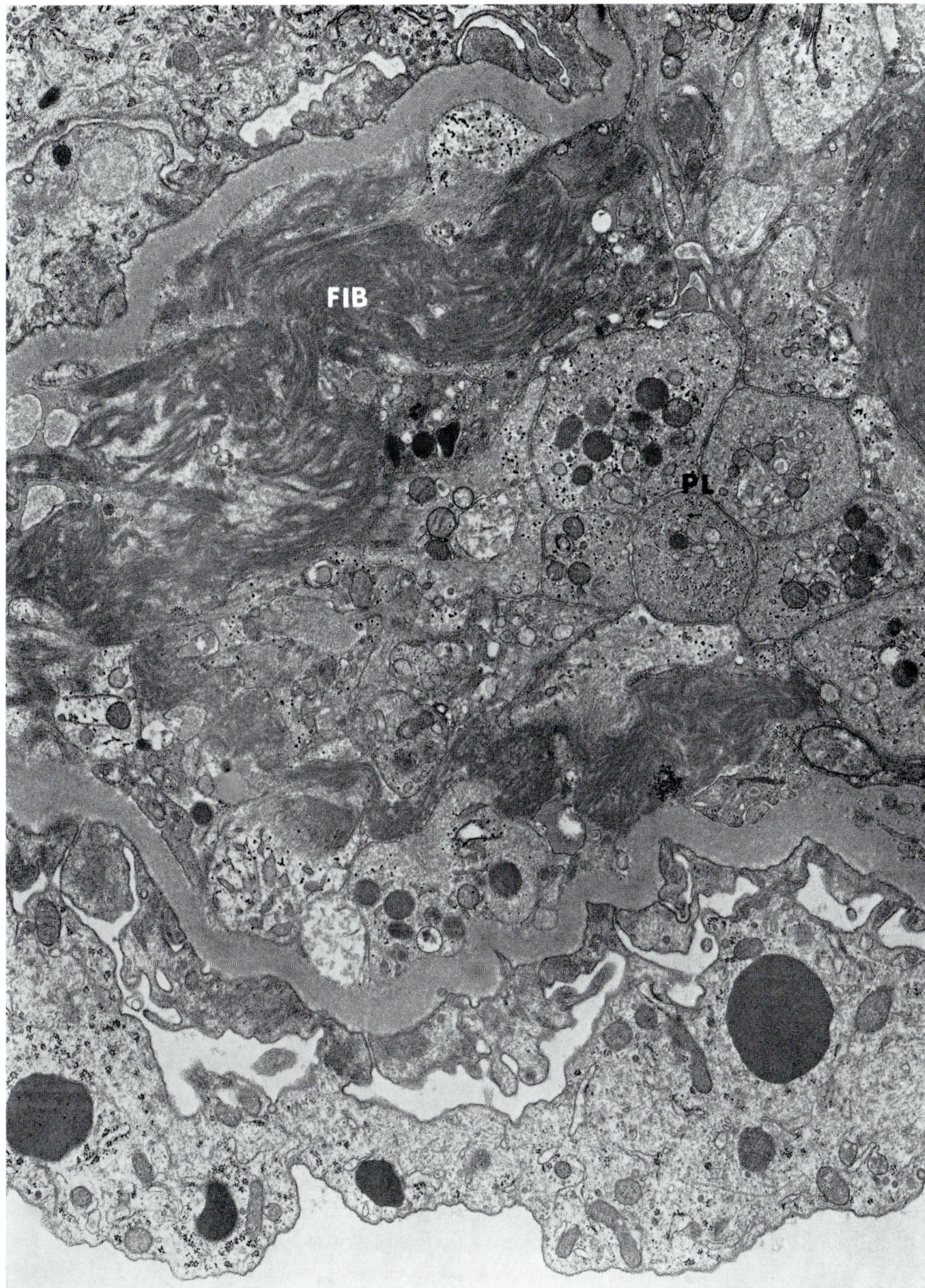

Fig. 5-3 First phase of rat Masugi nephritis (6 hours after injection of rabbit NTAb). A capillary portion occluded by platelet (PL)-fibrin (FIB) aggregates. Broad fusion of epithelial foot processes is present. ×14,000.

seen [165].   Scattered glomeruli still show thrombotic occlusion of the segmental area. In the persistent thrombi definite strands of fibrin tend to be obscured, undergoing a dense amorphous or finely granular fibrinoid mass.   The fibrionoid deposits are seen not only in the lumen but also in the mesangium and subendothelial space.   They frequently occur between the intercellular space so irregularly as to mimic a basement membrane-like material.   The capillary lumens are also occluded by large macrophages derived from blood monocytes [165].   Fibrinoid material is often present enclosed within phagosomes of the macrophages.   By contrast, phagocytic activity of glomerular cells is far less prominent.   After the subsidence of the acute changes, the mesangium is still widened due to swelling and increase of cytoplasmic processes of mesangial cells and of matrix.   The GBM shows localized splitting, wrinkling, and subendothelial thickening.   Fusion of epithelial foot processes has persisted at this reparatory stage and sometimes becomes even more prominent.   In general the podocytes are swollen and contain a number of dense granules. Interestingly at the site of intraluminal deposition of fibrinoid, a similar dense material is seen in the urinary space or in the cytoplasmic vacuoles of podocytes.   The GBM exhibits an increased density apparently insudated by the fibrinoid material.   These findings imply that the fibrinoid deposits in the lumen are in part filtered into the urinary space under the condition of increased GBM permeability and entrapped by the podocytes.

After 72 hours the recovery may further progress.   Fibrinoid deposits are rare and macrophages are decreased in number.   It is thus clear that the glomerular alterations in the first phase are reversible unless the glomeruli have been severely affected by the thrombotic process.   The changes for the most part consist of an intraluminal event and proliferative responses of glomerular cells are minimal, if present.

b. The second phase

The second phase develops several days after the injection relevant to the host antibody formation to the heterologous NTAb.   The autologous antibody along with C3 fixed to the GBM can be visualized in immunofluorescence as a continuous, linear fluorescence [66, 145, 162].   The precise onset of the second phase is not readily recognizable morphologically due to gradual formation and fixation of the host antibody to the GBM-bound NTAbs.   It was shown that, in rats tolerant to rabbit γ-globulin and incapable of producing antibodies against the rabbit NTAb, the first phase was reversible and morphologic as well as functional recovery was ascertained within 4 weeks [45, 66].   In contrast, the second phase may be irreversible in general.   The glomerular changes seen in the early second phase may be a remnant of the first phase rather than the actual initiation of a new inflammatory process.   Many of conflicting descriptions in the previous reports are attributable to the fact that the authors were not strictly aware of the distinction between the first and the second phases.   With this in mind, Feldman et al. examined ultrastructural changes in the second phase developing from 5 to 7 days after the injection [43, 45].   The predominant finding was the appearance of dense, granular subendothelial deposits intimately applied to the peripheral GBM.   In the most severe lesions, the abundant deposits, together with swelling and increase in the number of intraluminal as well as mesangial cells led to almost complete occlusion of the capillary loops.   Swelling and proliferation of endothelial cells, which regressed within 3 weeks, were also noted by Fujimoto et al. [48].   As mentioned before, a weak rabbit NTAb does not induce the first phase at all but does induce the second phase.   Shigematsu and Kobayashi observed glomerular changes limited to the second phase by using such a weak NTAb [166].   The first noticeable change was seen at the 4th day associated with glomerular localization of rat IgG. The GBM showed mottling with subendothelial deposition of an amorphous or finely granular substance.   Similar deposition was also present within the mesangium.   With

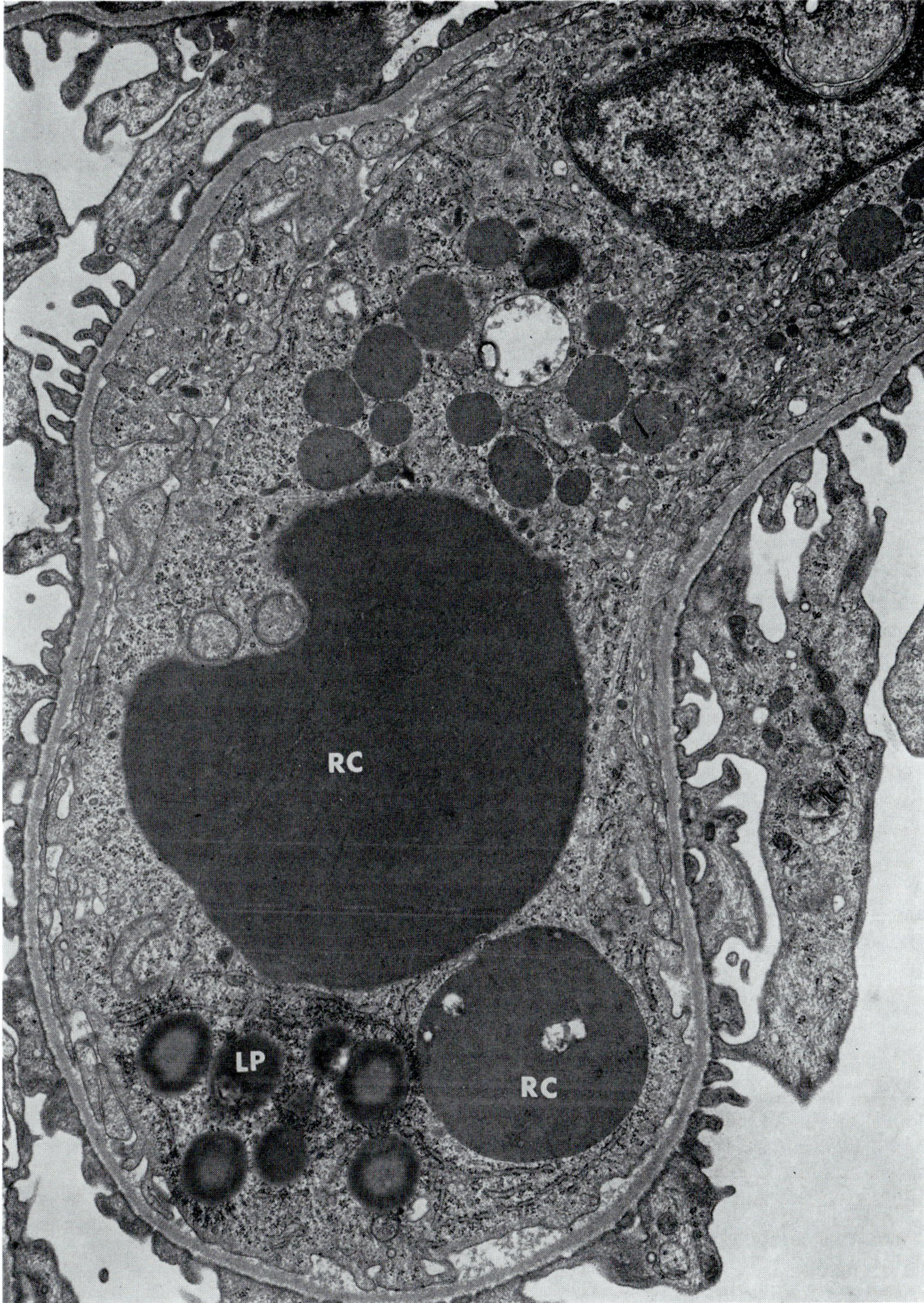

Fig. 5-4 Fist phase of rat Masugi nephritis (24 hours after injection of rabbit NTAb). A huge monocytic macrophage obliterating a capillary lumen. Numerous dense phagosomes, lipid granules (LP), and two red blood cells (RC) are present within the cytoplasm.   ×13,000.

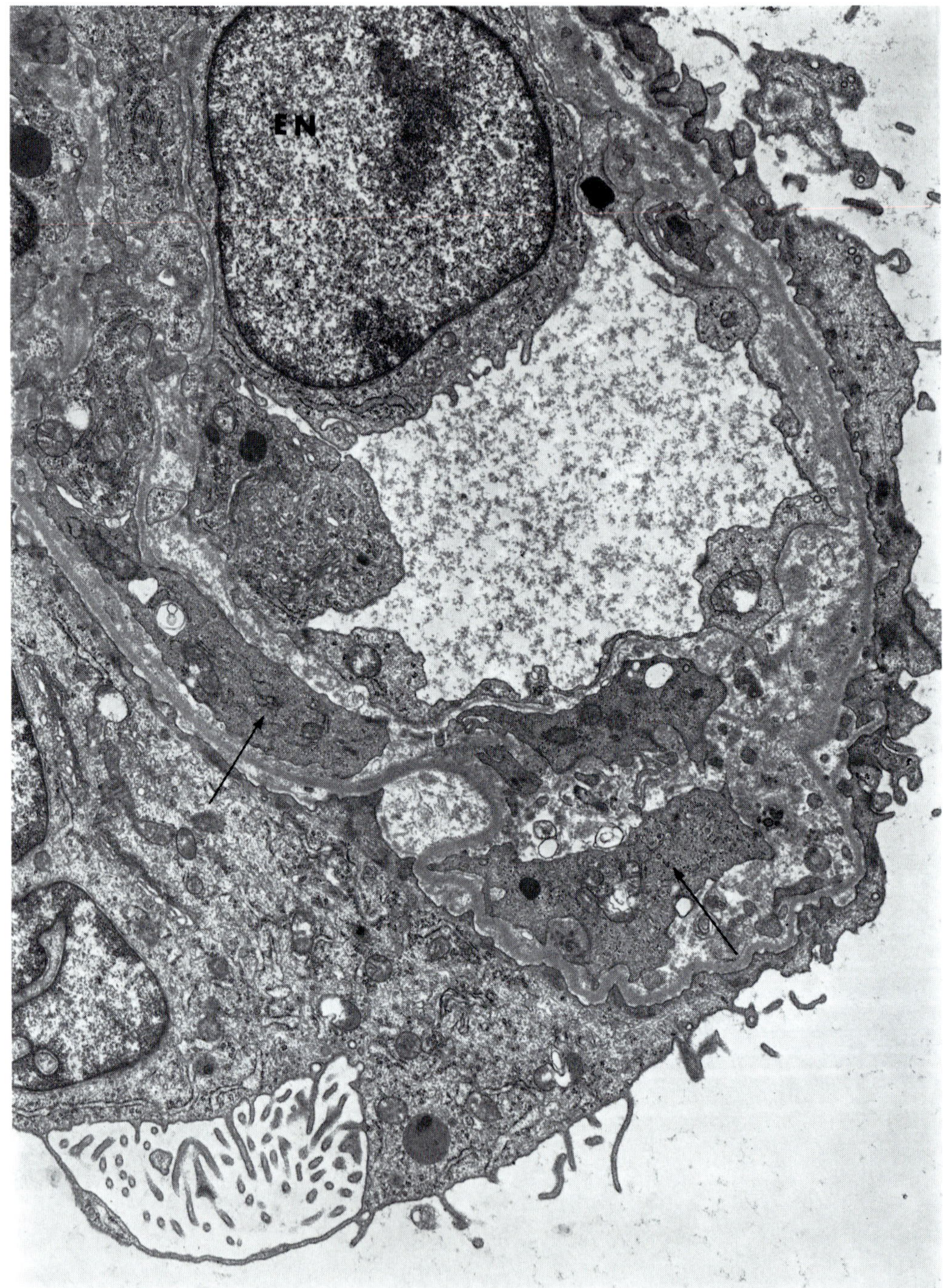

Fig. 5-5 Second phase of rat Masugi nephritis (7 days after injection of rabbit NTAb). Note prominent widening of the subendothelial space and peripheral interposition of mesangial cytoplasm (arrows). Swelling of an endothelial cell (EN) and diffuse fusion of epithelial foot processes are also seen.   ×3,200.

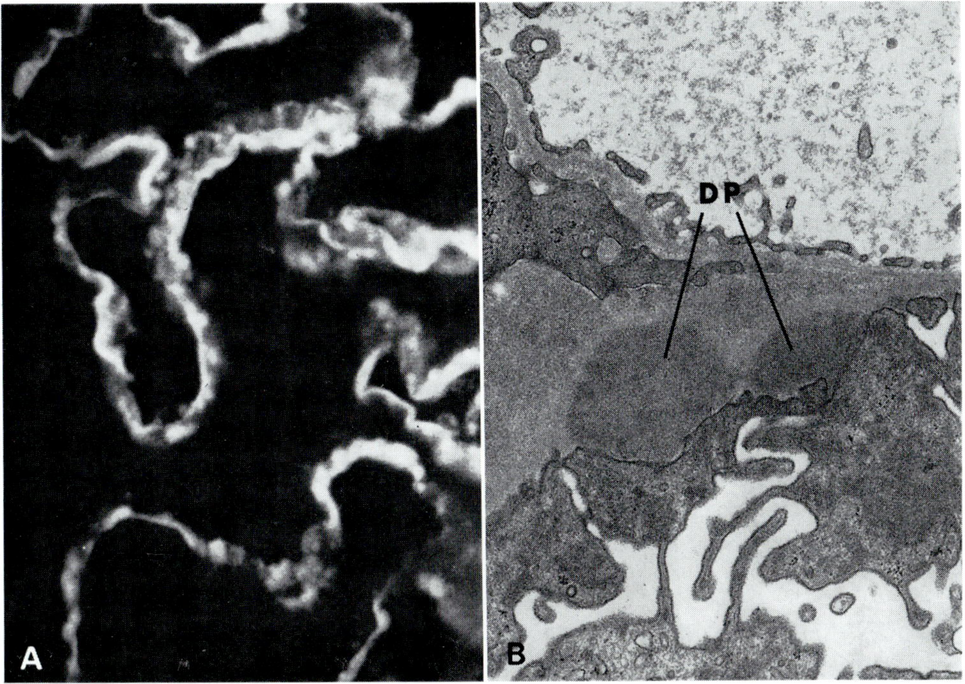

Fig. 5-6   Rat Masugi nephritis produced by injection of a large dose of a weak NTAb. Possible coexistence of immune complex-mechansim. *A*: Characteristic immunofluorescent feature exhibiting mixed linear and granular localization pattern of rat IgG. 30 days after injection of rabbit NTAb. (From Shigematsu, H. and Kobayashi, Y.: *Virchows Arch. Abt. B 8*: 83–95, 1971) *B*: Subepithelial dense deposits (DP). 11 days after injection of goat NTAb.   × 10,000.

the onset of proteinuria, which appeared more than 7 days later, dense deposits occurred at the subepithelial aspect of the GBM, increased in numbers, and became aggregated. Large numbers of mononuclear cells (monocytes) accumulated in the lumen associated with the GBM deposits.   Their role for the removal of the deposits was suggested by their in-timate contact to the GBM.   The subepithelial deposits were gradually diminished and incorporated into the GBM resulting in irregular GBM thickening.   Infiltration of PMNs was minimal in contrast to the first phase.   Irregular protrusions of the GBM were also noted by Morita et al. but they observed no dense subepithelial deposits [127].   The second phase was further investigated by Shigematsu and Kobayashi using duck NTAb [167]. The rat received a simultaneous injection of normal duck γ-globulin with adjuvant to enhance the host antibody response as suggested by Unanue and Dixon [189].   As com-pared to their previous report, marked disorganizing alterations developed in the rats thus treated.   The glomerular tufts often showed a ballooning or globular transformation in which fibrinoid material and numerous monocytic cells were included.   The endo-thelial layer diffusely disappeared and mesangial matrix was severely destroyed.   The extremely dilated tufts eventually ruptured resulting in the loss of some lobuli and forma-tion of a crescent.   Obviously the immunization was crucial in inducing the disorganizing glomerulonephritis, indicating that the intensity of the glomerular changes in the second phase was largely dependent upon that of the host immune response.

It is worthy of note that emigration of PMNs is not remarkable and mononuclear pha-gocytes predominate in the cellular exudation.   In addition cellular proliferation of the

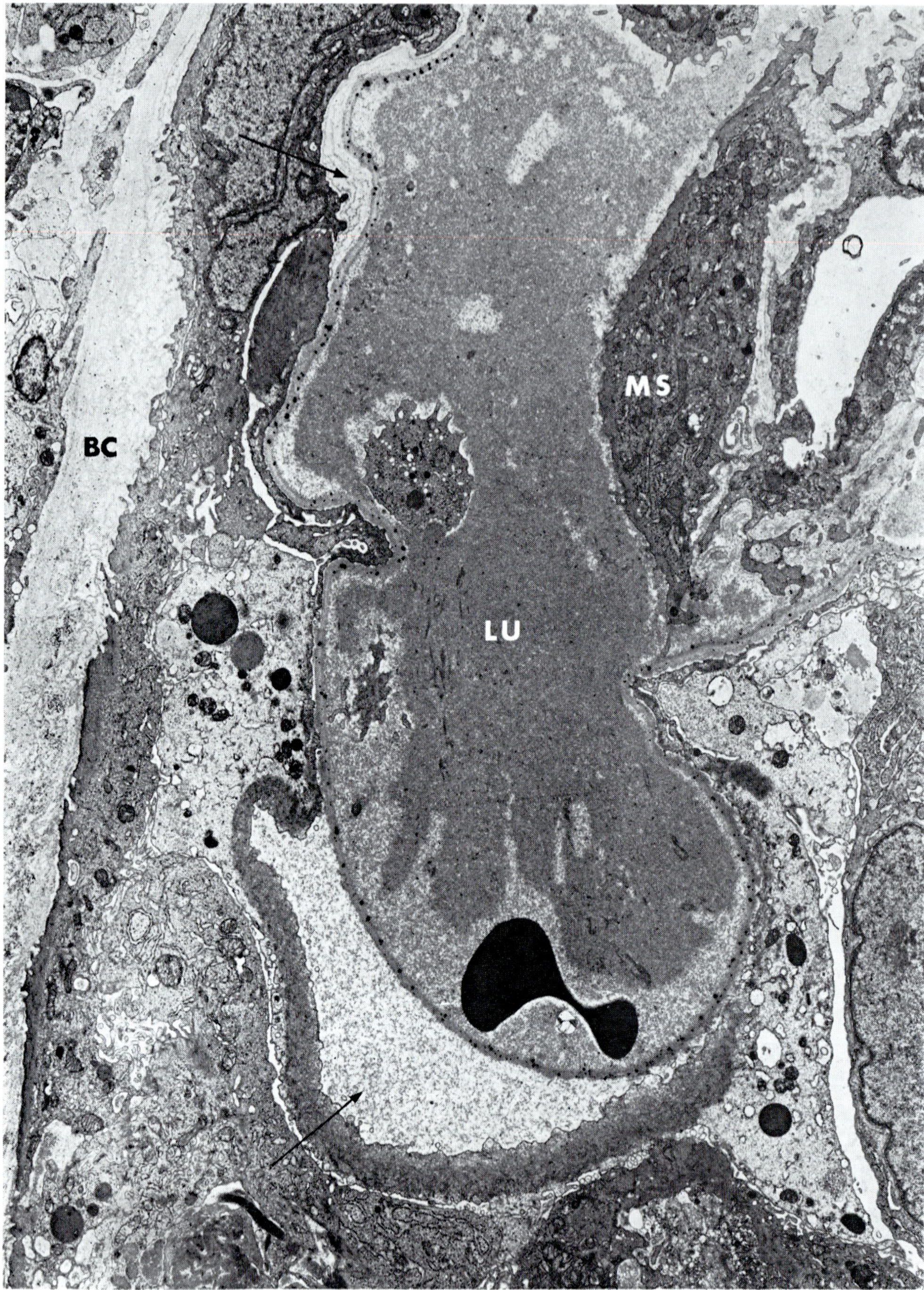

Fig. 5-7 Second phase of rat Masugi nephritis (22 days after injection of duck NTAb). Disorganizing change consisting of diffuse loss of endothelial lining, obliteration of capillary lumen (LU) with fibrinoid deposit, and detachment of epithelium from the GBM (arrows). Mesangial matrix is loosened and a mesangial cell (MS) is directly exposed to the blood stream. Capsular basement membrane (BC) is mottled. The GBM is labeled with AgNO₃.   ×17,000. (From Shigematsu, H. and Kobayashi, Y.: *Virchows Arch. Abt. B 14*: 313–328, 1973)

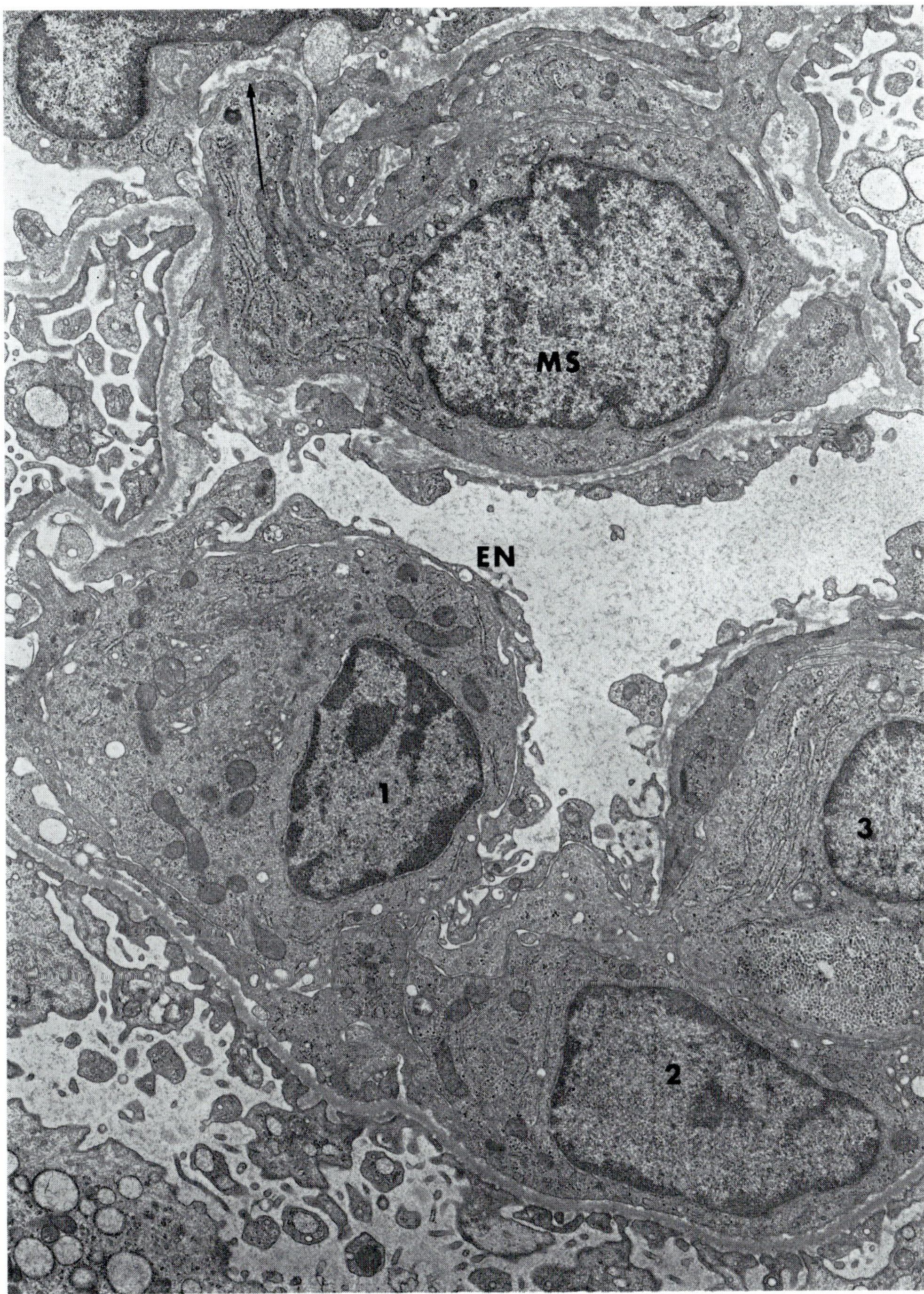

Fig. 5-10   Rabbit Masugi nephritis (12 days after injection of duck NTAb). Three monocytes (1, 2, and 3) migrated under endothelial lining (EN). A mesangial cell (MS) extends its cytoplasm beneath the endothelial cell body (arrow).   ×8,300.

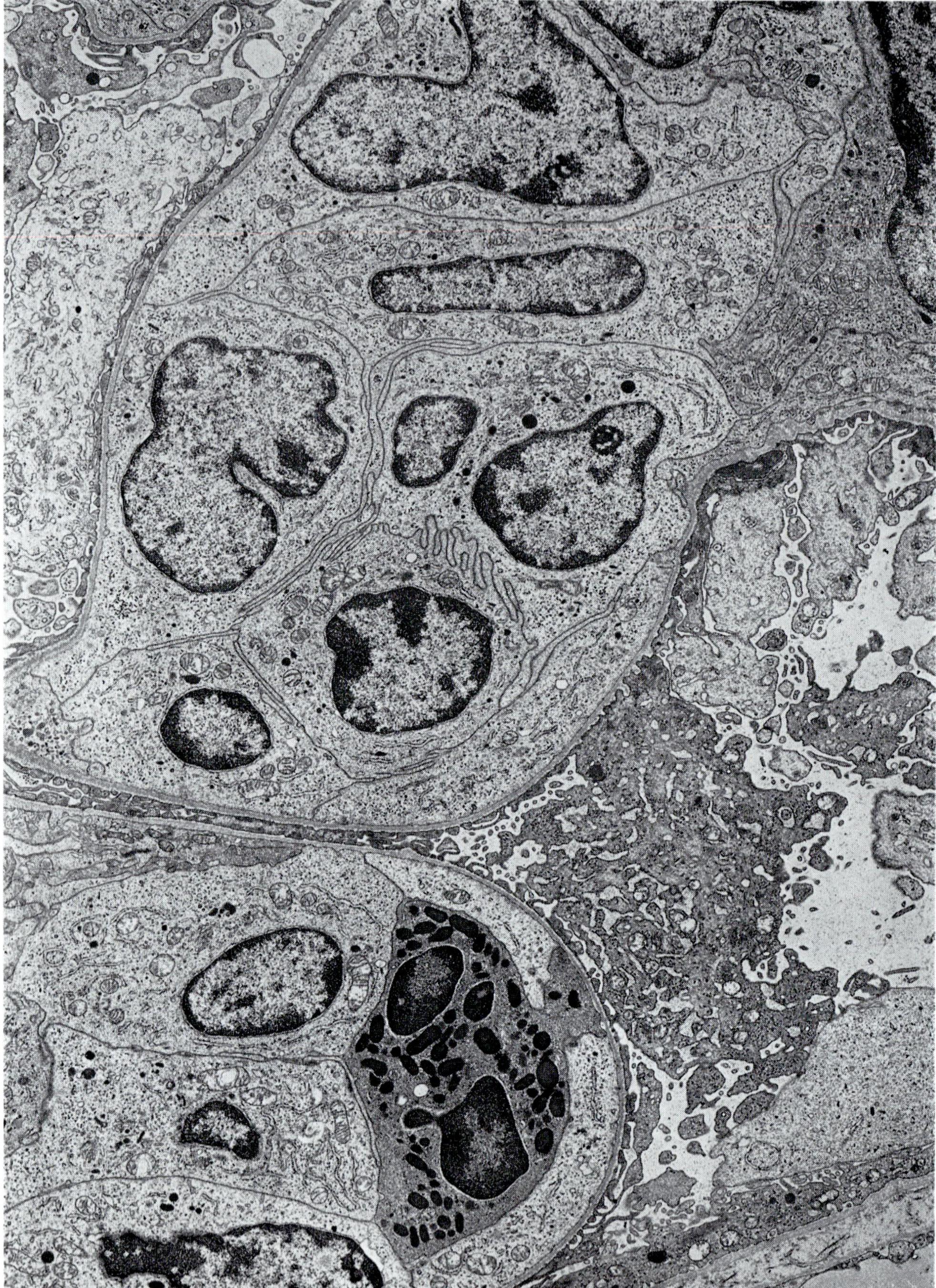

Fig. 5-11   Rabbit Masugi nephritis (8 days after injection of duck NTAb).   Glomerular tufts are completely obliterated by massive accumulation of clear monocytic cells (epithelioid cells).   Note broad disappearance of endothelial lining.   In general, this kind of change is reversible. A PMN is also seen attached to the GBM.   ×6,000.

monocytic accumulation. If fixed glomerular cells proliferated so extensively as to completely obliterate the capillary lumens, this rapid recovery could not be achieved. In any case, the restored capillaries are entirely covered by the thin endothelial layer. The GBM, however, shows considerable irregularity consisting of splitting, mottling, and wrinkling. Especially widening of the subendothelial space is noticeable. These GBM abnormalities may to some extent result from a rapid contraction of the dilated tufts and represent an inadequate adaptation to the restored blood circulation. The mesangial matrix is edematous whereas in some portions dense basement membrane-like material and collagen fibers are produced. Around the juxtamesangial areas, cytoplasmic processes of mesangial cells may be found to be inserted into the subendothelial space. Fusion of epithelial foot processes is significantly improved.

It appears that the persistent changes do not regress promptly, though these are not related to any known clinical abnormalities at least during the several months observed so far. Throughout the course of the disease fibrin deposition is not remarkable except in scattered glomeruli. Infiltration of PMNs is minimal, differing from an immediate rabbit Masugi nephritis induced by injection with a potent sheep NTAb in which the development of glomerular injury is PMN-dependent [67].

b. Progressive changes

Whenever the amount of duck NTAb is increased, a severe, often fatal glomerulonephritis may develop. In this progressive glomerulonephritis moderate proliferation of endothelial cells and prominent accumulation of monocytic cells are similarly observed as in reversible glomerulonephritis. In addition, serious injuries involving the mesangium and GBM are usually observed. Of these most characteristic are loss of the supporting mesangium and rupture of the GBM [94].

Ultrastructurally swelling, disarrangement, and fragmentation of mesangial matrix (mesangiolysis) may be seen from the early stage [95]. Hypertrophy and proliferation of mesangial cells then follow. The proliferated mesangial cells exhibit conspicuous Golgi areas and numerous profiles of granular endoplasmic reticulum thereby resembling active fibroblasts. Subsequent to the mesangiolysis the mesangial cells extend their cytoplasmic processes along the subendothelial space, or into the capillary lumens. The capillaries are narrowed, distorted, and even subdivided into branches by this random mobilization of the mesangial cells [95]. The extremely loosened mesangium is infiltrated by numerous monocytic cells and a few PMNs. Accordingly the normal mesangio-capillary organization is entirely obscured, resulting in transformation of a tuft into a dilated sac filled with proliferated glomerular cells (mostly mesangial cells), migrated blood cells, and clotting material. An attempt to reconstruct the damaged matrix is evident at this florid stage as shown by formation of basement membrane-like material around the proliferated mesangial cells. Strands of collagen fibers are seen within the newly formed matrix.

Another change of special note is GBM rupture. Hypercellularity in the tufts, together with some lytic lesions, may cause the GBM to become increasingly stretched and virtually interrupted. This is apparently enhanced by a necrotizing process evoked by fibrin deposition. In fact, Vassalli and McCluskey [195] and Watanabe and Tanaka [205] are of the opinion that intravascular coagulation is largely responsible for the induction of severe glomerular injury. It is suggested that the GBM rupture is crucial in producing crescentic glomerulonephritis [94]. Following local or wide spread destruction of the GBM, there is massive influx of blood cells and proteinaceous substances into Bowman's space. The migrated cells are mostly monocytic epithelioid cells with a few multinucleated giant cells. Simultaneously there is a proliferation of podocytes and capsular epithelial cells, the latter being more prominent. The podocytes are swollen, often binucleated, and reveal a

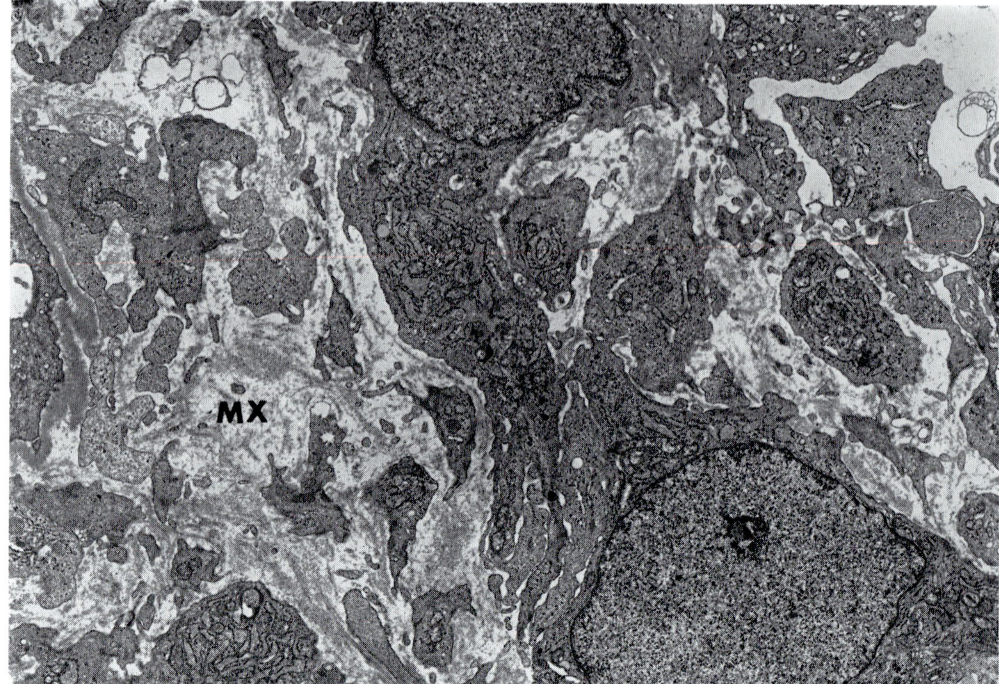

Fig. 5-12   Rabbit Masugi nephritis (9 days after injection of duck NTAb). An early manifestation of progressive glomerular changes. Note marked swelling or lysis of mesangial matrix (MX).   ×6,300. (From Okabayashi, A. et al.: *Curr. Topics Path. 61*: 1–43, 1976)

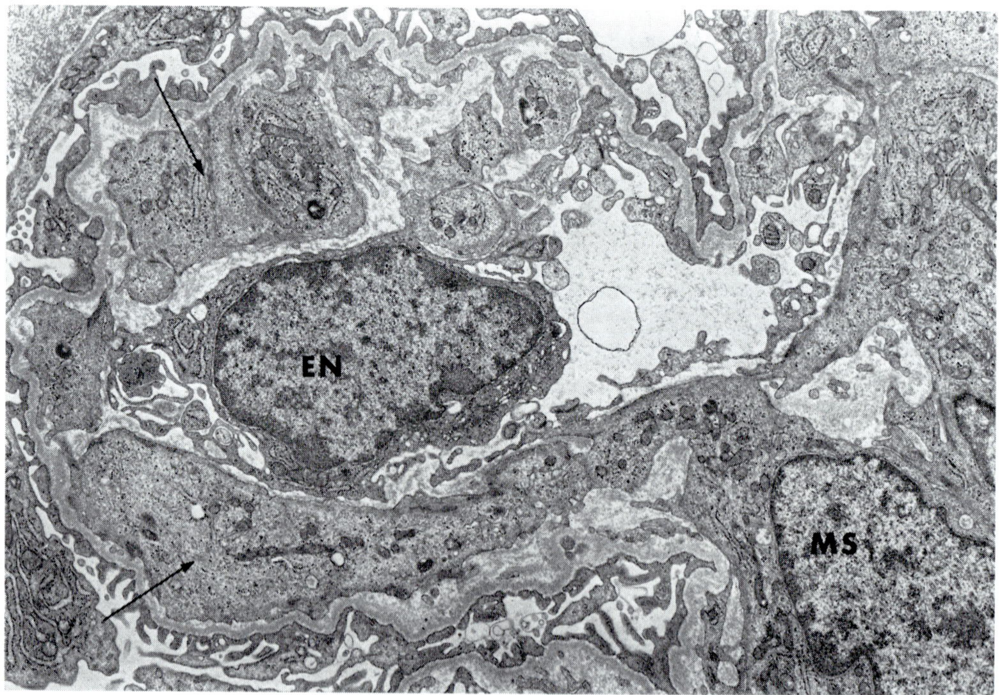

Fig. 5-13   Rabbit Masugi nephritis (9 days after injection of duck NTAb). Early peripheral interposition (arrows) of a mesangial cell (MS) subsequent to mesangiolysis. EN; endothelial cell.   ×7,700. (From Kondo, Y. et al.: *Lab. Invest. 34*: 363–371, 1976)

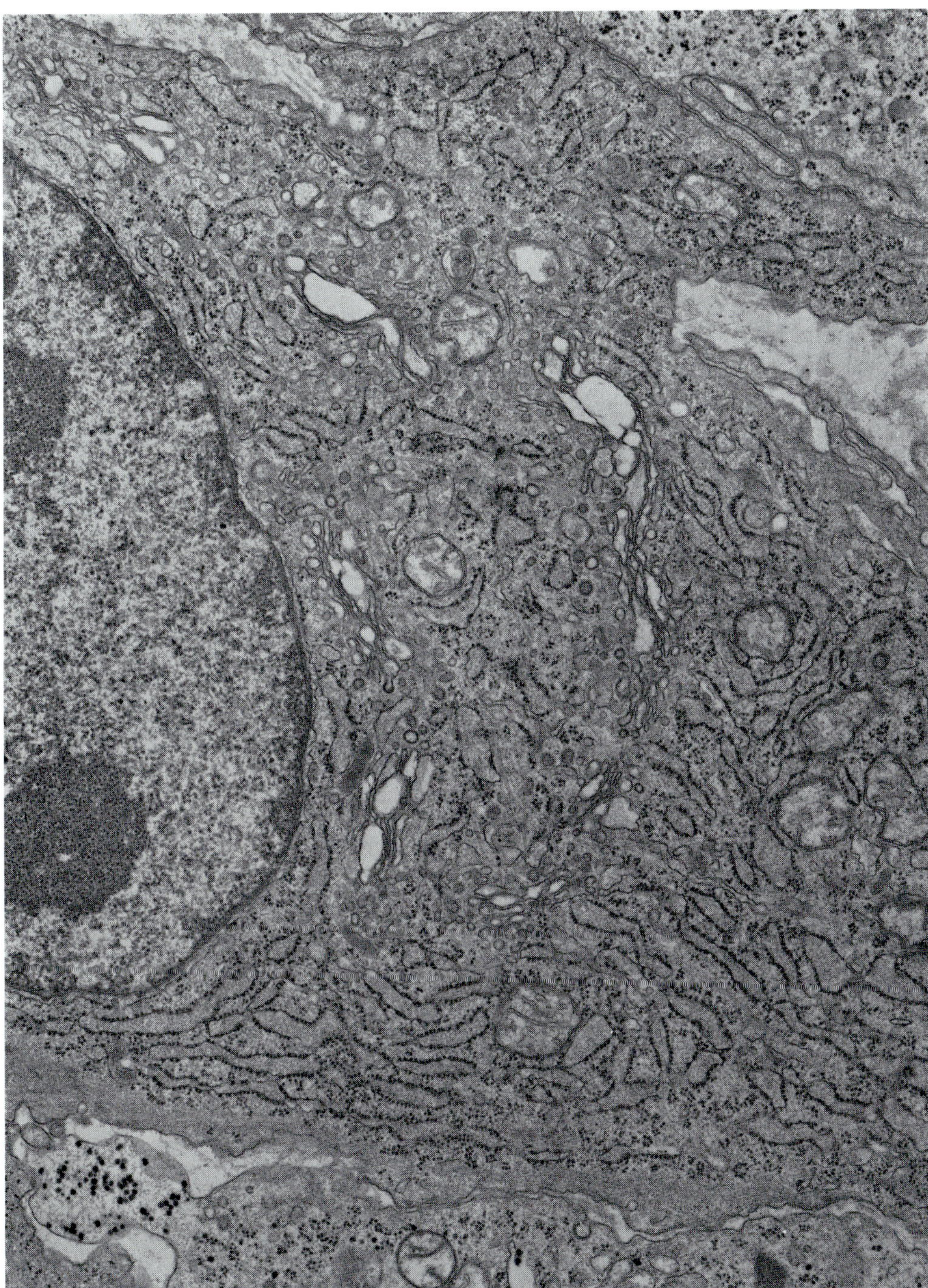

Fig. 5-14 Rabbit Masugi nephritis (13 days after injection of duck NTAb). A portion of an activated mesangial cell. Note prominent Golgi area and numerous profiles of granular endoplasmic reticulum. Nucleus is clear and nucleoli are distinct. ×21,000.

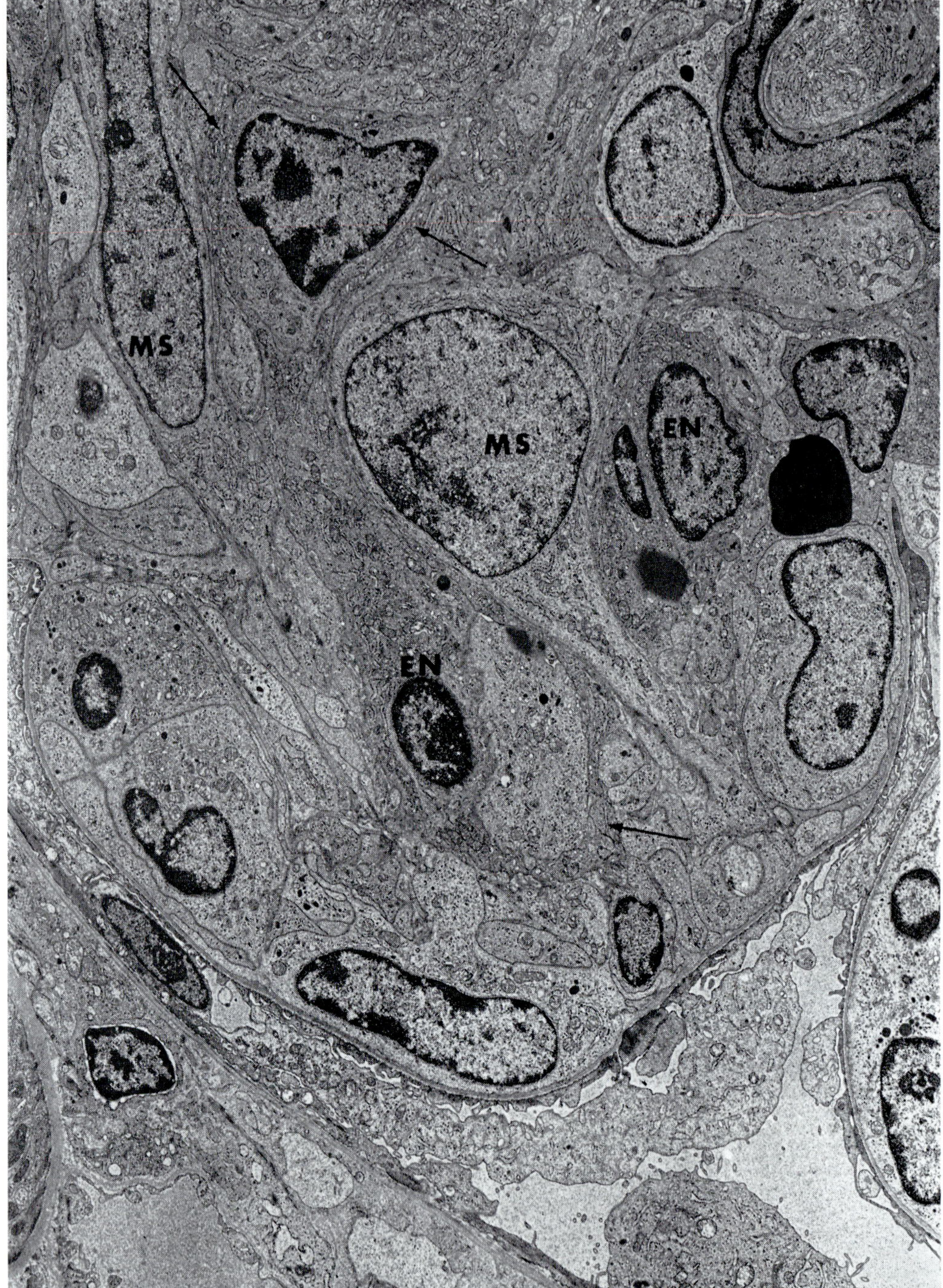

Fig. 5-15 Rabbit Masugi nephritis (8 days after injection of duck NTAb). A ballon-like distortion of a tuft filled with numerous monocytic cells, mesangial cells (MS), and endothelial cells (EN). Endothelial linings are indicated by arrows. ×4,500. (From Okabayashi, A. et al.: *Curr. Topics Path. 61*: 1–43, 1976)

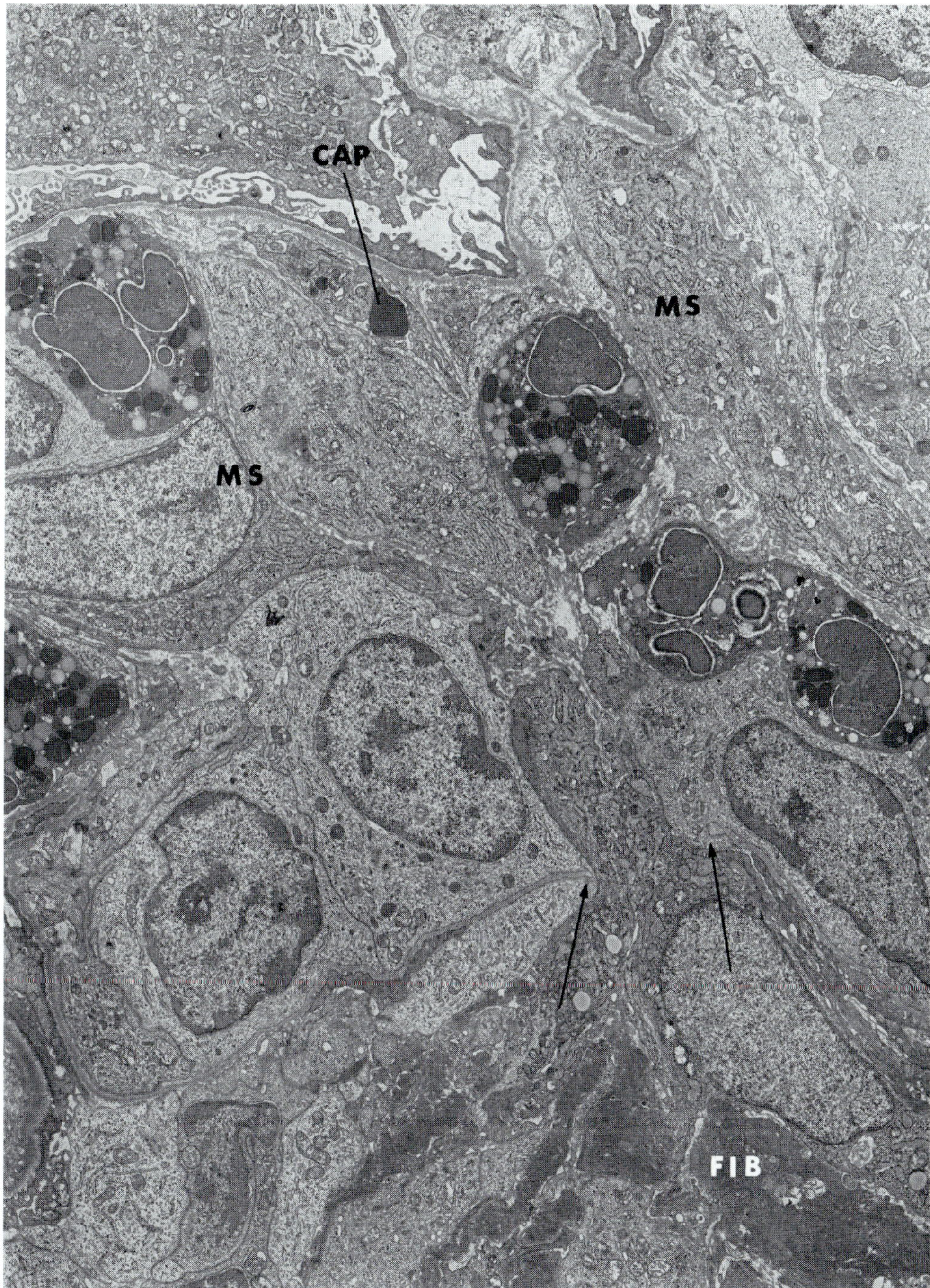

Fig. 5-16 Rabbit Masugi nephritis (9 days after injection of duck NATb). A mesangial portion showing proliferation and swelling of mesangial cells (MS), emigration of monocytes and PMNs, and apparent rupture of the GBM (arrows). A capillary (CAP) is confined to a very limited area. Fibrin deposition (FIB) is seen in Bowman's space associated with GBM rupture. ×6,000. (From Kondo, Y. et al.: *Lab. Invest.* *27*: 620–631, 1972)

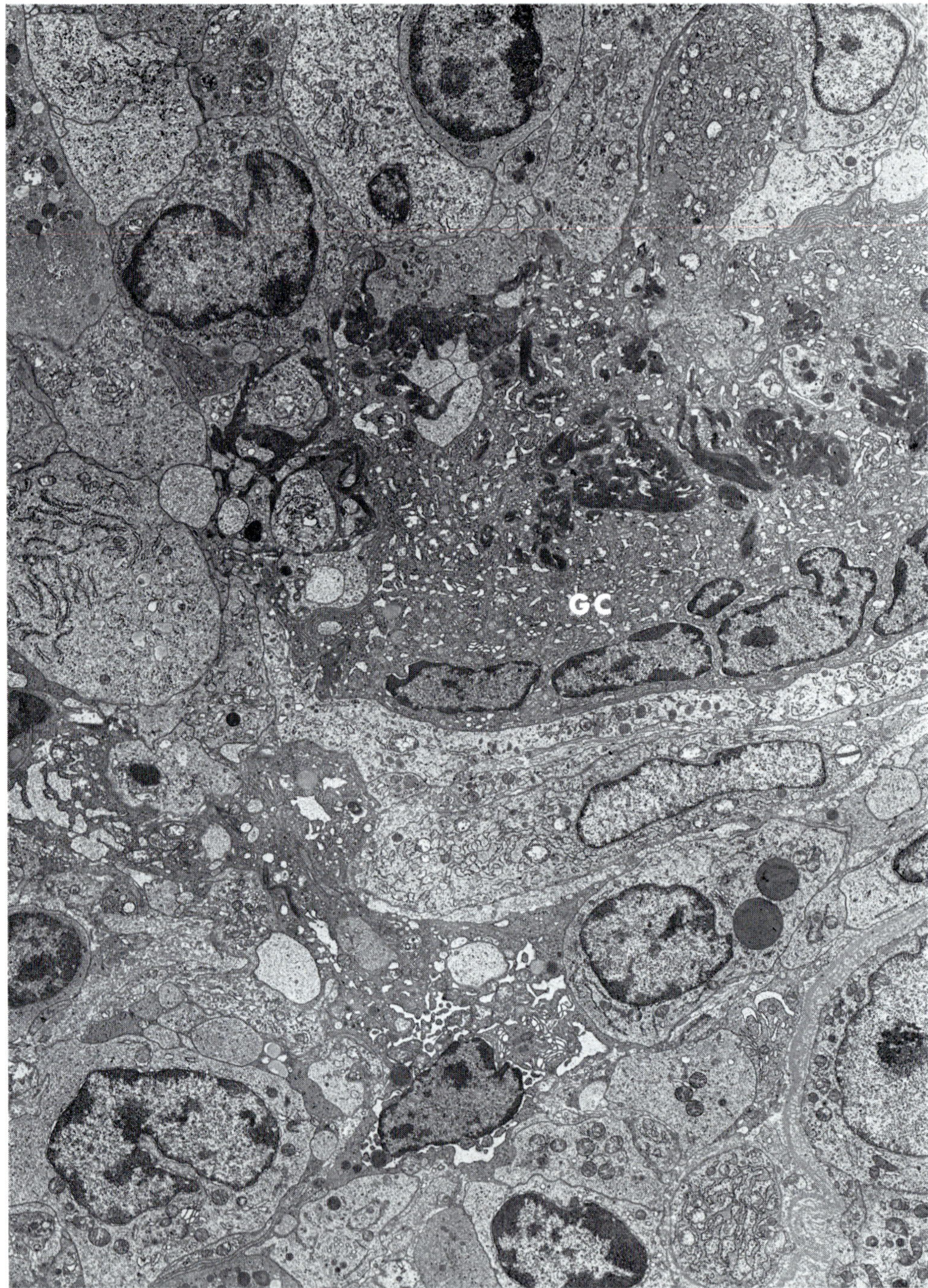

Fig. 5-17   Rabbit Masugi nephritis (27 days after injection of duck NTAb). A portion of Bowman's space filled with inflammatory mononuclear cells (monocytic crescent). A multinucleated giant cell (GC) is enclosing strands of fibrin.   ×4,200.

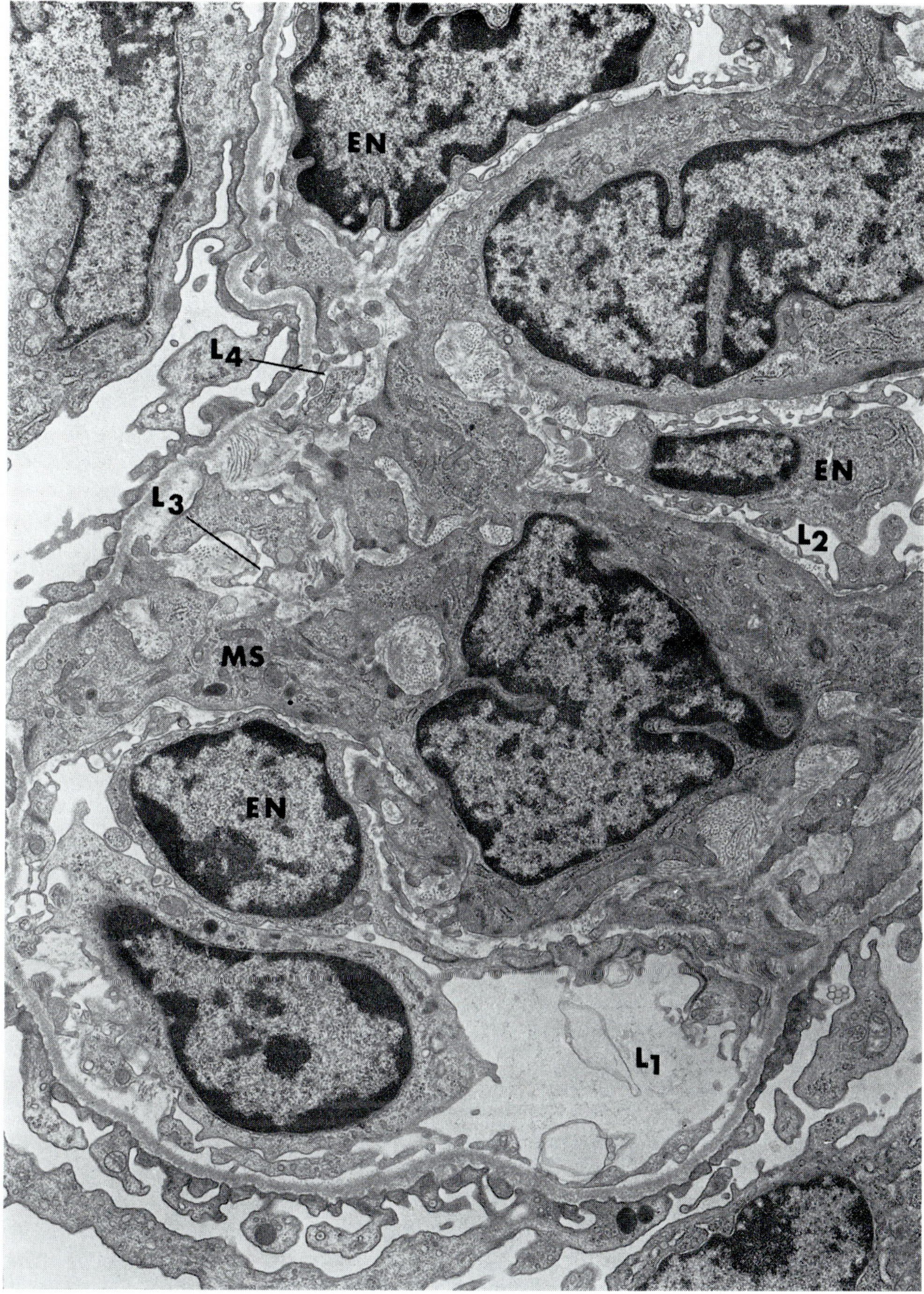

Fig. 5-18 Rabbit Masugi nephritis (27 days after injection of duck NTAb). Persistent golmerular changes. Subdivision of a capillary (L₁ to L₄) caused by mesangial bridge formation (MS). EN; endothelial cells. ×8,300. (From Kondo, Y. et al.: *Lab. Invest. 34*: 363–371, 1976)

marked increase in cytoplasmic organelles such as granular endoplasmic reticulum, Golgi complexes, and mitochondria. Large vacuoles are sometimes present. The capsular epithelial cells are also swollen and may be arranged in several layers. The inflammatory process often extends beyond the capsular basement membrane. Not infrequently localized GBM rupture may terminate in rapid collapse of the tuft or segmental capsular adhesion without any crescentic changes. In the collapsed tuft, migrant cells have disappeared and the glomerular cells are shrunken with GBM folding. Within two weeks resolution of the acute inflammation may occur unless the glomeruli had been diffusely destroyed. The characteristic findings of this stage are reminiscent of antecedent mesangiolysis and mesangial proliferation. Mesangial hypercellularity with peripheral interposition is still present but the mesangial cells generally show a decreased activity as suggested by their shrunken nucleus and cytoplasm containing fewer organelles. As mentioned before, mesangial cells do divide a capillary tuft into branches in the early stage. Some of these mesangial bridges now become solid due to new matrix formation including abundant collagen fibers [95]. The capillaries are narrowed by centrifugal expansion of the mesangium on the one hand and are subdivided into several branches by the mesangial bridges, on the other. Although the ultimate outcome of these persistent changes is unknown, a complete recovery may hardly be expected, at least in any glomeruli involved in either of the above mentioned changes.

3. Masugi nephritis in other animal species

Movat et al. reported biphasic glomerulonephritis in the dog produced by rabbit or sheep NTAbs [128]. In the first phase, "quellung" and splitting of the GBM were seen. In the second phase, there was proliferation of glomerular intracapillary cells with scattered dense deposits applied to the intercellular space as well as subendothelial space. Battifora and Markowitz observed monkey Masugi nephritis induced by rabbit or sheep NTAbs [5]. The early changes consisted of foot process fusions of podocytes and rare subendothelial deposits. In the second phase, swelling and proliferation of glomerular cells were observed. The proliferative changes regressed later while various GBM alterations began to appear. The GBM acquired increased density diffusely with subepithelial dense deposits. The lamina densa was irregularly thickened and split. There were true gaps of the GBM, forming ultrastructural aneurysms. These changes persisted for several months.

4. Autologous antiGBM nephritis (Steblay)

It has been known that autologous antiGBM antibodies are produced in experimental animals by immunization with homologous or heterologous GBM antigens in Freund's complete adjuvant. Steblay originally reported the induction of fatal, fulminant glomerulonephritis in sheep employing this experimental procedure [177]. The sheep glomerulonephritis is characterized by a severe extracapillary proliferation with crescent formation. There might be variable proliferation of intracapillary cells, infiltration of PMNs, and areas of necrosis [102, 177]. Lerner and Dixon demonstrated diffuse fluorescent localization of sheep immunoglobulins and C3 along the GBM and tubular basement membranes [102]. Transfer of induced nephritis was successfully carried out by using serum obtained from nephrectomized nephritic donors. Moreover Steblay and Rudofsky revealed that immunoglobulins eluted from the GBM of the nephritic sheep reacted with sheep GBM in vitro [179]. The antibody also reacted with lamb GBM in vivo with an immediate onset of glomerular injury. It is thus firmly established that the sheep immunized with heterologous GBM do produce antibody directed against autologous GBM. The pathologic process leading to crescentic glomerulonephritis has not been fully elucidated. Germuth et al. [53] and Ohnuki [138] described a frequent occurrence of GBM rupture in the glomeruli with crescent formation. It is likely that influx of the blood cells and plasma from such GBM gaps into Bowman's space is largely responsible for the initiation of fulminating extracapillary inflammation. By using a similar immunization method, autologous antiGBM antibodies could be produced in monkeys [148, 178], rabbits [191, 192], and guinea pigs [28, 30]. The glomerular changes seen in these animals other than sheep or goat are usually mild with rare crescent formation, though definite linear localization of immunoglobulins is demonstrated by immunofluorescence. In these instances, complement [28] or fibrin [148] does not appear to be a necessary concomitant of antiGBM glomerulonephritis.

Shibata et al. have recently reported that with a single injection of purified GBM antigen, a progressive glomerulonephritis develops in rats [164]. With immunofluorescence host immunoglobulins were found to be deposited in the mesangium at the beginning stage but later diffusely along the capillary walls in a granular fashion, distinct from other antiGBM nephritis.

5. Acute immune complex nephritis

a. Acute serum sickness nephritis in rabbits

In addition to the above mentioned antiGBM nephritis, there is an alternative prototype of immunologically induced glomerulonephritis, namely immune complex nephritis. Undoubtedly the pathogenesis of immune complex nephritis has been elucidated through studies on experimental serum sickness [37, 52, 68, 153, 154]. Classical "one-shot" serum sickness develops in animals, especially in rabbits, after single intravenous injection of large amount of purified protein antigen such as bovine serum albumin (BSA). The onset of a wide variety of serum sickness diseases including proliferative glomerulonephritis is seen at a crucial phase of antigen elimination referred to as the immune phase of antigen elimination [37, 52]. The severity of the induced tissue lesions in acute serum sickness may be intensified by one or more successive injections of the same antigen either before or after the antigen elimination (accelerated serum sickness) [168]. It has been shown that glomerular lesions develop subsequent to depositions of the non-glomerular, soluble antigen-antibody complexes that have been produced in the circulation in an antigen excess situation [37, 52]. The glomerular localization of antigen, antibody, and C3 is visualized in immunofluorescence as discrete, granular deposits of fluorescence along the capillary walls and within the mesangium [37, 46]. The granular fluorescent pattern is in sharp contrast to a continuous linear pattern observed in antiGBM nephritis.

Feldman first examined ultrastructural lesions in acute serum sickness in rabbits developing a few days after complete antigen (BSA) elimination [42]. The most striking and extensive change was swelling and proliferation of endothelial cells, presumably as a consequence of direct or indirect action of immune complexes. The capillaries were obliterated by the endothelial cell increase but PMNs or other blood mononuclear cells were rare, if present. The GBM was for the most part unaffected. There were, however, segmental thickenings and excrescences of the GBM, and deposits of an electron dense material which blended into the GBM. The deposits were most often seen at the subendothelial aspect but some were also present at the subepithelial aspect. Interestingly the number and size of the GBM abnormalities did not correspond to the quality and distribution of antigen and IgG which were seen by immunofluorescence to be abundantly fixed to the

GBM [44].   Robertson and More focused attention toward the behavior of the mesangium in rabbit serum sickness nephritis [157].   In the florid stage of the glomerular inflammation the glomerular capillaries were obliterated by masses of swollen cells, making it virtually impossible to identify the origin of these increased cells.   However, mesangial cells contained the very prominent endoplasmic reticulum which was sparse in endothelial cells. They therefore concluded that the mesangial cells increased in number in the early lesions, while endothelial cells did not.   Later extracellular fibrils with a main periodicity of about 424Å were found in relation to the increased cells.   Observing acute serum sickness nephritis induced in rabbits by one or two injections of large doses of BSA, Fish and associates noted the occurrence of large dense subepithelial deposits compatible with those seen in acute poststreptococcal glomerulonephritis in humans [46].   The earliest abnormality detected in the glomeruli consisted of narrowing of the capillary lumens due to swelling and proliferation of endothelial and mesangial cells.   Occasionally PMNs and circulating macrophages were seen.   The PMNs contained numerous lysosomes in varying stages of degranulation.   Later, besides these alterations, characteristic dense deposits appeared at the subepithelial side of the GBM, usually a few days after antigen elimination.   With progression of nephritis the deposits became fewer but much larger.   Correlated fluorescent and electron microscopic studies disclosed that the dense deposits did not always correspond to the localization sites of antigen, host IgG, or C3.   Similar subepithelial deposits were also observed by Arakawa and Kimmelstiel in one-shot serum sickness [3]. In the early stage endothelial and mesangial cells both participated by proliferation in obliterating the capillary lumens.   With time only the mesangial cells seemed to be increased in number.   They apparently showed morphologic evidence of enhanced metabolic activities such as enlarged Golgi complex and increase in free and membrane-bound ribosomes.   The mesangial cells were widely separated from each other by an electron-translucent material which was mixed with few irregular, poorly-defined, rather dark spots, giving rise to a speckled appearance.   As the process continued, the matrix was narrowed, became electron dense, and underwent a trabecular structure containing fine fibrillar substances.   At no stage was an increase of PMNs noted.   The GBM *per se* was for the most part preserved.   Characteristic dense subepithelial deposits (hump or its variants) were seen in all rabbits examined, generally after antigen elimination.   The mesangial changes did not resolve within 4 weeks, nor did the dense deposits.   There was no correlation between the severity and the number and size of the deposits.   They again emphasized a close resemblance between the rabbit glomerulonephritis and human poststreptococcal glomerulonephritis in terms of dense subepithelial deposits and the behavior of mesangial cells.

Additional observations of interest have recently been made by Shigematsu and Kobayashi in rabbit serum sickness nephritis [168].   Transient but marked proliferative glomerulonephritis was induced by a single injection of a large dose of BSA in rabbits having been preimmunized with a small dose of BSA and Freund's complete adjuvant. It was for the first time clarified that the increased cellularity was the result of intracapillary accumulation of migrant blood monocytes (macrophages).   In contrast to the previous reports, proliferation of endothelial and mesangial cells was mild and did not appear to be a major factor that contributed to the cellularity.   The macrophages often showed a direct contact with the inner surface of the GBM following local exfoliation of the endothelial lining.   They sometimes migrated into the mesangium thereby accentuating lobulation of the glomerular structure.   The capillary lumens were also occluded by fibrin or fibrinoid material and a varying number of PMNs.   The clotting material and other cellular debris were engulfed and removed by macrophages.   The changes resolved within a few weeks

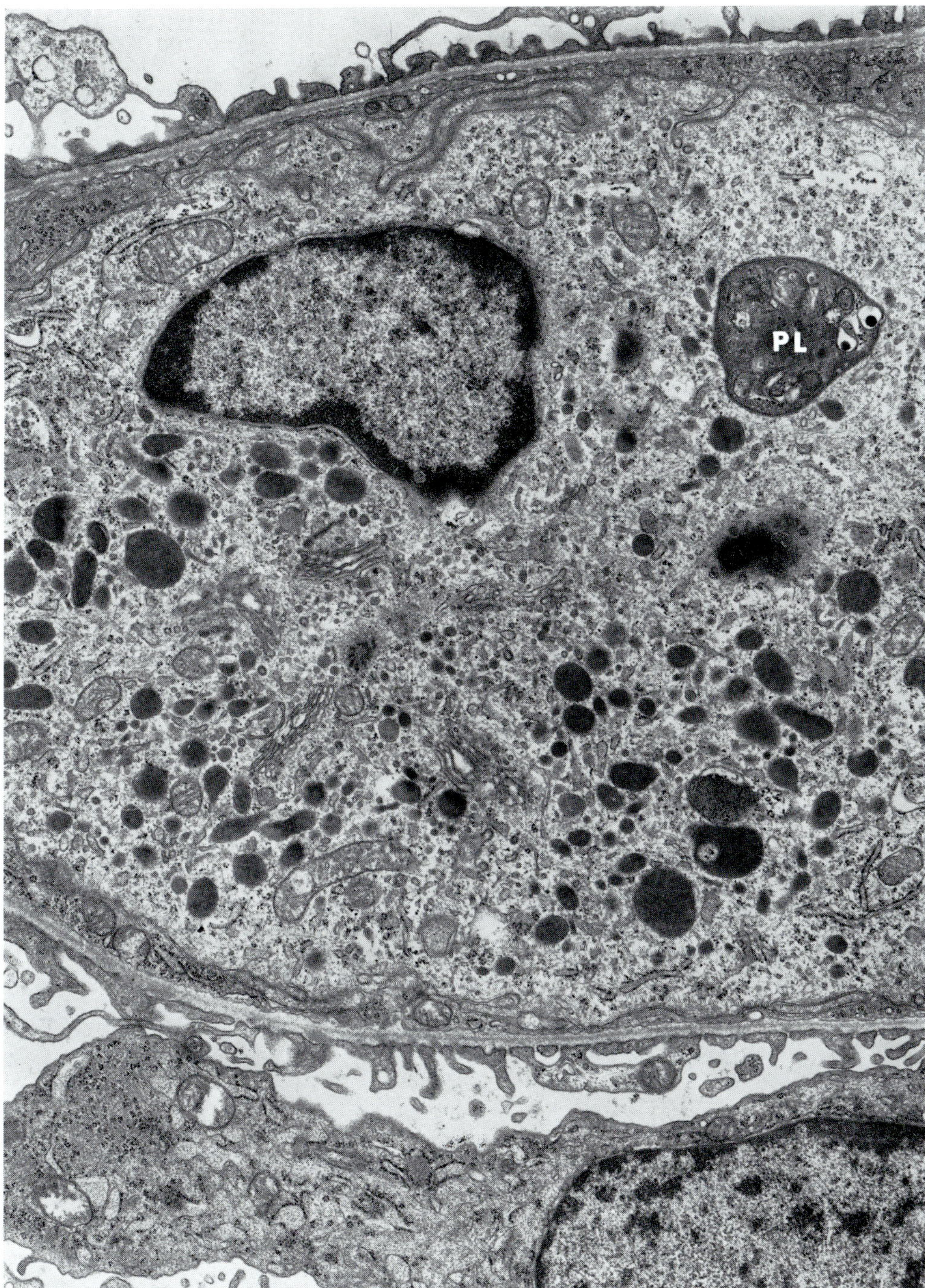

Fig. 5-19 Acute serum sickness nephritis in a rabbit (12 days after injection of 250 mg/kg of BSA). A high-power view of monocytic macrophage. Numerous lysosomal granules are seen around Golgi area. A platelet (PL) is also seen in the cytoplasm.   ×13,000.

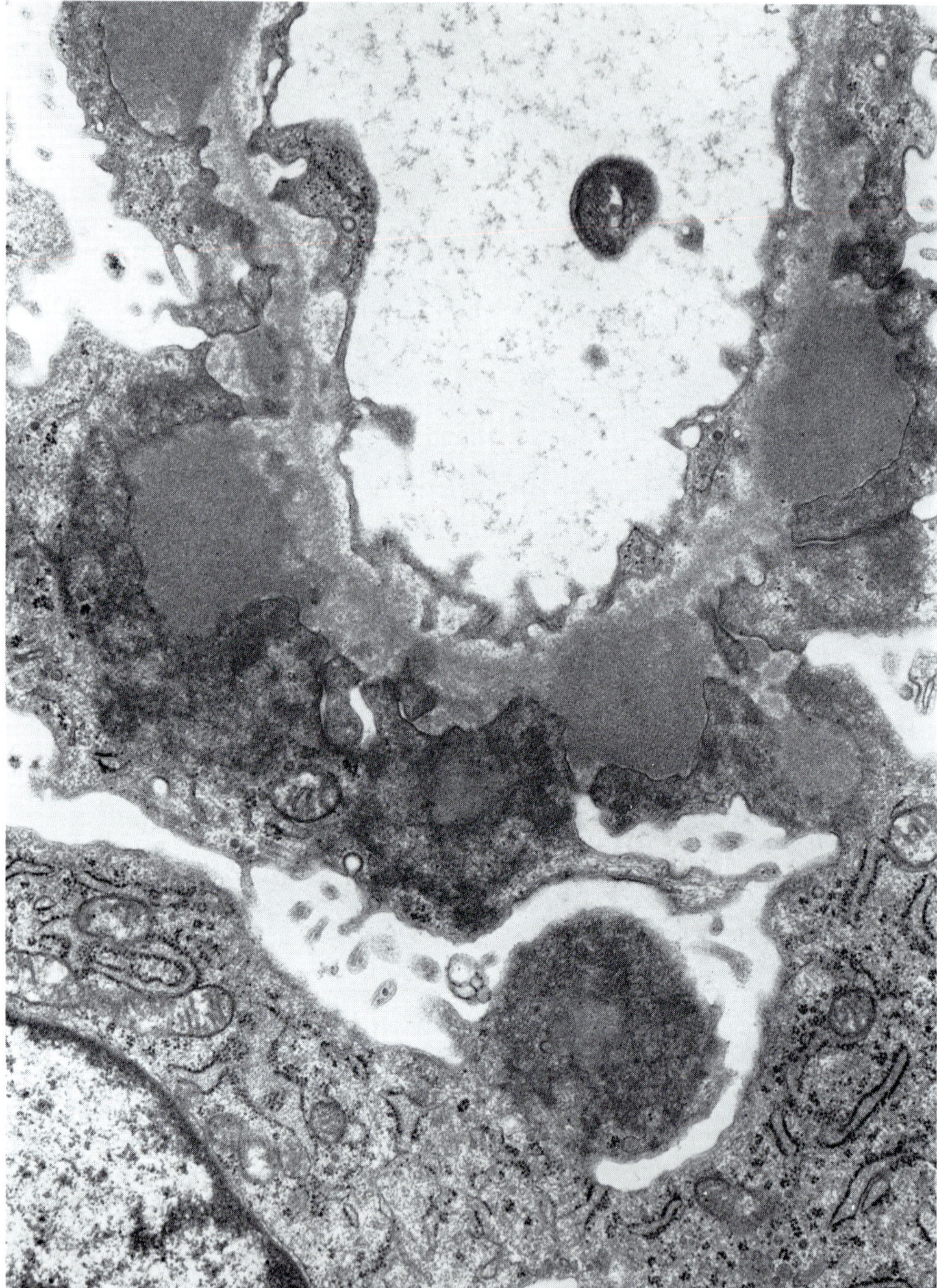

Fig. 5-20 Acute serum sickness nephritis in a rabbit (19 days after injection of 250 mg/kg of BSA). A glomerular portion showing occurrence of large subepithelial deposits after resolution of acute inflammatory changes. Note broad, inrregular fusion of epithelial foot processes.   ×21,000.

and the histologic organization of the glomeruli was fairly well restored. At this stage large dense deposits occurred in some animals localized at the subepithelial side of the GBM which were rare in the florid stage of the inflammation. If rabbits received a second large injection of BSA 7 days after the first injection (accelerated serum sickness), there developed disorganizing glomerular changes. The disorganizing process was evoked by a conspicuous flood of proteinaceous material into the subendothelial space and mesangium. This led to a diffuse loss of the endothelial lining and lysis of the mesangial matrix. In the most severely involved segments, the endothelium and mesangial matrix disappeared almost completely so that the mesangiocapillary organization was no longer discernible. The tufts were converted into a balloon-like structure that contained mesangial cells and other cellular fragments floating in excess electron-translucent, proteinaceous material. The affected tufts showed rapid collapse and scarring obsolescence with capsular adhesions. In some other segments accumulation of macrophages and formation of fibrin or fibrinoid thrombi were prominent. The lytic process along with massive thromboses often caused rupture of the GBM, resulting in crescent formation. These features were much like those observed in progressive Masugi nephritis in the rabbit. The mechanism leading to such pronounced lytic changes was unknown. Dense subepithelial deposits were rare at any stages of the observation. It was suggested that in this disorganizing glomerulonephritis, the GBM failed to trap immune complexes under the condition of its very increased permeability. The role of blood monocytes in rabbit serum sickness nephritis was reconfirmed in a similar series of experiments. Sano described the ultrastructural hallmarks and behavior of the accumulating macrophages in more detail [160]. Their phagocytosis was clearly shown by uptake of carbon particles injected while such activities were very limited in endothelial and mesangial cells.

b. Passive serum sickness nephritis

Since the role of soluble immune complexes was well established in acute "active" serum sickness in the rabbit, McCluskey and associates attempted to produce similar inflammations by a passive administration of antigen-excess, soluble immune complexes prepared in vitro [113, 114]. They reported that proliferative glomerulonephritis developed in mice following glomerular deposition of the preformed complexes. More recently Okumura et al. reinvestigated this passive serum sickness nephritis with the aid of electron microscopy [144]. It was revealed that preformed, soluble complexes (BSA-rabbit antiBSA) were localized predominantly within the mesangium and capillary lumens but the deposition was rare around the GBM. The complexes were then engulfed by numerous emigrating macrophages and PMNs. The mesangium was infiltrated by the phagocytes and was therefore enlarged enormously. Endothelial and mesangial cells did not show any notable phagocytosis of the deposits. They emphasized an outstanding difference in the localization of immune complexes between active and passive serum sickness nephritis. Haakenstad et al. prepared soluble immune complexes composed of human serum albumin and specific rabbit antibodies in vitro [65]. It was found that the complexes prepared with reduced and alkylated antibodies rather persistently circulated in the blood and were deposited in the mesangium of mouse glomeruli. Electron microscopy revealed dense deposits localized within the mesangium. Mesangial cells, however, did not show any definite phagocytosis for the deposits. They suggested that the deposits were possibly removed by migrant phagocytes. Gabbiani et al. examined "Arthus-type" glomerular reactions [49]. They immunized rabbits with horse ferritin and injected the antigen into the aorta or renal artery. Large aggregates of insoluble, presumably antibody excess complexes were soon produced within the glomerular capillary lumens. The deposits were mostly removed by infiltrating PMNs.   Associated with the formation of the insoluble complexes, severe thrombotic lesions were seen.   As compared to usual serum sickness nephritis, the glomerular events resembled the vascular changes taking place in the skin in the Arthus reaction.   Later focal areas of mesangial proliferation and sclerosis appeared, suggesting that insoluble complexes were responsible for the induction of focal nephritis.

It seems that under certain circumstances, an antigen is first deposited in the glomerulus and then reacts with circulating antibody, producing a peculiar immune complex nephritis. Mauer et al. devised a unique experimental system to prove this [112].   A donor rabbit received antigen injection (aggregated human IgG or albumin).   The antigen was deposited predominantly in the glomerular mesangium.   The kidney was removed and transplanted.   The recipient then received a passive injection of antibody.   The antibody was found to specifically react with antigen deposited in the mesangium and acute mesangioproliferative glomerulonephritis developed in the transplanted kidney but not in the recipient's own kidney.

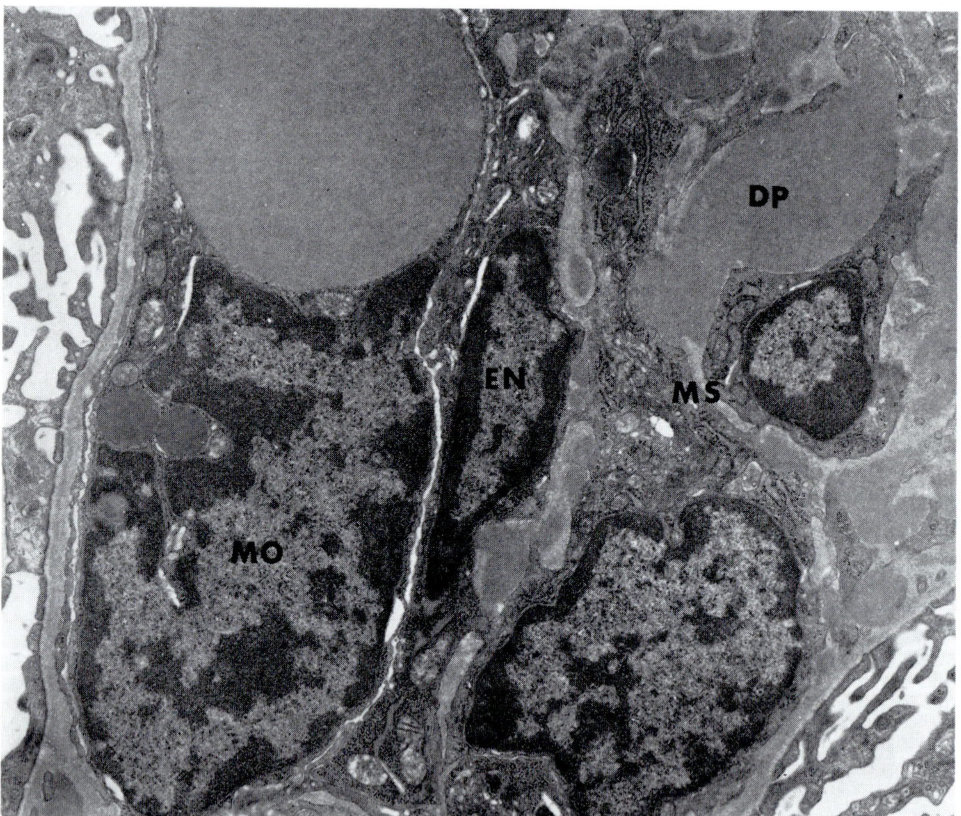

Fig. 5-21   Passive serum sickness nephritis in a mouse produced by three injections of preformed BSA-antiBSA (rabbit) complexes. Large aggregates of immune complexes (DP) are seen within mesangium. An interaluminal monocyte (MO) is engulfiing deposit whereas neither mesangial cells (MS) nor endothelial cell (EN) exhibit such an activity.   × 11,000.

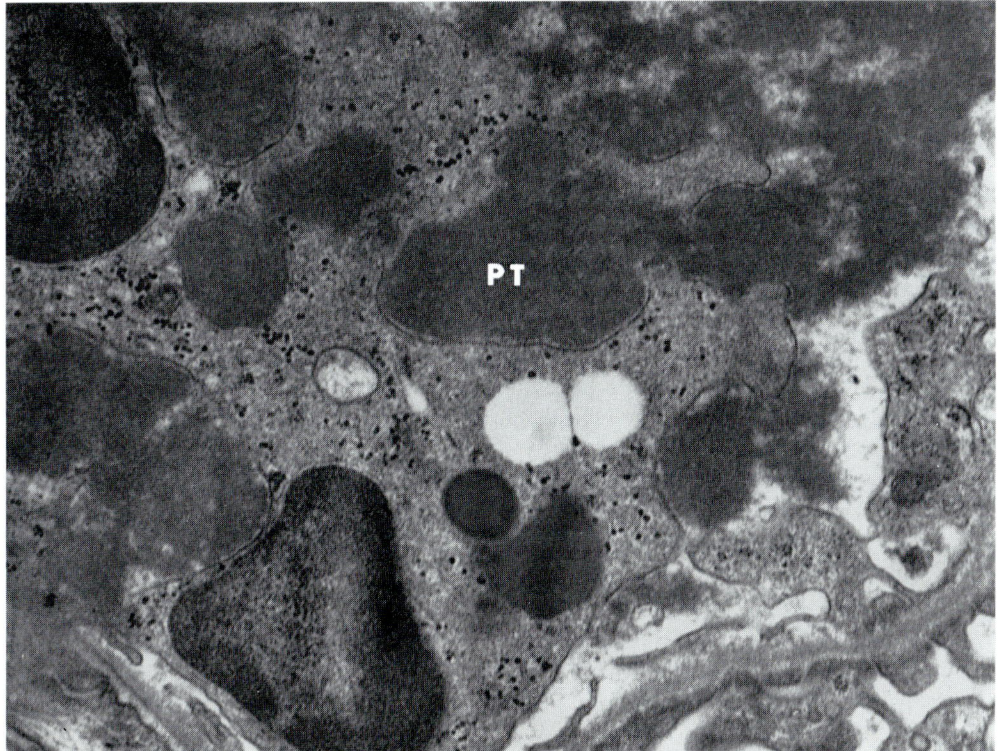

Fig. 5-22 Glomerulonephritis produced by injection of antigen (BSA) into the renal artery of a hyper-immune rabbit. A PMN showing endocytosis of antigen-antibody precipitates (PT) in the glomerular capillary lumen. ×10,000.

6. Chronic immune complex nephritis

a. Chronic serum sickness nephritis

Repeated injections of protein antigens via various parenteral routes over a period of many weeks or months may result in the induction of chronic glomerular diseases in experimental animals. The first detailed studies on the immunologic and morphologic events in this chronic serum sickness nephritis were made by Dixon and associates [34]. In rabbits that received daily intravenous injections of variable amounts of BSA or other foreign serum protein antigens, there was a frequent occurrence of chronic glomerulonephritis. They found that an equivalence range of antigen-antibody interaction in the circulation was the most consistent immunologic characteristic of the rabbits that developed a chronic glomerular disease. Morphologically the glomerular changes basically consisted of diffuse thickening of the GBM. In some instances the GBM thickening was not complicated by other severe glomerular changes and resembled human membranous nephropathy. More commonly, however, advanced GBM thickening was associated with lobulation of the tufts and proliferation of endothelial, mesangial, and epithelial cells. These inflammatory reactions often resulted in scarring obliteration of the glomeruli. Dense deposits that corresponded with antigen and rabbit IgG by immunofluorescence were observed on the GBM which varied in localization during the early stage. Following the progress of the disease the deposits were beaded numerously along the outer surface of the GBM. Present occasionally in the glomerular capillaries were PMNs and mononuclear cells containing immune complexes. In the most advanced lesions the capillaries were filled with proliferated cells and leukocytes making it impossible to differentiate each cell type. In addition the GBM was wrinkled or fragmented resulting in extensive capsular adhesions. There was still yet another type of chronic glomerulonephritis found in the rabbits that developed proteinuria during antigen excess; a few rabbits showed principally a proliferation of the mesangial stalk cells with little evidence of GBM and other changes. The GBM of these rabbits contained few or no immune complexes. Morphologic repair after cessation of antigen injections was inconspicuous in all rabbits as evaluated by light microscopy, implicating that chronic glomerulonephritis once developed could persist without further depositions of immune complexes.

Chronic serum sickness-type nephritis could also be induced in mice. Moppelt and Fresen immunized mice by repeated intraperitoneal injections of egg albumin over several weeks [126]. Antigen and mouse globulin were found within the mesangium and along limited areas of the GBM. There was widening of the mesangium due to increase of basement membrane-like material with or without dense deposits. In the nephritic mice proliferation and swelling of endothelial and mesangial cells were present together with leukocytic infiltration and fibrin deposits. Glomerular changes taking place in the mice undergoing prolonged intraperitoneal immunization with horse ferritin were examined by Stilmant et al. [181]. The mice had a proliferative glomerular lesion with mesangial hypercellularity and matrix increase. Antigen, IgG, and C3 were localized mainly in the mesangium. By electron microscopy there were marked deposits of ferritin complexes in an expanded mesangium and mesangial interposition. The deposits were to some extent present at the subendothelial and subepithelial aspects of the GBM, the latter localization being more frequent. Ferritin-containing, membrane-limited vacuoles were seen within the mesangial cell cytoplasm but, compared with the large amount of ferritin deposited in the matrix, the quantity of intracytoplasmic ferritin was unimpressive.

It seems that in chronic mouse glomerulonephritis the mesangium is the primary site of deposits for immune complexes whereas in no instances are beaded, subepithelial deposits present. The reason why typical membranous nephropathy does not develop in mice has not been clarified in these studies.

b. Autologous immune complex nephritis (Heymann)

Heymann et al. first reported that rats immunized with homologous renal tissue in Freund's complete adjuvant developed severe proteinuric glomerulonephritis [77], which has been referred to as autologous immune complex nephritis. The rat glomerular disease exhibits many features in common with those of human membranous nephropathy. Both autologous immunoglobulin and C3 are found to be localized diffusely along the capillary walls in a granular fashion [36, 142]. Several weeks after repeated antigen injections, subepithelial deposition of dense granular material is observed with the start of proteinuria [2, 12, 43, 97, 182]. The deposition is progressive and accompanied by a marked GBM thickening which is recognizable with light microscopy as numerous spiky projections of the GBM [12]. In general there are no inflammatory reactions in the glomeruli, e.g., cellular emigration and proliferation except extension of mesangial cytoplasm toward the peripheral loops or into the capillary lumen. In view of these findings, many investigators are inclined to believe that rat nephropathy is an example of chronic immune complex nephritis. This has been clearly proved by Edgington et al. [39]. They separated the renal tissue components and were able to purify an antigenic constituent of the nephritogenic complexes which was derived from the brush border of the proximal tubules. Only one injection of a very small amount of this purified antigen in

Freund's complete adjuvant was capable of inducing typical Heymann nephritis in the rat. It was further clarified that the tubular antigen, autologous IgG, and C3 were deposited in the glomeruli [58].   When a nephritic rat received a syngeneic kidney transplantation, circulating immune complexes were deposited in the transplanted kidney [40].   Moreover Grupe and Kaplan showed that elutable immunoglobulin from the diseased kidney specifically reacted with the brush border of the proximal tubules [63].   As to the pathogenesis of Heymann nephritis, it is thus realized that with antigenic stimulation, specific rat antibody is produced which then interacts with tubular antigen normally circulating in the blood; the tubular antigen-antibody complexes are deposited in renal glomeruli to induce nephropathy.

It has also been reported that immunization of rats with a modification of Heymann's original method resulted in the production of multiple renal lesions.   Klassen et al. observed tubular changes associated with localizations of IgG and C3 in addition to immune complex glomerulonephritis [88].   The tubular lesions were often accompanied by massive lymphocytic infiltration, suggesting the participation of cell-mediated mechanisms. Passive transfer of this disease has been a matter of controversy.   Sugisaki et al. were able to transfer it by means of serum from the nephritic rat [182].   They postulated that the recipient lesions resulted not from transfer of immune complexes but rather of free antibody which might combine with circulating antigen to form soluble, antibody excess complexes. The presence of tubular antigens in the circulation is reconfirmed by Feenstra et al. [41]. They produced membranous nephropathy in the rat with passive injection of rabbit antibody directed against tubular antigens and found that the tubular antigen-heterologous antibody complexes were deposited in glomeruli as early as 3 hours after the injection.

c. Glomerulonephritis in New Zealand (NZ) strain mice

Among many naturally occurring diseases in experimental animals, glomerulonephritis developing in NZB mice, along with various other autoimmune phenomena, is outstanding in its high incidence and resemblance to nephropathy in human SLE [80, 122].   In the F_1 hybrid NZB/NZW, the glomerular involvement has been found to be more frequent [71] which is manifested at an earlier age than in NZB mice and is usually fatal, especially in females.   Immunofluorescent studies have revealed progressive granular or lumpy deposition of mouse immunoglobulins in the mesangium and along the GBM, indicating that the disease is an immune complex nephritis [1, 25, 78, 116, 121, 133].   Although there is a broad resemblance between NZB and NZB/NZW F_1 mice with respect to the glomerular lesions, proliferative changes with crescent formation may more frequently be encountered in the latter [133].   With electron microscopy, Channing et al. observed abundant subendothelial deposits of fibrinoid material in the glomeruli of NZB/NZW F_1 mice [16].   A complicated, bizarre basement membrane-like material appeared within the mesangium which contained scattered dense deposits.   Dense subepithelial deposits were also present but less abundantly.   Shimizu et al. found finger print-like deposits in the mesangium [170], resembling characteristic organized deposits detected in human SLE [62].   The prominent subendothelial distribution of the dense deposits has been confirmed by other investigators.   McGiven and Lynraven investigated the disease process from the early stage [117].   By the age of 1 month, glomerular deposits of dense material on the epithelial side of the GBM were recognizable in electron microscopy, while no abnormalities were detectable by light microscopy and immunofluorescence.   With age the deposits were seen most markedly at the subendothelial space often in the region of the mesangial stalk.   Marked glomerular distortion was gradually brought about by the continued deposition and proliferation of intracapillary cells which later resulted in hyaline obliteration of the affected loops.   The process may further be exaggerated by concomitant

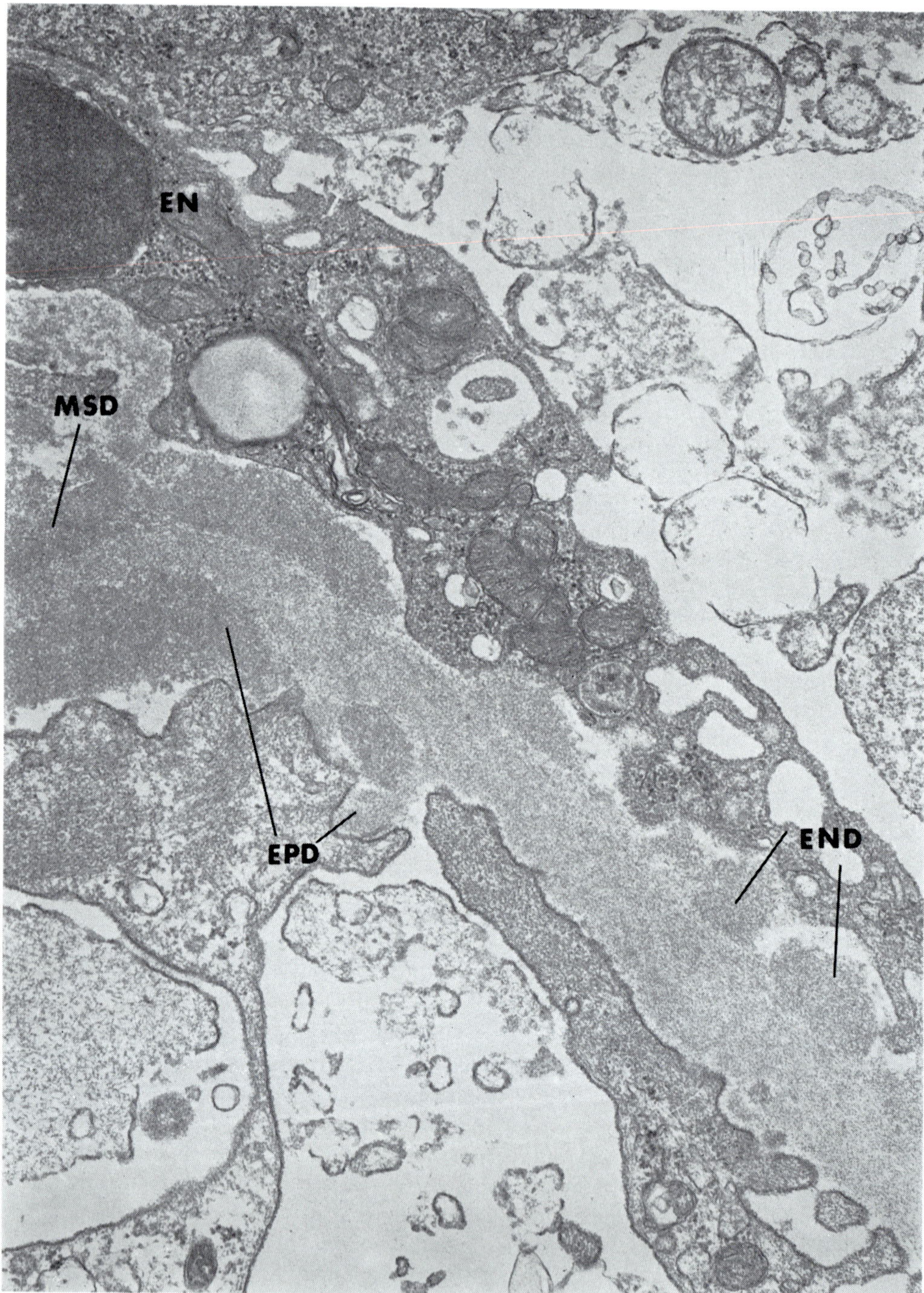

Fig. 5-23 Glomerulonephritis of a NZB mouse. Dense deposits are seen at the subendothelial (END) and subepithelial (EPD) aspects of the GBM. Mesangial deposits (MSD) are also present. Note marked thickening of the GBM. EN; endothelial cell.   ×28,000. (Courtesy of Drs M. Imamura and S. Shirai)

exudative lesions, namely deposits of plasma proteins [116, 133]. Occasionally, however, there are mice with features of membranous nephropathy. Kelly and Cavallo showed that glomerular lesions of these proteinuric mice were characterized by abundant epimembranous deposits [86]. Various changes of epithelial cells (podocytes) were seen associated with the deposition such as distortions or loss of slit diaphragm and formation of occluding junctional complexes in residual slits.

Two somewhat controversial concepts accounting for the pathogenesis of glomerulonephritis in NZ strain mice have been presented. First, it has been demonstrated that NZ mice possess a high susceptibility to murine leukemia virus and produce natural antibody against the viral antigen [123]. Since glomerulonephritis developed in association with immune elimination of the antigen from the circulation and since the antigen and mouse immunoglobulins deposited in the diseased glomeruli, Mellors and collaborators concluded that viral antigen-antibody complexes were the major causative factor in producing the mouse glomerulonephritis [124]. Second, Lambert and Dixon analyzed acid eluates from the nephritic kidneys and found that elutable immune complexes were composed of nuclear antigens and antinuclear antibodies [98]. Moreover in a quantitative assay, they disclosed that the antibody activity of elutable IgG was for the most part directed to nuclear protein but partly to viral antigens [35], implicating that nuclear antigen-antibody complexes were of causative immune complexes. Recently Yoshiki et al. have presented evidence in favor of the first concept [212]. It was found that the tissues and serum of NZ mice contained a remarkably high concentration of glycoprotien antigen, gp 69/71, derived from the envelope of murine leukemia virus. With NZB and NZB/NZW F_1 mice, gp 69/71 was found to be specifically localized in the glomeruli as shown by immunofluorescence. The distribution pattern was similar to that of mouse immunoglobulins. Elution studies of the perfused kidneys further confirmed that gp 69/71 and immunoglobulins deposited in the form of immune complexes.

The unusually high concentration of viral envelope antigen and the enhanced antibody response to this antigen strongly suggest that there exists dysfunction of the immune system in NZ mice. The fact that the incidence of the mice disease is increased by thymectomy could be accounted for by the decrease of T lymphocytes that suppress immune responses [4]. Shirai and Mellors have recently reported that NZ mice produced natural thymocytotoxic antibody which was increased with age [171]. It may well be that the thymocytotoxic antibody is, at least in part, responsible for a turbulence of the immune response from which exaggerated antibody formation against viral antigens, nuclear antigens, and other exogenous or endogenous antigens ensues. Many of the immunologic abnormalities in this unique mouse strain would be manifestations of characteristic gene controls to which recent investigators have directed their attention.

d. Glomerulonephritis in Aleutian disease of mink

The similarities between the glomerular lesions in NZ mice and mink bearing Aleutian disease have been pointed out in regard to the occurrence of lupus-like nephropathy of possible viral etiology. In the mink infected spontaneously or experimentally with Aleutian disease virus, a fatal glomerulonephritis usually develops which is characterized by mesangial and peripheral deposition of eosinophilic, PAS positive material and proliferation of mesangial cells [75, 147]. Focal necrosis and dilation of Bowman's space are also present [87]. The deposition is increasingly prominent with time and eventually results in diffuse obsolescence of the glomeruli. Capsular adhesion and crescent formation may occur occasionally [147]. Immunofluorescent localization of mink immunoglobulins and complement is well correlated with amorphous eosinophilic deposits [74, 147]. Fibrinogen and albumin are present in some severely involved glomeruli [74, 147]. Tests for antibody activity against nuclear proteins and GBM performed by using glomerular eluates are negative [147].

The most consistent finding by electron microscopy is abundant dense subendothelial deposits corresponding to wire-loop lesions in light microscopy [74, 87, 146, 147]. Similar deposits could be found within the mesangium and, less frequently, within the GBM or subepithelial space. Pan et al. suggested that the deposits were transported into subendothelial space via cytoplasmic channels of endothelial cells [146]. Endothelial cells were swollen, moderately increased, and sometimes detached from the GBM [75, 146]. In addition there is a pronounced lesions in the mesangium. Henson and associates reported that cellular proliferation as well as increase in matrix of the mesangium was seen from the early stage in keeping with mesangial and subendothelial depositions of dense material [75, 76]. Increase in size and number of cytoplasmic projections of the mesangial cells and infiltration of macrophages also contributed to diffuse enlargement of the mesangial area. The cellular elements were separated by serpentine strands of the matrix. The mesangial cells and macrophages often contained dense material. It was proposed that the progressive deposition of dense material, most likely immune complexes, might stimulate mesangial cells to proliferate [76], but an overwhelming deposition might result in diffuse degenerative lesions with cellular necrosis [146]. The GBM *per se* does not seem to be the primary site of involvement, though marked distortion of the GBM was usually seen at the later stage [75, 76]. In studying various coagulation parameters of the diseased mink, McKay et al. found the presence of a process of episodic, incomplete intravascular coagulation [120]. They speculated that intravascular coagulation was an intermediate mechanism for the development of the mink disease and that the deposits might represent a mixture of incompletely polymerized fibrin, albumin, and globulin.

The pathogenesis of glomerulonephritis in Aleutian disease of mink has not yet been elucidated, though morphologic observations have strongly indicated that the disease is initiated by glomerular deposition of circulating immune complexes. Porter et al. revealed that viral antigen-antibody complexes were circulating in the mink blood and the induction of glomerulonephritis was apparently related to the formation of the complexes [151, 152]. Unfortunately, however, they could demonstrate very faint localization of viral antigen(s) in the glomeruli of only a few animals [152].

7. Prolonged antigenic stimulation and glomerulonephritis

As mentioned before, in chronic serum sickness nephritis, glomerular changes manifested are not uniform. It has been implied that one of the factors related to the different morphologic manifestations of the involved glomeruli is the nature of antibody included in nephritogenic complexes [96]. It is not unlikely that continued antigen administration may somehow affect the immune system to exert an altered antibody formation. Employing various antigens, Okabayashi has performed a series of experiments in rabbits to demonstrate sequential changes taking place in the immune system under the condition of prolonged antigenic stimulation [139, 140]. It was found that the lymph nodes and other antibody forming tissues were virtually depleted at the later stage of the experiments. The alteration of the immune system was reflected by the unusual antibody response and degenerative conversion of hypersensitivity inflammation.

For example, Kuriyama reported occurrence of a chronic, degenerative glomerular disease in rabbits undergoing prolonged antigenic stimulation [96]. By weekly intramuscular immunization of egg albumin with Freund's incomplete adjuvant, these rabbits developed membranous glomerular changes characterized by granular fluorescence con-

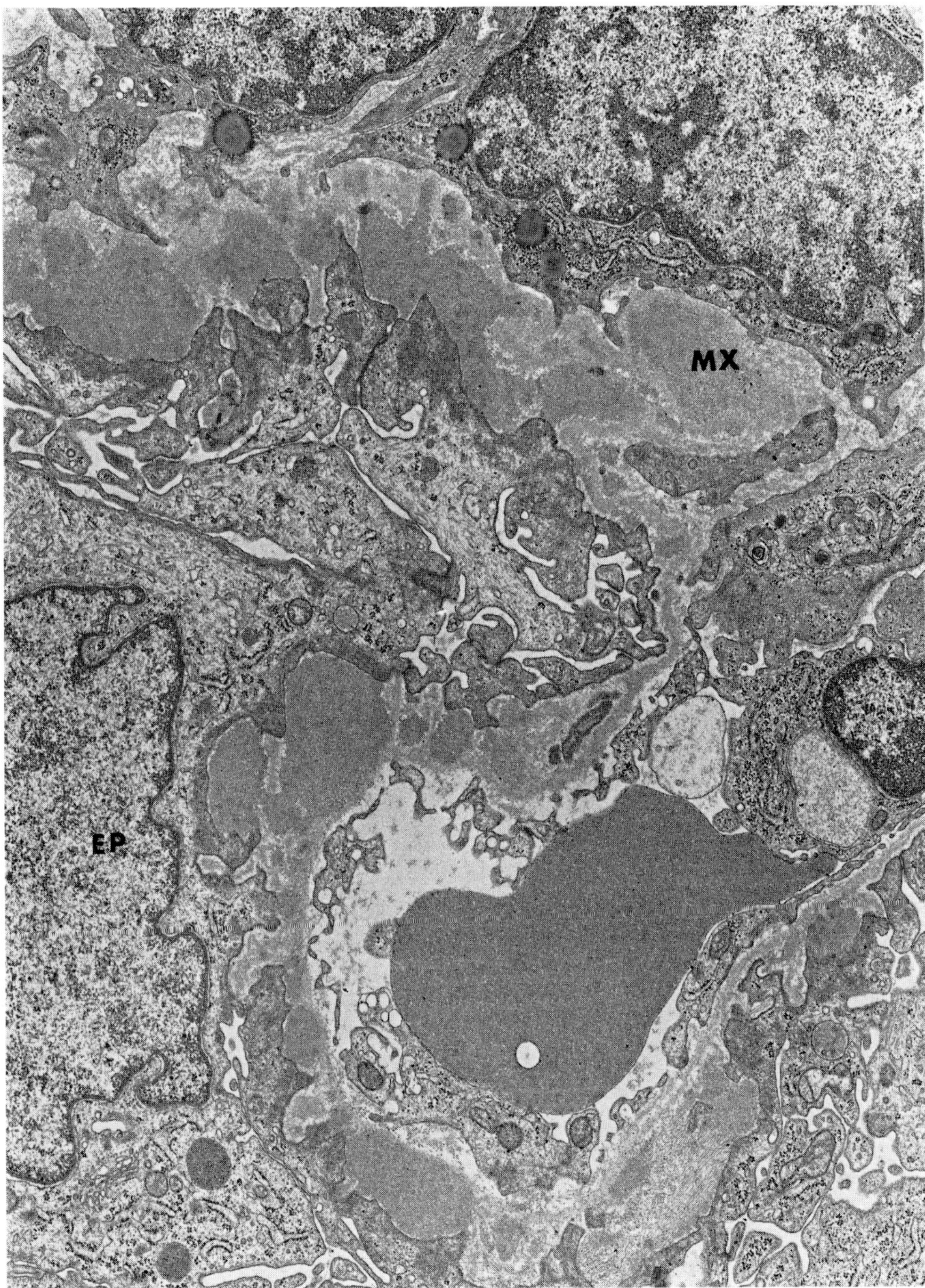

Fig. 5-24 Prolonged antigenic stimulation and rabbit membranous nephropathy. Note numerous dense subepithelial deposits and irregular thickening of the GBM. Similar deposits are also present in mesangial area (MX). Epithelial cell (EP) is swollen and foot processes are fused. ×13,000.

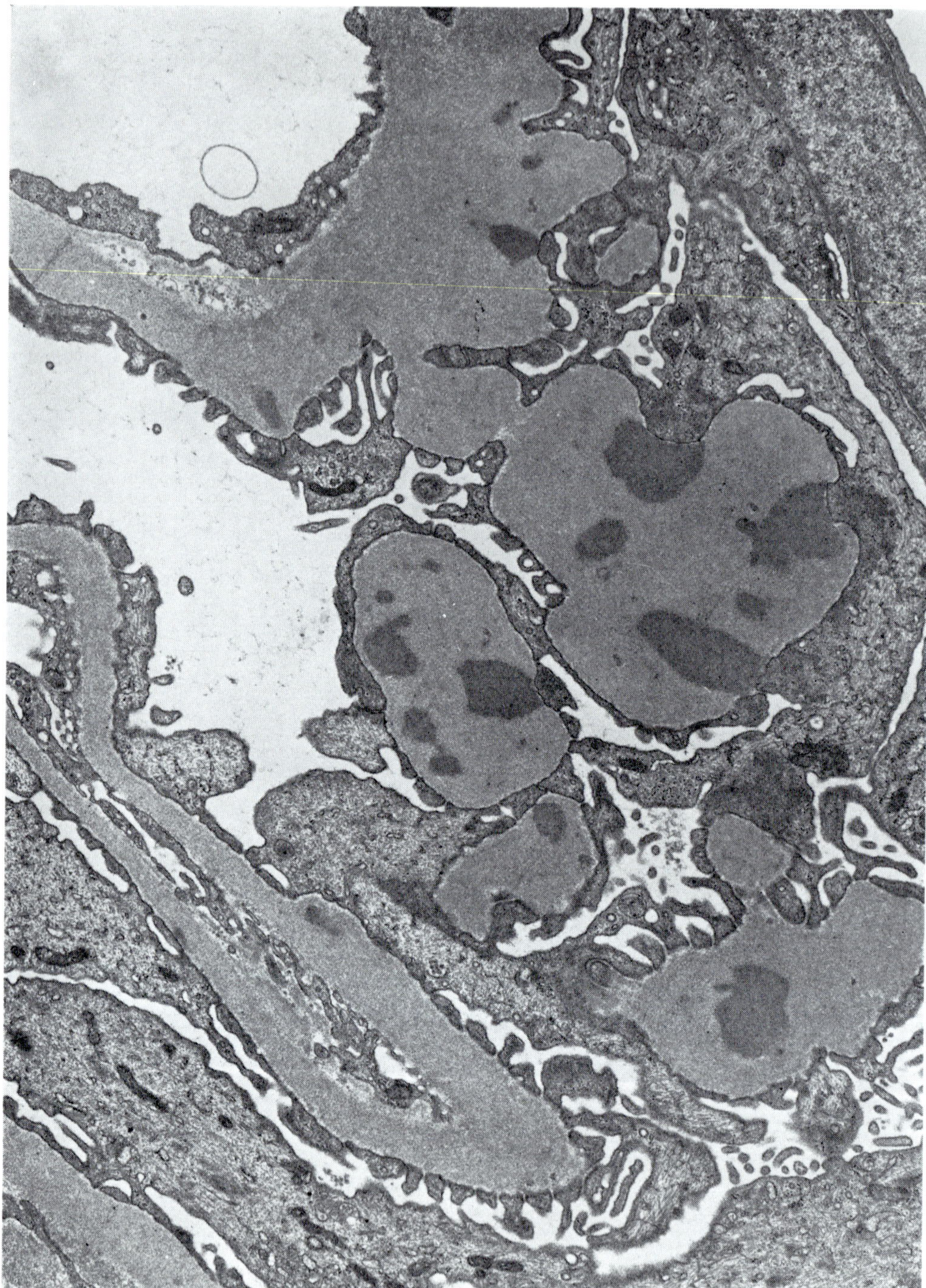

Fig. 5-25   A glomerular portion of a mouse received prolonged antigenic stimulation. Electron dense deposits are seen within or subepithelial side of the GBM.   ×12,000. (From Okumura, K.: *Acta Path. Jap.* *23*: 695, 1973)

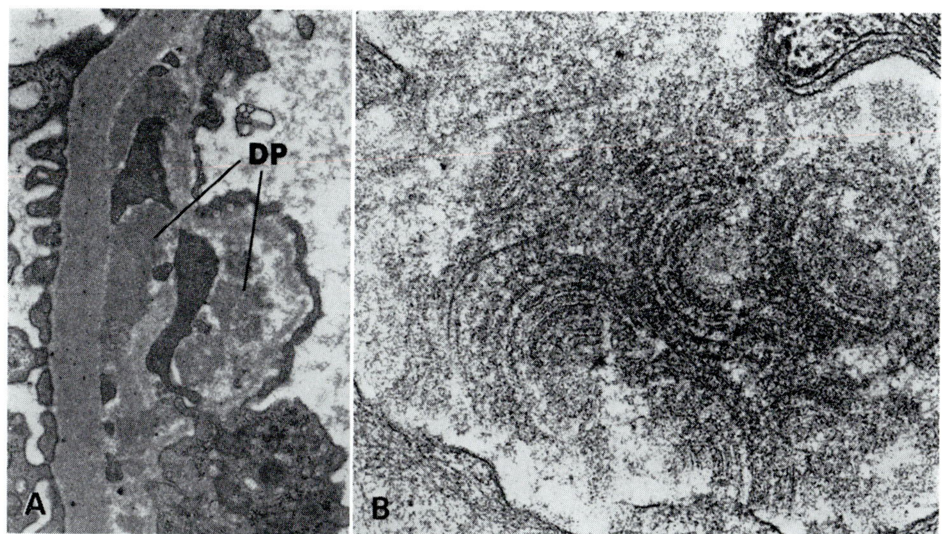

Fig. 5-26   Lupus-like glomerulonephritis observed in the later stage of prolonged antigenic stimulation in the mouse. *A*: Electron dense deposits (DP) are mostly seen at the subendothelial side of the GBM. ×18,000. *B*: Characteristic finger print-like deposits found in the mesangium. ×55,000. (From Okumura, K.: *Acta Path. Jap. 23*: 695–704, 1973)

sisting of antigen, rabbit IgG, and C3 along the GBM and within the mesangium.   These deposits, especially antigen, were rather sparse at the onset of proteinuria but were increasingly abundant thereafter.   From the results of the sequential immunofluorescent and ultrastructural observations, it was proposed that the immune complexes were first deposited beneath the endotheilum as a flocculent, ill-defined material and then migrated and aggregated at the subepithelial site.   Interestingly most rabbits were found to produce antibody with low avidity.   It was therefore suggested that the formation of complexes consisting of antigen and non-precipitating antibody might be essential in inducing membranous nephropathy.

Some rabbits on the other hand showed chronic, proliferative glomerular changes.   In these animals, IgG and C3 were mainly localized in the mesangial stalk areas but antigen was actually absent.   Dense deposits were present within the mesangium but not around the GBM.   The proliferative change resulted from proliferation of mesangial cells and of unclassified mononuclear cells.   The rabbits produced precipitating antibody with high avidity, in contrast to those with membranous nephropathy.

Moreover, in the later experimental stage, Okabayashi showed that wire-loop glomerular lesions developed in some animals associated with production of autoantibodies directed against blood cells, nuclear antigens, and tissue constituents [139].   Okumura also performed prolonged antigenic stimulation in mice with intramuscular injection of egg albumin [143].   After several months, chronic proliferative glomerulonephritis developed in mice with glomerular localization of antigen and mouse IgG.   Interestingly some other mice had a large amount of circulating antinuclear antibody.   Lumpy deposits of IgG were conspicuous in the glomeruli in these mice while antigen was absent.   Electron microscopy revealed abundant dense deposits localized within the mesangium and at the both sides of the GBM.   In addition, peculiar finger print-like deposits, similar to those observed in NZ mice [170] and human SLE [62] were detected in the mesangium.   It was thus assumed that in the later stage of the experiment, two different types of glomerulonephritis could be induced in animals, i.e., chronic serum sickness nephritis and lupus-like nephritis.

Correlation between tissue lesions and immune system alterations is thorougly discussed in Chapter 6.

III. Mechanisms of Glomerular Injury

Although tissue injury often develops on the basis of antigen-antibody interaction, it has not been determined that this interaction *per se* provides a deleterious effect on the tissue involved.   Evidence so far obtained suggests that the initiation of hypersensitivity inflammation is usually mediated by various substances derived from the blood and tissue constituents which are mobilized or activated via the antigen-antibody interaction.   This may also be the case in immunologically induced glomerulonephritis and, indeed, a number of mediators claimed to produce glomerular lesions have been reported.   Since publications dealing with the mechanisms of inflammation in general are vast, our discussion will be limited to those concerned with the pathogenesis of glomerulonephritis.   For further information regarding the pathogenesis of glomerular diseases many excellent reviews cited are available.

1. Masugi nephritis

Morphologic manifestations of Masugi nephritis are quite variable depending upon the source and dose of NTAbs injected, and animal species used as reviewed by Unanue and Dixon [190].   In addition the following immunologic or nonimmunologic participants have been thought to be important in determining the nature of glomerulonephritis induced.

a. Complement

Complement has been regarded as a powerful candidate contributing to the clinical and pathologic events in Masugi nephritis.   Many attempts have been made to elucidate the role of complement in mediating glomerular injury, using either enzymatically digested NTAbs, which still have an affinity for the GBM but have little or no ability to fix complement, or animals being decomplemented [190].   The result is similar in terms of the prevention of the immediate onset of glomerular lesions, indicating that the first phase of Masugi nephritis could be greatly influenced by the presence or absence of complement. This could be reconfirmed by using duck NTAb which fixes little, if any, complement of the host.   No immediate glomerular events have been recognized in the rat so far examined after injection of a moderate dose of the NTAb [66].   The cytolytic destruction of cell membranes is the hallmark of complement action and a consequence of activation of the terminal sequence [130, 137].   It is unknown whether such a sequence of complement activation occurs similarly in glomerulonephritis induced by immunologic means which causes the constituents of the glomerulus to be destroyed.   Gang et al. showed that some alteration in the chemical composition of the GBM occurred within 1 hour accompanying increased permeability [50].   Since the early change was PMN-independent, they speculated that immune reactants themselves were the triggering factor.

Some products of complement components have been known to be related to altered vascular permeability; for instance, anaphylatoxins, the cleavage peptides of C3 and C5, cause increased permeability via release of histamine from mast cells [130, 137].   It is unlikely that complement fixed on the GBM contributes in this way to proteinuria.   Other actions of complement should be more seriously considered to account for actual injury of the glomerulus.   Cochrane and collaborators showed that massive accumulation of PMNs and proteinuria in acute rat Masugi nephritis were mediated by complement fixation [26]. The PMN accumulation could not be seen when animals were decomplemented, although the injected NTAb was fixed to the GBM as usual. Complement-derived factors such as C3a, C5a, or C567 complex have been known to be chemotactic for PMNs [201, 202, 203]. Cleavage products of complement, e.g., C5a might be likewise chemotactic for mononuclear cells [175]. In acute rat nephritis, these chemotactic factors would be produced on the GBM during a cascade of complement fixation with a resultant accumulation of the blood cells. It has been revealed that blood cells of certain animal species also attach to complement-bound immune complexes by their receptors for C3 (immune adherence phenomenon; [135]). Besides leukocytes rabbit or rat platelets are aggregated by immune complexes coated with C3b [130, 137]. This would account for, at least in part, the mechanisms by which platelet aggregation and intravascular coagulation are brought about at the early stage of Masugi nephritis. That certain components of complement participate in the coagulation process has recently been demonstrated [130]. These observations favor the view that complement is important in producing acute glomerular injury. However, there are several lines of evidence to the contrary. It has been observed that when a large dose of duck NTAb was injected, glomerular injury occurred immediately in rats without any participation of complement [66, 190]. In rat nephritis induced by nephrotoxic guinea pig IgG$_1$, Kobayashi et al. reported that proteinuria developed immediately after the injection without significant complement fixation [91]. Ultrastructurally marked endothelial desquamation with thromboses was observed. Moreover F (ab')$_2$ of this NTAb was also effective in producing immediate proteinuria and endothelial damage, though fibrin thrombi were rare [92]. There is other evidence to indicate that structural abnormalities with increased permeability do occur in the first and the second phase, independent of participation of complement component [29, 173, 185].

Masugi nephritis induced in animals with a congenital deficiency in the complement system is of interest in this respect. Lindberg and Rosenberg found no distinct difference between normal and some strains of mice that lacked hemolytic component(s) of complement with respect to the glomerular morphology during the first phase [103]. In the second phase glomerular changes were almost identical in both groups [193]. In rabbits with congenital deficiency of C6, the changes in the second phase were seen to occur in the same fashion as in normal rabbits [158], suggesting that the terminal complement sequence was not involved. In brief, the issue regarding the role of the complement system in the mediation of glomerular injury is still conflicting. It may be that in addition to known functions of complement, other mediators are also operative in the inflammatory process in the glomerulus.

b. Polymorphonuclear leukocytes and mononuclear phagocytes

In general PMNs are the most integral part of cellular exudates in many acute inflammatory reactions and are intimately connected with tissue injury. This is particularly prominent in the Arthus reaction as reviewed by Cochrane and Janoff [24]. The process is interpreted as follows; the PMNs accumulated in the subcutaneous tissue engulf antigen-antibody complexes, release injurious substances included in their granules, and the Arthus inflammation develops. The sequence has been thought to be principally mediated by complement. In acute Masugi nephritis in the rat, PMNs accumulate in the glomerular capillaries exhibiting broad contacts with the GBM [26, 165]. The characteristic behavior of the PMNs can be best explained by the presence of substances, being chemotactic for PMNs. Although a number of substances capable of attracting PMNs have been reported, complement is the most likely candidate accounting for the pathogenesis of massive PMN infiltration in immunologic disease as discussed before. GBM-bound com-

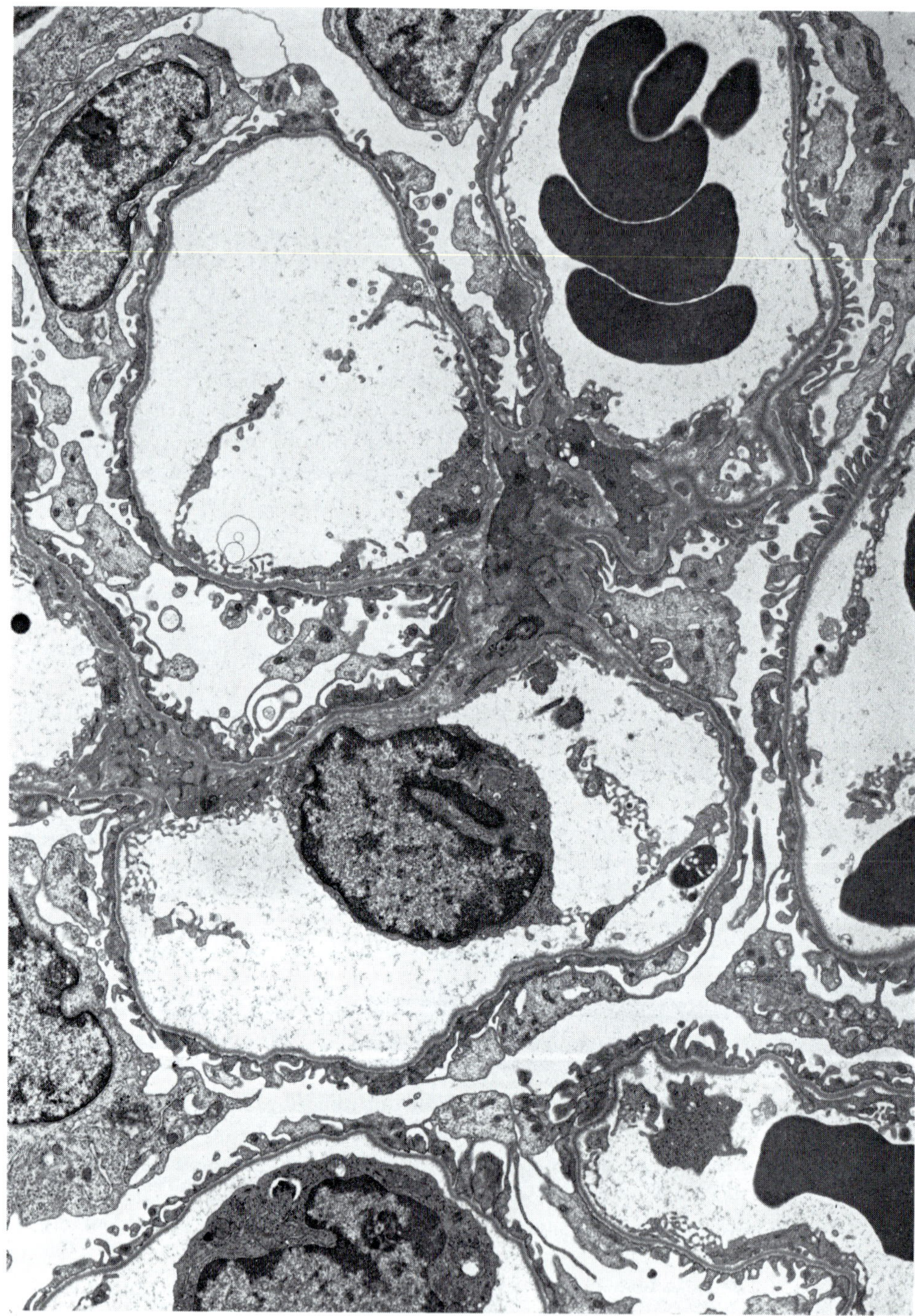

Fig. 5-27   Complement-independent glomerular lesion produced by injection of F (ab')$_2$ of nephrotoxic guinea pig IgG$_1$ in a rat. Diffuse detachment and exfoliation of the endothelium are seen.   ×7,200. (From Kobayashi, Y. et al.: *Virchows Arth. Abt. B15*: 35–44, 1973)

plement (C3) may also attract PMNs by immune adherence mechanisms [22].   Hayashi et al. have recently isolated a very effective chemotactic factor from the inflamed tissue of rabbit skin [69, 70].   It was found that this factor was derived from an IgG fragment including Fc portion which was produced by the action of SH-protease on native IgG molecules.   The protease was relaeased from mononuclear cells adjacent to the blood vessels.   Human myeloma IgG was also effective in mediating chemotaxis in vivo after enzymatic digestion.   It is possible that heterologous or autologous IgG localized along the GBM is modified in this way to produce a chemotactic factor.   In any case, the maximal activity of these possible chemotactic factors may be self-limited since PMN accumulation is usually transient in Masugi nephritis.

The next problem concerns how PMNs damage the glomerular tissue.   There is evidence to indicate that proteinuria develops on the basis of GBM alteration brought about by an accumulation of PMNs.   At the time when PMNs attached to the GBM, proteinuria developed in the rat while depletion of circulating PMNs prior to injection of rabbit NTAb prevented immediate proteinuria despite glomerular fixation of the NTAb and complement [26].   In rabbit Masugi nephritis induced by sheep NTAb, PMN-depletion resulted in no glomerular injury [67].   When animals received graded doses of homologous PMNs the severity of the injury was directly related to the number of the PMNs passively injected. Large molecular proteins, e.g., IgG and fragments of the GBM could be found in the urine only when PMNs participated in the glomerular injury.   Simultaneously both acid proteins (cathepsin) and cationic proteins, derivatives of PMN granules, were also excreted in the urine [67].   Since the use of conventional electron microscopy sometimes failed to show any substantial GBM changes during PMN infiltration, Gang et al. appreciated the value of lanthanum to disclose GBM alterations [51].   Focal dense concentrations of lanthanum, a manifestation of increased GBM permeability, were seen at areas where the GBM was contiguous with a PMN.   The occurrence of these concentrations corresponded in time to the onset of excretion of the GBM-like material and to the beginning of excretion of all classes of serum globulins.   At this stage there was a striking change in distribution of glomerular sialoprotein (GSP), the major antigenic component of the GBM [17].   The normal linear distribution of GSP was disrupted and dispersed, suggesting that the GSP might be removed from its normal position and redistributed within the glomerulus due to the action of infiltrating PMNs.

Obviously the role of PMNs in acute inflammation is to phagocytose various phlogogenic materials and/or inflammatory products.   The phagocytosis, in turn, stimulates the PMNs to release injurious substances.   It is now established that lysosomes confined within PMN granules are composed of hydrolytic enzymes [24, 27, 59].   These lysosomal enzymes are capable of digesting phagocytic material and, along with other non-lysosomal enzymes, exhibit a deleterious effect to the tissue upon their release into extracellular sites. The first step of PMN activation starts with attachment of PMNs to a target by virtue of chemotactic factors or PMN receptors as discussed before.   The endocytosed material is then fused with PMN granules to make secondary lysosomes (phagolysosomes).   This process leads to loss of the granules but is by no means injurious to tissues unless the PMNs release the lysosomal enzymes.   Under certain circumstances, however, granular constituents are able to gain acess to the extracellular environment without any lysis of the cell membrane.   Several possible pathways by which such a secretory reaction of PMNs is induced have been presented by Henson [72] and Weisman et al. [206].   Of particular interest is that PMNs attached to the surface of a non-phagocytosable substance discharged their granules along the adherent cell membrane.   This suggests that solid tissue components such as GBM containing immune reactants are digested by action of PMNs in situ.

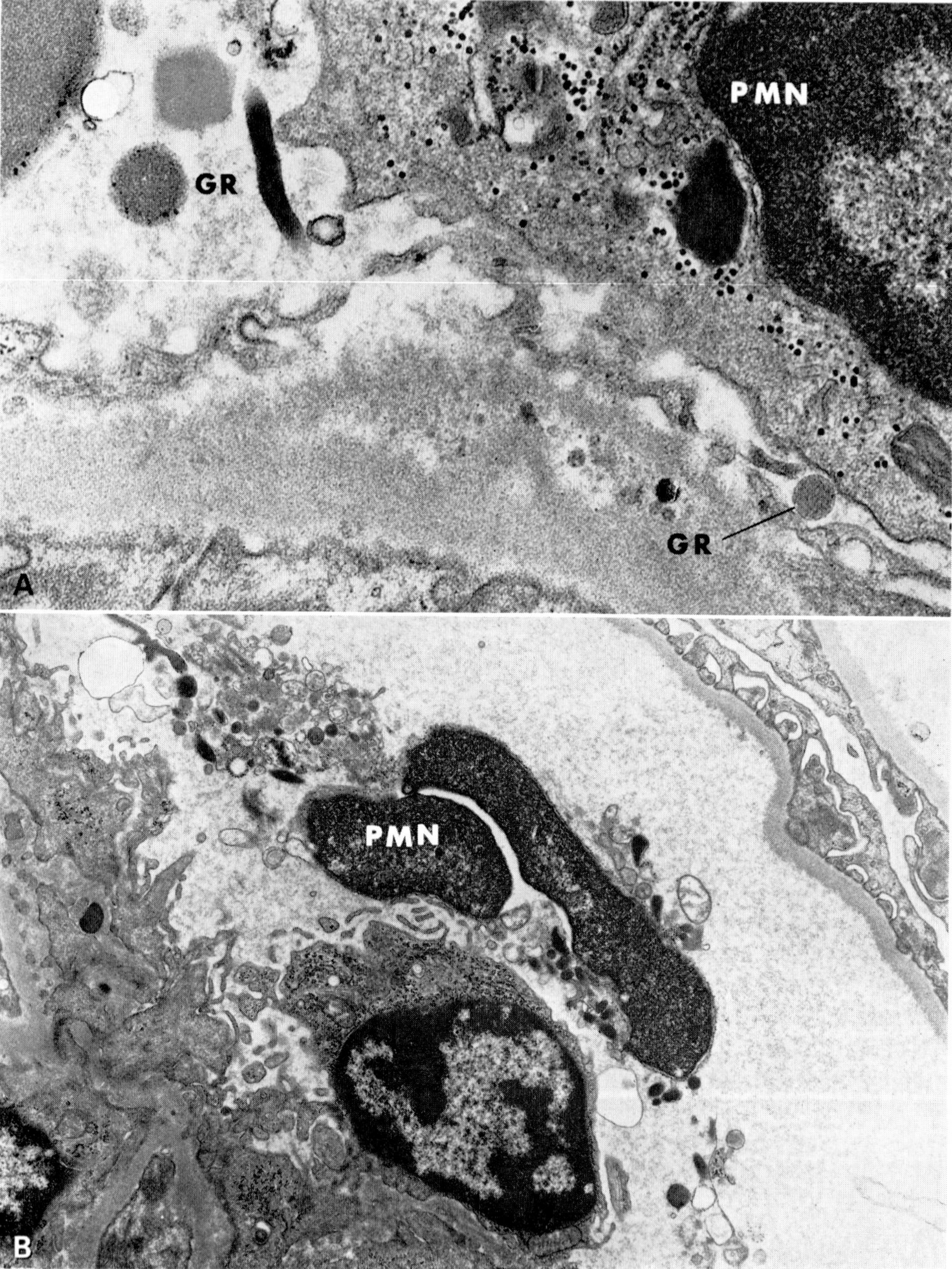

Fig. 5-28   PMN granules discharged in the glomerular capillary lumen (rat Masugi nephritis; 6 hours after injection of rabbit NTAb). *A*: Graunles (GR) released from an intact PMN.   ×39,000.   *B*: Discharge of granules associated with cell lysis of PMN.   ×8,600.

That PMN granules are themselves injurious for tissues was first demonstrated in the Arthus reaction [184]. With intradermal injection of isolated PMN granules, rabbit skin reactivity to the reversed passive Arthus reaction was enhanced. The reaction also appeared upon the same injection into PMN-depleted animals. Lysates from rabbit PMN granules injected into rats produced glomerular alteration [106]. Any of the known lysosomal enzymes included in PMN granules may exert a digestive action in vivo possibly in concert with others. However, little is known about the exact role of these enzymes in an inflamed tissue. Cochrane and Aikins showed that acid proteases (cathepsins D and E) digested GBM in vitro at pH 3.4 and 2.5 [21]. Whether such an extreme pH condition can be present in the diseased glomerulus is questionable. Other proteases operating at neutral or alkaline pH ranges have also been found in PMN lysosomes [206]. Of these a specific collagenase [99, 100] active at neutral pH may be mentioned with respect to its ability to digest the interstitial tissue, e.g., vascular basement membranes. Non-enzymatic mediators are another important consituents of PMN granules. Cationic proteins are a heterogeneous population of proteins and presumably play a role in the production of the acute inflammatory reaction [24]. Their biological activities are diverse, including; permeability effects, mast cell degranulation, chemotaxis for mononuclear cells, pro- and anti-coagulant effects, and others. In addition various other substances of PMN origin have been implicated to behave as a mediator for inflammation [24].

In acute inflammation infiltration of PMNs is usually followed by that of mononuclear phagocytes. Blood monocytes emigrated into extravascular sites may undergo transition to macrophages [199, 200]. This sequence of cellular exudates can also be seen even in the delayed-type of skin reactions mediated by cellular immunity [186]. Obviously many previous investigators were unaware of the possibility that a similar cellular event may occur in acute glomerulonephritis. Glomerular hypercellularity observed in experimental as well as human glomerulonephritis has been thus ascribed to proliferation of fixed glomerular cells. Jones for the first time emphasized that the hypercellularity was basically brought about by accumulation of migrant mononuclear cells within the glomerulus [82, 83]. In the first phase of rat Masugi nephritis, it was revealed that the inflammatory process taking place in the glomerulus resembled in many respects that observed in other tissues [165]. Subsequent studies on various types of experimental glomerulonephritis have reconfirmed this observation that migrant monocytes (predominantly monocytic phagocytes) are often the major cell line appearing in the acute stage, rather than fixed glomerular cells [93–95, 127, 141, 144, 160, 167, 168, 205]. In the second phase of rabbit Masugi nephritis induced by duck NTAb, the monocytic phagocytes predominated from the early stage while PMNs were rare throughout the course [93]. It would appear that the monocytes specifically accumulate in response to some factors localized in the GBM. A number of endogenous and exogenous substances have been reported to be capable of attracting mononuclear cells in vitro [175, 176]. Some of the chemotactic factors for mononuclear cells act directly on the cells while others do so indirectly by stimulating mediators in plasma or serum [176]. Antigen-antibody complexes may become chemotactic in the latter manner. It is not unlikely that immune reactants localized along the GBM are similarly effective to activate the plasma mediators thereby attracting mononuclear cells. The mechanisms of glomerular accumulation of mononuclear phagocytes could also be explained in the following ways; mononuclear cells may specifically interact with immune complexes since receptors for IgG and C3 are equipped on their cell surface [81]; cytophilic antibodies fixed on the cell membrane may be similarly effective for their attachment to antigens [136]; they may accumulate in glomeruli as a consequence of cell mediated immunity. It has been well realized that sensitized lymphocytes release, during interaction with specific antigen, various soluble mediators including a factor capable of aggregating macrophages referred to as macrophage migration inhbition factor (MIF) [11, 31, 186].   If lymphocytes specific for antigen (e.g., NTAb) are circulating and react with the GBM bound antigen, a working hypothesis may be considered that migrated monocytes are attached and spread along the GBM by the mediation of MIF.   By the present time, however, the participation of cellular immunity in mediating glomerular lesions has not been confirmed in antiGBM nephritis.

The biological behavior of macrophages derived from the bone marrow precursor has been documented in great detail [180].   Their participation in inflammation of delayed hypersensitivity [104, 105, 186, 209] as well as immune complex diseases [168, 169] has been clarified beyond dispute.   Nonetheless, it is poorly understood whether or not macrophages are actually concerned in producing tissue injury.   They are generally regarded to act only as scavengers.   However, in view of the fact that macrophages contain abundant lysosomal enzymes which are tremendously increased associated with phagocytosis [180], it seems unlikely that they accumulate solely for phagocytosis and repair of the damaged tissue.   It can be assumed that the macrophages play a comparable role with PMNs in inflammatory sites by releasing these enzymes or other phlogogenic material. Several reports to support this possibility have recently been published.   Under certain circumstances, macrophages cultured in vitro released various substances which might be potentially related to inflammation, those including lysosomal hydrolase [32], cytolytic factors [118], elastase [208], and collagenase [207].

c. Platelets and intravascular coagulation

Platelets are another important participant of acute glomerulonephritis induced by immunologic means and are often seen in close connection with fibrin deposition (intravascular coagulation).   Conceivably several conditions favoring platelet aggregation are present in the diseased glomerulus.   As mentioned before, the early glomerular changes in Masugi nephritis are characterized by desquamation of the capillary endothelium.   It is known that platelets flowing in the blood can adhere to collagen of connective tissue and vascular basement membranes after desquamation of the endothelium [213].   The next important factor is the presence of immune reactants around the vascular walls.   Siqueira and Nelson observed that rabbit platelets aggregated with antigen-antibody complexes in the presence of plasma [174].   Platelet receptor for C3 is necessary to induce this type of reaction (immune adherence) in some animal species but not in others.   Immune complexes then stimulate platelets to release a number of substances for blood coagulation and inflammation, e.g., histamine and serotonin, with or without the intervention of complement [6].   Movat and associates showed that immune complexes formed in the vascular lumen were phagocytosed by platelets and that during this process their degranulation occurred with release of lysosomal enzymes [129].   In addition to their known role in the blood coagulation, platelets thus contribute to the inflammatory process in two other ways, namely as a source of vasoactive amines and lysosomal enzymes.   In Masugi nephritis, however, there is no evidence to indicate the participation of vasoactive amines as a mediator of inflammation.   The precise role of platelet-derived lysosomes is also unknown.

Platelets are important in the intrinsic pathway of coagulation since they are main source of phospholipid and other material [131].   The mechanisms that trigger coagulation of the blood are still puzzling.   Among possible factors, immune complexes, complement, platelets, leukocytes, activation of Hageman factor due to endothelial desquamation, release of thromboplastin from damaged tissues, and circulatory disturbances may all play a direct or indirect role in the initiation and promotion of intravascular coagulation.

Whatever the mechanisms, the importance of intravascular coagulation has been emphasized for production of noticeable glomerular alterations [115]. The glomerular response to the clotting is not uniform depending upon its intensity. A fully-developed clotting caused by antigen-antibody interaction, for example, may give rise to a typical picture of the generalized Shwartzman reaction. Whereas in more mild situations, there may ensue glomerular changes other than massive thromboses. Vassalli et al. revealed that some agents accelerating blood coagulation caused a variety of glomerular changes upon intravenous injection into the rabbits, compatible with those features observed in acute and chronic glomerulonephritis [197]. Vassalli and McCluskey evaluated the role of the coagulation process in the pathogenesis of rabbit Masugi nephritis [195]. A severe proliferative glomerulonephritis developed with injection of sheep NTAb, often associated with the deposition of fibrin and fibrinoid substance. The presence of these fibrinogen derivatives was clearly demonstrated by immunofluorescence but not by electron microscopy with the same frequency. When large deposits of fibrin were present, cellular proliferation was mild or absent. The clotting material was also seen in Bowman's capsular space with concurrent proliferation of epithelial cells (crescent formation). These changes could be significantly prevented by treatment of anticoagulant (Warfarin). It was concluded that the coagulation process initiated by the immune reaction within the glomeruli was the major cause of cellular proliferation, crescent formation, and rapid destruction of the glomeruli. They explained that swelling and proliferation of intracapillary cells were the result of phagocytosis of the clotting material. Recently these results have been further extended by Watanabe and Tanaka [205]. They showed that fibrinolytic activity of the glomerulus in rabbit Masugi nephritis was found to be accelerated in rather mild glomerulonephritis whereas it was almost abolished in severely damaged cases with massive fibrin deposition. It was also found that the predominant cells accounting for the increased cellularity were monocytic phagocytes which might play a role in disposing of various substances formed during the clotting process. These observations imply that the coagulation process is pathogenetically related to the occurrence of cellular and tissue alteration in glomerular diseases, which can be activated by immunologic as well as non-immunologic stimuli. Besides the acute injurious effect of fibrin deposits, it is also likely that the persistence of the clotting material incorporated within the subendothelial space, GBM, and mesangial area is responsible for the deposition of additional basement membrane-like material or hyalin resulting in gradual obsolescence of the affected glomeruli [196].

Impairment of fibrinolytic activities in damaged local areas is another factor influencing the coagulation process. In general thrombotic material can be removed by either cellular phagocytosis or enhanced fibrinolysis. There is evidence to indicate that both mononuclear phagocytes and PMNs are important in resolution of thrombi via these two ways. It has been proved that monocytes and PMNs attached to a thrombus phagocytose platelets, fibrin, and other cellular debris [14, 15, 79, 84, 172]. Fibrin and fibrinoid material were presumed to be removed to some extent by vascular endothelium [119, 197].

Whenever fibrin is deposited, plasminogen is readily absorbed by fibrin, possibly to initiate fibrinolysis [119]. Plasminogen requires an activator contained in the endothelium and other cells or tissues to be converted into plasmin, a powerful fibrinolytic substance. Employing the skin window method, Riddle and Barnhart showed that PMNs were important cellular agents for removal of fibrin in inflammatory sites [155]. It was found that exudative PMNs participated in extra- and intracellular dissolution of fibrin, in both cases PMN granules being actively involved. Characteristically an increasing loss of typical fibrin structure was seen around the PMNs associated with release of their granules.

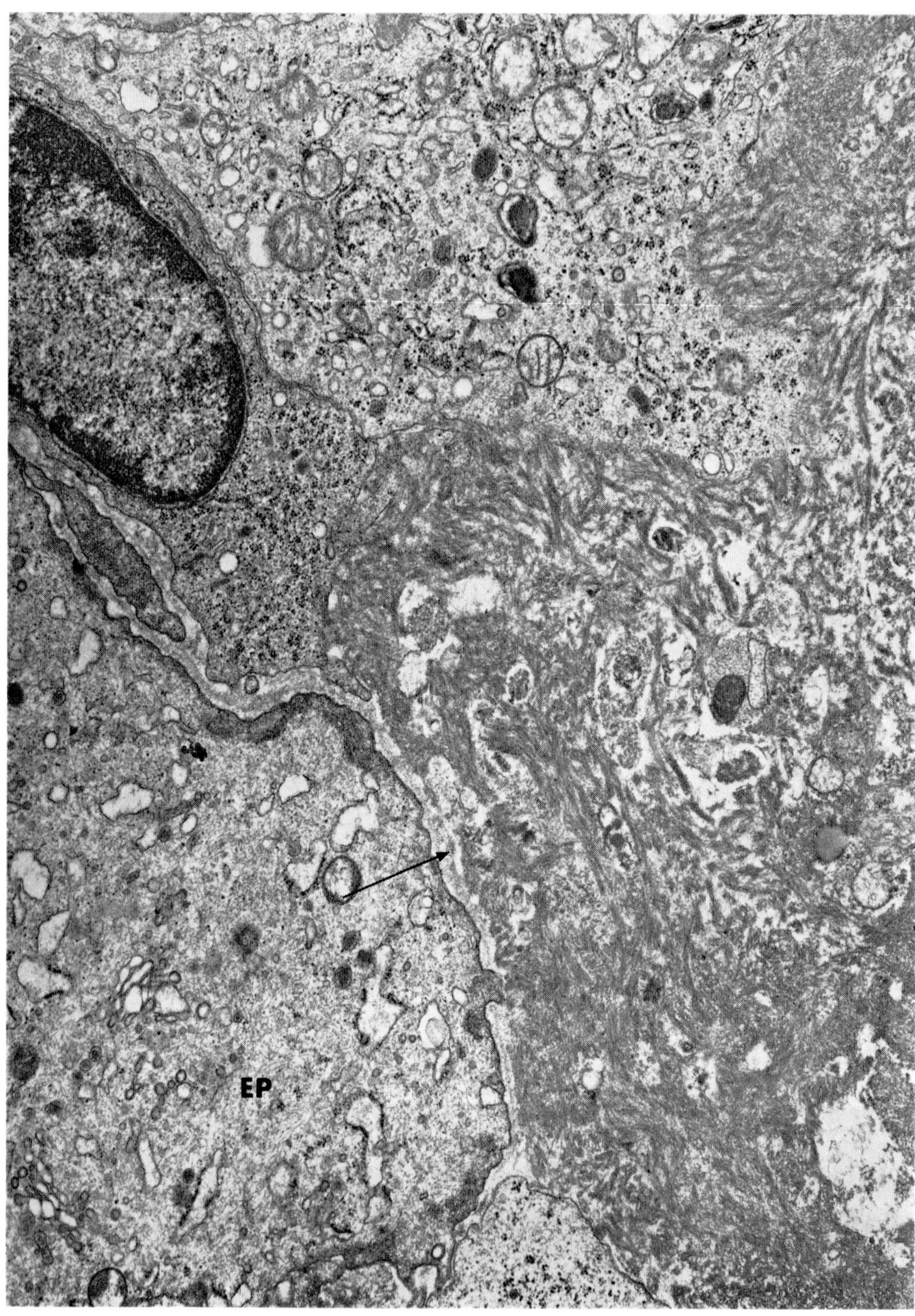

Fig. 5-29   Lysis or fragmentation of the GBM (arrow) is seen correlated with massive fibrin deposition. Epithelial cytoplasm (EP) is attached to intraluminal mass of fibrin (rabbit Masugi nephritis; 13 days after injection of duck NTAb).   ×19,000.

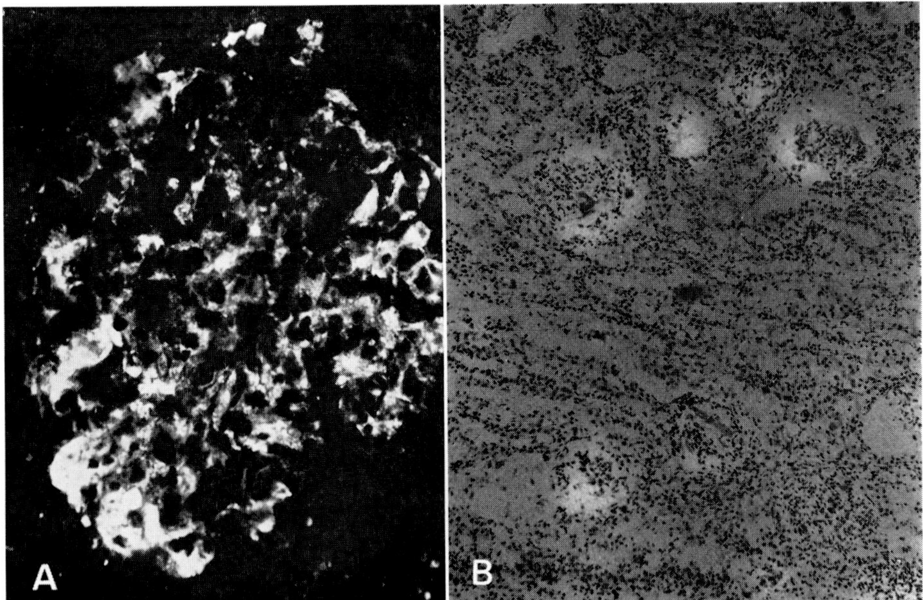

Fig. 5-30 Glomerular deposition and lysis of fibrin (rabbit Masugi nephritis produced by injection of duck NTAb). *A*: Prominent deposit of fibrin visualized by immunofluorescence. *B*: Fibrinolysis autography of a rather mild glomerulonephritis showing a definite glomerular activity of fibrinolysis. (From Watanabe, T. and Tanaka, K.: *Acta Path. Jap. 26*: 147–165, 1976)

Since PMN granules contain plasminogen as well as plasminogen activator [60, 111], it is not surprising that fibrin deposits are dissolved by the PMN-discharged granules.   Recently it has also been revealed that monocytes release plasminogen activators in vitro [61, 194]. The extent of fibrinolysis to which these cellular activities contribute, however, has not been exactly assessed.

Fibrinolytic activity has been found to be present in the vascular endothelium including renal glomeruli.   Plasminogen activator was supposed to be released from endothelial lysosomes [204].   Whenever this endothelial activity is preserved, fibrin deposited in the glomerular lumen could be promptly removed, whereas under the condition of lesser endothelial activity, enhanced thrombosis may ensue.   This may well account for a high susceptibility in the rabbit to the Shwartzman reaction as compared to the rat [10, 132]. Endothelial damage frequently encountered in glomerular diseases may accelerate fibrin deposition by stimulating the clotting mechanisms on the one hand and, on the other, by decreasing the local fibrinolytic activity.

2. Immune complex nephritis

In Masugi nephritis heterologous NTAbs specifically react with the GBM of a recipient animal and therefore the severity of glomerular injury is entirely relevant to the amount and nature of the kidney fixing antibody (NTAb) injected and the intensity of the host immune response.   In immune complex nephritis, however, a number of other factors should be considered since the complexes have no specific affinity for the glomerular constituents. The mechanisms leading to the initiation of immune complex diseases have recently been reviewed [25, 55, 101, 115, 141, 190].   The following discussion will be limited to possible mechanisms of serum sickness-type of glomerulonephritis induced by using purified protein antigens.

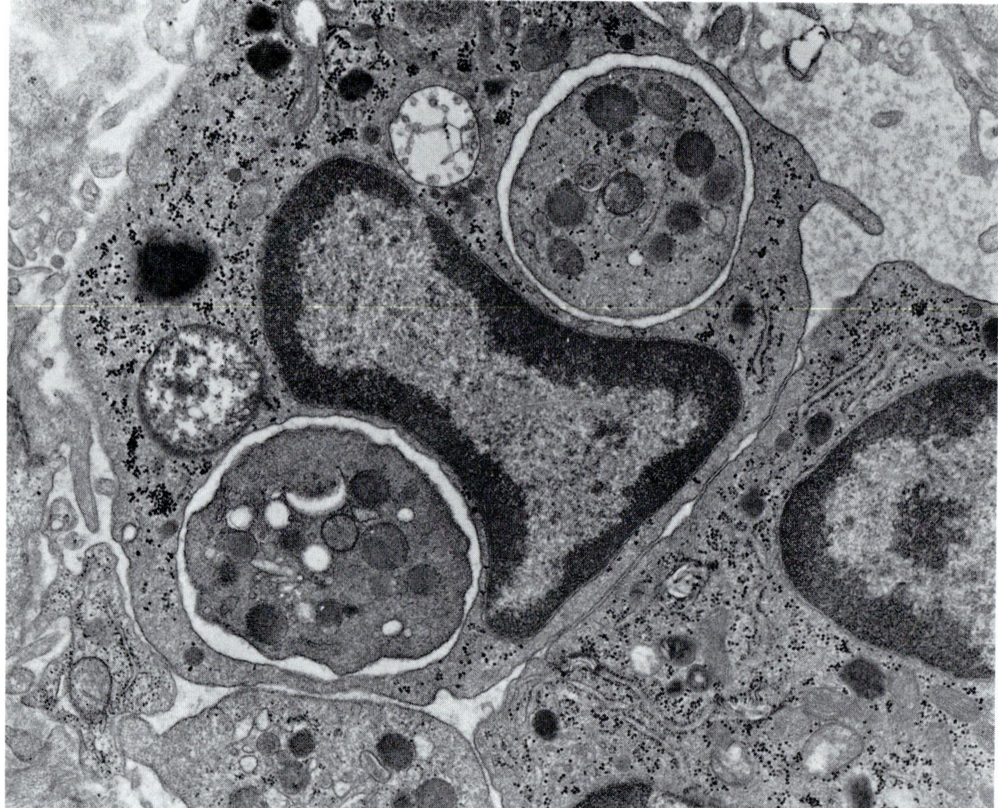

Fig. 5-31   Phagocytosis of platelets by a PMN (rat Masugi nephritis; 6 hours after injection of rabbit NTAb).   ×16,000.

a. Formation of nephritogenic immune complexes

It has been well established that in acute serum sickness in the rabbit, the injected antigen is eliminated from the circulation in three phases consisting of; (1) an equilibration of the antigen between the intravascular and extravascular fluid spaces, (2) non-immune catabolism by the host, and (3) a rapid elimination resulting from the formation of antigen-antibody complexes [37, 52].   As cited before, acute serum sickness diseases are apparently evoked by tissue depositions of antigen excess and soluble immune complexes produced during the third phase of antigen elimination [37, 52].   The peak incidence of glomerulonephritis is found shortly after complete elimination and it may tend to resolve at the time when free antibody appears in the circulation.   In fact animals exhibiting a rapid rate of immune elimination usually develop severe glomerulonephritis whereas those exhibiting a slower rate do not [55, 210].   It was shown that circulating immune complexes were for the most part entrapped and catabolized by the reticuloendothelial system, particularly in the liver, and were deposited in the renal glomeruli in a very limited proportion [8, 107, 211].   Some modifications of classical one-shot serum sickness have been reported with an attempt to enhance the host immune response and, accordingly, to increase the incidence of glomerulonephritis [89, 168].   However, some rabbits may not show any of manifestations of serum sickness despite a good antibody response [55], indicating that the immune elimination is not always correlated to the induction of serum sickness diseases.

Possible factors governing the incidence have been investigated and, of these, the size of immune complexes has been thought to be the most important factor.   Cochrane and Hawkins examined the relationship between the size and tissue localization of immune complexes [23].   Among various sizes of soluble complexes prepared in vitro, only those having a sedimentation rate greater than 19S readily localized in arteries of guinea pigs. Increased vascular permeability (histamine injection) was crucial for the deposition but complement was found to have no effect on the ability of circulating complexes to localize in vessel walls.   In acute one-shot serum sickness in rabbits, it was again confirmed that rabbits having heavy or rapidly sedimenting BSA-antiBSA complexes (more than 19S in size) developed severe arterial and glomerular lesions whereas those with light or slowly sedimenting complexes did not.   Although both groups similarly showed marked depletion of hemolytic complement activity, immunofluorescence demonstrated glomerular localization of the complexes only in the former group.   They concluded that the ability of circulating immune complexes to become deposited in the tissue site was related essentially to the size of the complexes rather than to other factors.   A similar size of complexes might be circulating in rabbits with chronic serum sickness nephritis [211].   Although larger complexes are generally nephritogenic, very large complexes are often aggregated within the capillaries resulting in aggregate anaphylaxis of animals before the development of inflammation [101].   Dreesman and Germuth analyzed the nature of nephritogenic complexes in acute serum sickness [38].   The size of BSA-antiBSA complexes circulating in rabbits bearing proliferative glomerulonephritis was calculated to be 3–5×10^5 daltons. This suggested that since the complexes were formed in the presence of excess antigen, the molecular composition of the complexes ranged from $Ag_2 Ab$ to $Ag_3 Ab_2$, if it is correct to assume that the complexes are solely composed of BSA and IgG antibody.   The antiBSA antibody was indeed of the IgG class with a low avidity.   Occasionally complexes consisting of IgM antibody were produced which caused lytic-necrotizing glomerular changes with mesangial proliferation.

It was reported that antigen excess, soluble complexes were also pathogenetic for the development of chronic serum sickness nephritis [34].   Germuth et al. investigated the interrelationship between immune complex composition and size, site of immune complex localization within the glomerulus, and the character of the glomerular injury, employing chronic BSA-rabbit system [56].   With daily injections of a fixed amount of BSA (12.5 mg), the antibody response was variable in each animal.   The high responder quickly cleared injected BSA without the development of any glomerular abnormalities.   In rabbits exhibiting an intermediate immune response, immune complexes and complement were found to be localized in the mesangium.   The size of the complexes was estimated to be 1×10^6 daltons or greater, which might be too large to penetrate the GBM.   The mesangial deposits were less harmful to the glomerulus unless the deposition was so extreme as to exhaust the sequestration capability of the mesangium.   The diposits disappeared within a few days following cessation of antigen injection.   Severe proliferative glomerulonephritis was observed only in those animals exhibiting low antibody responses.   The immune complexes were composed of highly avid IgG antibody and persisted in the circulation for as long as 24 hours after antigen injection.   Their size ranged from 5 to 7×10^5 daltons which corresponded to $Ag_3 Ab_2$ or $Ag_4 Ag_3$.   The complexes were deposited across the GBM at the subepithelial regions.   The occurrence of membranous nephropathy was also found in this low responder group, mostly in the animals receiving a dose of antigen smaller than 12.5 mg [57].   They suggested that with injections of the smaller doses of antigen, a slow and gradual deposition of the complexes in the glomerulus might follow with a minimal lytic, inflammatory change.

The mechanism of the induction of membranous nephropathy has been interpreted by other investigators in somewhat different ways.   Pincus et al. clarified that in addition to quantity of antibody, quality of antibody might play an important role in the development of chronic serum sickness [150].   With daily injections of 10 mg of BSA over a period of 10 weeks, chronic glomerulonephritis was observed only in rabbits forming complexes composed of non-precipitating antibody.   Animals with membranous nephropathy has a low molecular weight complex while those with proliferative glomerulonephritis had a complex heavier than 19S.   They concluded that complexes formed with non-precipitating antibody, which were less rapidly removed from the circulation, would have a greater opportunity to deposit in glomeruli and induce glomerulonephritis.   Kuriyama [96] and Nakabayashi [134] also reported that membranous nephropathy developed in rabbits showing a decline of precipitating efficiency of antibody and the production of antibody of low avidity in the later stage of antigenic stimulation.   In contrast, in other rabbits showing a continuous synthesis of antibody of high avidity, mesangioproliferative glomerulonephritis developed.

b. Deposition mechanisms of circulating immune complexes

Circulating immune complexes, likewise carbon or other foreign materials, are entrapped mostly by the cells of the RES.   Benacerraf et al. revealed that unusual depositions of carbon particles occurred in mice subsequent to the RES blockade by thorotrast or administrations of vasoactive amines [7].   Injection of preformed immune complexes was also effective for this by possible activation of vasoactive amines.   There might be at least two factors influencing tissue depositon of immune complexes, the state of RES function and the participation of vasoactive amines respectively.   It is reasonable to expect that dysfunction of the RES enables immune complexes to circulate more persistently in the blood and, accordingly, enhances glomerular deposition.   On the other hand, it was suggested that the nature of antibody was important in determining the tissue localization of immune complexes.   Haakenstad et al. prepared immune complexes with reduced and alkylated antibodies in vitro [64, 65].   They showed that these complexes persisted longer in the circulation than complexes prepared with intact antibodies upon intravenous injection into mice.   The persistence was attributed to decreased hepatic RES localization of the complexes.   Interestingly this led to increased, persistent localization of the complexes in renal glomeruli.

The fact that tissue deposition of immune complexes is not a process of simple diffusion but an active process mediated by many factors, notably by vasoactive amines, has been emphasized by Cochrane et al. [20, 23, 25, 90].   In acute serum sickness in rabbits, a state of increased vascular permeability existed during the time immune complexes were depositing from the circulation.   Antagonists of vasoactive amines given at the time immune complexes appeared in the circulation, prevented in great part their deposition in tissue sites [25].   Moreover when rabbit platelets, the most important reservoir of vasoactive amines (histamine and serotonin) were depleted, deposition of immune complexes was markedly suppressed.   In studying the release mechanism of vasoactive amines from platelets, they proposed a basophil-dependent pathway [25, 90], as follows; basophilic leukocytes with adherent IgE antibody release a soluble intermediary upon interaction with antigen; the intermediary then activates platelets to clump and to release vasoactive amines, initiating an increase in vascular permeability whereby immune complexes enter and become entrapped along filtering membrane of the vessel wall to induce injury.

It has been known that the movement of macromolecules from the capillary lumen into and across the GBM is influenced by their electrical charge.   Cationized ferritins, for example, gained access more easily into all layers of the GBM than native anionic ferritin [156].   Conversely abnormal glomerular filtration of anionic polymer (dextran sulfate) was observed in nephritic rats in keeping with the reduction of the content of GBM sialoprotein [9].   In view of these results it appears that the electric charge of circulating immune complexes would be a factor that influences their deposition into the GBM, though this possibility could not be proved in previous study [23].   In any case, the question how such macromolecules as immune complexes gain across the GBM and are entrapped at the subepithelial sites remains to be answered.   The assumption that the fatigue of the phagocytic property of mesangial cells is responsible for GBM accumulation of immune complexes [211] is unlikely since the bulk of evidence obtained from the observations in passive serum sickness does not support it.   It is still probable that mesangial cells may somehow modulate deposition sites of immune complexes [55].   Also important are hydrodynamic factors that influence tissue deposition of immune complexes.   Arterial lesions in acute rabbit serum sickness were most frequently found at areas of blood turbulence, such as branches, bifurcations, and artificial coarctations [90].   In addition, hypertension apparently increased the incidence and severity of acute serum sickness lesions [47].   Either unilateral clamping of the renal artery or ligation of the ureter resulted in diminished deposition of circulating immune complexes [54].

c. Fate of immune complexes deposited

The first step of immune complex nephritis is undoubtedly glomerular deposition of antigen and antibody in the form of immune complexes.   Nonetheless, antigen or antibody may not always be demonstrated by immunofluorescence in an inflamed glomerulus.   Fish et al. stated that antigen could be visualized in immunofluorescence at the early limited stage and, later, only antibody and C3 were detectable as a discrete subepithelial mass [46].   By using I*BSA, Wilson and Dixon disclosed that the rabbit kidneys examined following 99% antigen elimination contained 1 to 35 μg of I*BSA, the detectable antigen in immunofluorescence being as little as 0.25 μg/g of kidney of I*BSA [210].   The I*BSA disappeared from the kidney with a half time of about 10 days.   Therefore the difficulty in demonstrating antigen was not attributable to a rapid catabolism of immune complexes deposited but to continued covering of antigenic site(s) by host antibody.   They speculated that antigen excess complexes just deposited were nephritogenic while those accumulated at the subepithelial site were no longer phlogogenic in spite of continued interaction with antibody and complement.   Not infrequently, however, there might be many other occasions in which no correlation could be ascertained between the immunofluorescent findings and the severity of glomerulonephritis [55].   In our limited experience, the localization of antigen and antibody was often minimal in the severest lytic, exudative glomerular injury.   Three possible pathways could account for the sparse presence of immune complexes in the glomeruli with florid inflammation.   First, the complexes are largely removed and catabolized by infiltrating PMNs or monocytes as has been shown in other experiments [25].   Second, the complexes are quickly dispersed into Bowman's space under the condition of greatly increased permeability of the GBM.   Third, the paucity of visible deposits is ascribed to formation of relatively small complexes, which tend to be dissolved during the immune phase of antigen elimination, rather than being later aggregated [55].   In general subepithelial dense deposits(humps) appear later in the course of acute serum sickness nephritis.   Although the deposits are regarded as an ultrastructural hallmark of immune complex nephritis, it has been agreed that the humps are by no means responsible for the initiation of active inflammation [3, 46, 168].

Our knowledge concerning the nephritogenic property and fate of immune deposits in chronic immune complex nephritis is also incomplete at present.   As mentioned before, some differences in the nature of immune complexes are important in determining their deposition sites and morphologic manifestations.   Apart from such considerations, it is clear that continued glomerular depositions of complexes inevitably lead to variable histologic as well as functional distrortion of the affected glomeruli.   Especially abundant subepithelial depositions are usually accompanied by GBM thickening and marked proteinuria. In studying chronic, progressive serum sickness nephritis in the rabbit produced by daily injections of BSA, Wilson and Dixon stated that the daily renal deposition rate of BSA was 0.04 per cent of the injected dose before the onset of proteinuria but, thereafter, it increased about 12–15-fold [211].   The half-disappearance rate of the renal-bound BSA was found to be about 5 days.   Injection of excess amounts of BSA resulted in a striking increase in the rate of this disappearance, suggesting that the deposited immune complexes were dissolved in the presence of excess antigen.   When the deposition of complexes in glomeruli was stopped by cessation of antigen injection, normal structure and function might slowly return [55].   This corresponded well to the decrease of deposits observed by immunofluorescence and electron microscopy.   It was revealed that the disappearance of antigen was first seen and then that of antibody followed, and C3 was detectable as long as 3 months [55].   Two to three months after cessation of antigen injection, typical dense subepithelial deposits were no longer detectable [34].   However, neither morphologic nor functional improvements were achieved in the glomeruli involved in severe inflammatory lesions, regardless of cessation of antigen injection.

d. Mediators of immune complex nephritis

In the Arthus reaction, it has been emphasized that antigen-antibody interaction *per se* is not injurious for tissues and that PMNs play a central role in initiating the inflammatory process [24].   In this concept immune complexes formed at the tissue sites merely act as a material capable of attracting PMNs via complement fixation.   The development of necrotizing angiitis involved in immune complex diseases might be mediated by a similar mechanism.   Either complement or PMN depletion resulted in marked suppression of the vascular lesion despite local deposition of immune complexes [89].   The observations imply that immune complexes deposited in glomeruli activate a number of mediators thereby inducing acute inflammation.   Unfortunately there is a notable difference in the situation between immune complex angiitis and glomerulonephritis.   It was found that acute serum sickness nephritis did occur even under the circumstance of PMN and complement depletion [73, 89].   If so, one might wonder about the role of complement fixed in the affected glomeruli of serum sickness nephritis.   In any case, it appears that PMN emigration is usually minimal in acute serum sickness nephritis.   An appreciable participation of PMNs has only been proved in passive serum sickness nephritis [49, 144].   In view of this fact, underlying mechanisms other than the PMN-dependent pathway should be considered to account for the pathogenesis of acute immune complex nephritis.   In brief, however, very little information is at hand as to the sequence of cellular and chemical events taking place subsequent to glomerular deposition of immune complexes, unless we accept an unlikely hypothesis that immune complexes are themselves injurious in the glomerulus but not in other tissue sites.   Presumably a number of mediators are also involved in immune complex nephritis as discussed in the previous section dealing with the pathogenesis of Masugi nephritis.

The mediation mechanisms of chronic immune complex nephritis are far more obscure, though the persistent presence of abundant complexes is belived to cause turbulence of structural and functional integrity of the glomerulus.

IV. Conclusions

A new era in the field of experimental glomerulonephritis has obviously started since the successful production of nephrotoxic nephritis by Masugi and associates. The high reproducibility of Masugi nephritis has virtually been furnishing us a bulk of opportunities to analyze morphologic and functional alterations of inflamed renal glomeruli. A tremendous advance in the pathology of glomerular disease has been achieved on the basis of investigations on Masugi nephritis and immune complex nephritis subsequently introduced. With the aid of electron microscopy, the nature of minute as well as highly complicated changes of various glomerular diseases has been clarified, making it possible to evaluate more precisely the relationship between the morphologic findings and functional disturbances. Underlying mechanisms leading to the development of glomerular injury along with localization sites of causative immune reactants can be determined by concurrent immunologic studies. The results of the investigations being performed currently are able to account for the basic pathogenesis and sequence of morphologic events of various types of experimental glomerulonephritis induced by immunologic means. Much of the evidence obtained may also be available for the consideration of human glomerulonephritis. Accordingly some old concepts based upon previous observations are now being replaced by new ones. The current studies, however, have yielded a number of important questions to be answered.

The inflammatory process taking place in renal glomeruli could not always be accounted for by the simple concept of immunologic inflammation. For example there is a definite difference in morphologic events between acute immune complex nephritis and Arthus inflammation, despite a common mechanism in terms of local deposition of immune complexes in the microvasculature. This suggests that in addition to amounts and properties of immune reactants, the structural organization of the tissue involved is important in determining the morphologic manifestations. On the contrary, there often exists a broad resemblance between antiGBM nephritis and immune complex nephritis relative to the acute glomerular inflammation manifested, implicating that both share common processes of inflammation despite the difference of the immune mechanisms. A number of factors have been claimed to govern the pathologic process in experimental glomerulonephritis as discussed in previous sections. Unfortunately very limited knowledge is at hand concerning intermediatories of inflammation which are presumed to be actually operative in producing glomerular injury. Complement components, a known inflammatory mediator, play a role in rat Masugi nephritis but in many other occasions do not. The behavior of PMNs and mononuclear phagocytes is diverse; they apparently contribute to the initiation of inflammation while at other times they play a role in tissue repair. These participants, in concert with others, may contribute to the induction, repair, or progression of glomerular inflammation and their role may be varied owing to the etiology and stage of the disease process.

In brief, there are a large number of questions to be settled to explain the entire problem of immunologic glomerular injury.

REFERENCES

1. Aarons, I.: Renal immunofluorescence in NZB/NZW mice. *Nature 203*: 1080–1081, 1964.
2. Alousi, M.A., Post, R.S., and Heymann, W.: Experimental autoimmune nephrosis in rats. *Amer. J.* Clin. *Path. 54*: 47–71, 1969.
3. Arakawa, M. and Kimmelstiel, P.: The glomerulonephritis of acute serum sickness. A study using light and electron microscopy. *Amer. J. Clin. Path. 54*: 60–70, 1970.
4. Barthold, D.R., Kysela, S., and Steinberg, A.D.: Decline in suppressor T cell function with age in female NZB mice. *J. Immunol. 112*: 9–16, 1974.
5. Battifora, H.A. and Markowitz, A.S.: Nephrotoxic nephritis in monkeys. Sequential light, immunofluorescence, and electron microscopic studies. *Amer. J. Path. 55*: 267–281, 1969.
6. Becker, E.L. and Henson, P.M.: In vitro studies of immunologically induced secretion of mediators from cells and related phenomena. *Adv. Immunol. 17*: 94–193, 1973.
7. Benacerraf, B., McCluskey, R.A., and Patras, D.: Localization of colloidal substances in vascular endothelium. A mechanism of tissue damage. I. Factors causing the pathologic deposition of colloidal carbon. *Amer. J. Path. 35*: 75–91, 1959.
8. Benacerraf, B., Sebestyen, M., and Cooper, N.S.: The clearance of antigen-antibody complexes from the blood by the reticuloendothelial system. *J. Immunol. 82*: 131–137, 1959.
9. Bennett, C.M., Glassock, R.J., Chang, R.L., Deen, W.M., Robertson, C.R., and Brenner, B.M.: Permselectivity of the glomerular capillary wall. Studies of experimental glomerulonephritis in the rat using dextran sulfate. *J. Clin. Invest. 57*: 1287–1294, 1976.
10. Bergstein, J.M., Hoyer, J.R., and Michael, A.F.: Glomerular fibrinolytic activity following endotoxin-induced glomerular fibrin deposition in the pregnant rat. *Amer. J. Path. 75*: 195–200, 1974.
11. Bloom, B.R.: In vitro approaches to the mechanism of cell-mediated immune reactions. *Adv. Immunol. 13*: 101–208, 1971.
12. Blozis, G.G., Spargo, B., and Rowley, D.A.: Glomerular basement membrane changes with the nephrotic syndrome in the rat by homologous kidney and Hemophilus pertussis vaccine. *Amer. J. Path. 40*: 153–165, 1962.
13. Burkholder, P.M.: Complement fixation in diseased tissues. I. Fixation of guinea pig complement in sections of kidney from human with membranous glomerulonephritis and rats injected with anti-rat kidney serum. *J. Exp. Med. 114*: 605–616, 1961.
14. Casley-Smith, J.R., Ardlie, N.G., and Schwartz, C.J.: Electron microscopical observations on the organization of artificial thrombi in the rabbit pulmonary artery. *Brit. J. Exp. Path. 48*: 501–506, 1967.
15. Chandler, A.B. and Hand, R.A.: Phagocytized platelets: a source of lipids in human thrombi and atherosclerotic plaques. *Science 134*: 946–947, 1961.
16. Channing, A.A., Kasuga, T., Horowitz, R.E., Dubois, E.L., and Demopoulos, H.B.: An ultrastructural study of spontaneous lupus nephritis in the NZB/NZW mouse. *Amer. J. Path. 47*: 677–694, 1965.
17. Chiu, J. and Drummond, K.N.: Chemical and histochemical studies of glomerular sialoprotein in nephrotoxic nephritis in rats. *Amer. J. Path. 68*: 391–406, 1972.
18. Churg, J., Grishman, E., and Mautner, W.: Nephrotoxic serum nephritis in the rat. Electron and light microscopic studies. *Amer. J. Path. 37*: 729–749, 1960.
19. Churg, J. and Sakaguchi, H.: Vascular lesions in anti-kidney serum nephritis of the rat. *Amer. J. Path. 47*: 953–963, 1965.
20. Cochrane, C.G.: Mechanisms involved in the deposition of immune complexes in tissues. *J. Exp. Med. 134*: 75s–89s, 1971.
21. Cochrane, C.G. and Aikins, B.S.: Polymorphonuclear leukocytes in immunologic reactions: The destruction of vascular basement membrane in vivo and in vitro. *J. Exp. Med. 124*: 733–752, 1966.
22. Cochrane, C.G. and Dixon, F.J.: Antigen-antibody complex induced disease. *In* Miescher, P.A. and Müller-Eberhard, H.J. (eds.): *Textbook of Immunopathology*, 2nd ed., Vol. 1, 137–156, Grune & Stratton, New York, San Francisco, and London, 1976.

23. Cochrane, C.G. and Hawkins, D.: Studies on circulating immune complexes. III. Factors governing the ability of circulating complexes to localize in blood vessels. *J. Exp. Med. 127*: 137–153, 1968.

24. Cochrane, C.G. and Janoff, A.: The Arthus reaction: A model of neutrophil and complement mediated injury. *In* Zweifach, B.W., Grant, L., and McCluskey, R.T. (eds.): *The Inflammatory Process*, 2nd ed., Vol. III, 85–162, Academic Press, New York and London, 1974.

25. Cochrane, C.G. and Koffler, D.: Immune complex disease in experimental animals and man. *Adv. Immunol. 16*: 185–164, 1973.

26. Cochrane, C.G., Unanue, E.R., and Dixon, F.J.: A role of polymorphonuclear leukocytes and complement in nephrotoxic nephritis. *J. Exp. Med. 122*: 99–116, 1965.

27. Cohn, Z.A. and Hirsch, J.G.: The isolation and properties of the specific cytoplasmic granules of rabbit polymorphonuclear leukocytes. *J. Exp. Med. 112*: 983–1004, 1960.

28. Couser, W.G., Spargo, B.H., Stilmant, M.M., and Lewis, E.J.: Experimental glomerulonephritis in the guinea pig. II. Ultrastructural lesions of the basement membrane associated with proteinuria. *Lab. Invest. 32*: 46–55, 1975.

29. Couser, M.G., Stilmant, M.M., and Jermanovich, N.B.: Complement-independent nephrotoxic nephritis in the guinea pig. *Kid. Intern. 11*: 170–180, 1977.

30. Couser, W.G., Stilmant, M.M., and Lewis, E.J.: Experimental glomerulonephritis in the guinea pig. I. Glomerular lesions associated with antiglomerular basement membrane antibody deposits. *Lab. Invest. 29*: 236–243, 1973.

31. David, J.R. and David, R.R.: Cellular hypersensitivity and immunity. *Progr. Allergy 16*: 300–449, 1972.

32. Davies, P., Page, R.C., and Allison, A.C.: Changes in cellular enzyme levels and extracellular release of lysosomal acid hydrolases in macrophages exposed to group A streptococcal cell wall substance. *J. Exp. Med. 139*: 1262–1282, 1974.

33. Dixon, F.J.: The pathogenesis of glomerulonephritis. *Amer. J. Med. 44*: 493–498, 1968.

34. Dixon, F.J., Feldman, J.D., and Vazquez, J.J.: Experimental glomerulonephritis. The pathogenesis of a laboratory model resembling the spectrum of human glomerulonephritis. *J. Exp. Med. 113*: 899–920, 1961.

35. Dixon, F.J., Oldstone, M.B.A., and Tonietti, G.: Pathogenesis of immune complex glomerulonephritis of New Zealand mice. *J. Exp. Med. 134*: 65s–71s, 1971.

36. Dixon, F.J., Unanue, E.R., and Watson, J.I.: Immunopathology of the kidney. *IVth Intern. Symp. Immunopath.* 363–373, 1965.

37. Dixon, F.J., Vazquez, J.J., Weigle, W.O., and Cochrane, C.G.: Pathogenesis of serum sickness. *Arch. Path. 65*: 18–28, 1958.

38. Dreesman, G.R. and Germuth, F.G.: Immune complex disease. IV. The nature of the circulating complexes associated with glomerulonephritis in the acute BSA-rabbit system. *Johns Hopkins Med. J. 130*: 335–343, 1972.

39. Edgington, T.S., Glassock, R.J., and Dixon, F.J.: Autologous immune complex nephritis induced with renal tubular antigen. I. Identification and isolation of the pathogenetic antigen. *J. Exp. Med. 127*: 555–572, 1968.

40. Edgington, T.S., Lee, S., and Dixon, F.J.: Persistence of the autoimmune pathogenetic process in experimental autologous immune complex nephritis. *J. Immunol. 103*: 528–536, 1969.

41. Feenstra, K., Lee, R.V.D., Breben, H.A., Arends, A., and Hoedemaeker, PH. J.: Experimental glomerulonephritis in the rat induced by antibodies directed against tubular antigens. I. The natural history: A histologic and immunohistologic study at the light microscopic and the ultrastructural level. *Lab. Invest. 32*: 235–242, 1975.

42. Feldman, J.D.: Electron microscopy of serum sickness nephritis. *J. Exp. Med. 28*: 108–962, 1958.

43. Feldman, J.D.: Pathogenesis of ultrastructural glomerular changes induced by immunologic means. *IIIrd Intern. Symp. Immunopath.* 263–281, 1963.

44. Feldman, J.D.: Ultrastructure of immunologic processes. *Adv. Immunol. 4*: 175–248, 1964.

45. Feldman, J.D., Hammer, D.K., and Dixon, F.J.: Experimental glomerulonephritis. III. Pathogenesis of glomerular ultrastructural lesions in nephrotoxic serum nephritis. *Lab. Invest. 12*: 748–763, 1963.

46. Fish, A.J., Michael, A.F., Vernier, R.L., and Good, R.A.: Acute serum sickness nephritis in the rabbit. An immune deposit disease. *Amer. J. Path. 49*: 997–1022, 1966.

47. Fisher, E.R. and Bark, J.: Effect of hypertension on vascular and other lesions of serum sickness. *Amer. J. Path. 39*: 665–679, 1961.

48. Fujimoto, T., Okada, M., Kondo, Y., and Tada, T.: The nature of Masugi nephritis. Histo- and immunopathological studies. *Acta Path. Jap. 14*: 275–310, 1964.

49. Gabbiani, G., Badonnel, M.-C., and Vassalli, P.: Experimental focal glomerular lesions elicited by insoluble immune complexes. Ultrastructural and immunofluorescent studies. *Lab. Invest. 32*: 33–45, 1975.

50. Gang, N.F., Mautner, W., and Kalant, N.: Nephrotoxic serum nephritis. II. Chemical, morphologic, and functional correlates of glomerular basement membrane at the onset of proteinuria. *Lab. Invest. 23*: 150–157, 1970.

51. Gang, N.F., Trachtenberg, E., Allerhand, J., Kalant, N., and Mautner, W.: Nephrotoxic serum nephritis. III. Correlation of proteinuria, excretion of the glomerular basement membrane-like protein, and changes in the ultrastructure of the glomerular basement membrane as visualized with lanthanum. *Lab. Invest. 23*: 436–441, 1970.

52. Germuth, F.G.: A comparative histologic and immunologic study in rabbits of induced hypersensitivity of the serum sickness type. *J. Exp. Med. 97*: 257–282, 1953.

53. Germuth, F.G., Choi, I., Taylor, J.J., and Rodriguez, E.: Antibasement membrane disease. I. The glomerular lesions of Goodpasture's disease and experimental disease in sheep. *Johns Hopkins Med. J. 131*: 367–384, 1972.

54. Germuth, F.G., Kelemen, W.A., and Pollack, A.O.: Immune complex disease. II. The role of circulatory dynamic and glomerular filtration in the development of experimental glomerulonephritis. *Johns Hopkins Med. J. 120*: 252–261, 1967.

55. Germuth, F.G. and Rodriguez, E.: *Immunopathology of the Renal Glomeruli*. Little, Brown and Company, Boston, 1973.

56. Germuth, F.G., Senterfit, L.B., and Dreesman, G.R.: Immune complex disease. V. The nature of the circulating complexes associated with glomerular alterations in the chronic BSA-rabbit system. *Johns Hopkins Med. J. 130*: 344–357, 1972.

57. Germuth, F.G., Senterfit, L.B., and Pollack, A.D.: Immune complex disease. I. Experimental acute and chronic glomerulonephritis. *Johns Hopkins Med. J. 120*: 225–251, 1967.

58. Glassock, R.J., Edgington, T.S., Watson, J.I., and Dixon, F.J.: Autologous immune complex nephritis induced with renal tubular antigen. II. The pathogenetic mechanism. *J. Exp. Med. 127*: 573–588, 1968.

59. Goldstein, I.M.: Lysosomal hydrolases and inflammatory materials. *In* Weissmann, G. (ed.): *Mediators of Inflammation*, 51–84, Plenum Press, New York and London, 1974.

60. Goldstein, I.M., Wunschmann, B., Astrup, T., and Henderson, E.S.: Effects of bacterial endotoxin on the fibrinolytic activity of normal human leukocytes. *Blood 37*: 447–462, 1971.

61. Gordon, S., Unkeless, J.C., and Cohn, Z.A.: Induction of macrophage plasminogen activator by endotoxin stimulation and phagocytosis. Evidence for a two-stage process. *J. Exp. Med. 140*: 995–1010, 1974.

62. Grishman, E., Porush, J.C., Rosen, S.M., and Churg, J.: Lupus nephritis with organized deposits in the kidneys. *Lab. Invest. 16*: 717–725, 1967.

63. Grupe, W.E. and Kaplan, M.H.: Demonstration of an antibody to proximal tubular antigen in the pathogenesis of experimental autoimmune nephrosis in rats. *J. Lab. Clin. Med. 74*: 400–409, 1969.

64. Haakenstad, A.O. and Mannik, M.: The disappearance kinetics of soluble immune complex prepared with reduced and alkylated antibodies and with intact antibodies in mice. *Lab. Invest. 35*: 283–292, 1976.

65. Haakenstad, A.O., Striker, G.E., and Mannik, M.: The glomerular deposition of soluble immune complex prepared with reduced and alkylated antibodies and with intact antibodies in mice. *Lab. Invest. 35*: 293–301, 1976.

66. Hammer, D.K. and Dixon, F.J.: Experimental glomerulonephritis. II. Immunologic events in the pathogenesis of nephrotoxic serum nephritis in the rat. *J. Exp. Med. 117*: 1019–1034, 1963.

67. Hawkins, D. and Cochrane, C.G.: Glomerular basement membrane damage in immunological glomerulonephritis. *Immunology 14*: 665–681, 1968.

68. Hawn, C.V.Z. and Janeway, C.A.: Histological and serological sequences in experimental hypersensitivity. *J. Exp. Med. 85*: 571–590, 1947.

69. Hayashi, H.: The intracellular neutral SH-dependent protease associated with inflammatory reactions. *Intern. Rev. Cytol. 40*: 101–151, 1975.

70. Hayashi, H., Yoshinaga, M., and Yamamoto, S.: The nature of a mediator of leucocyte chemotaxis in inflammation. *In* Sorkin, E. and Platz, D. (eds.): *Antibiotics and Chemotherapy*, Vol. 19, Chemotaxis: Its Biology and Biochemistry, 296–332, S. Kager, Basel, 1974.

71. Helyer, B.J. and Howie, J.B.: Renal disease associated with positive lupus erythematosus tests in a cross-bred strain of mice. *Nature 197*: 197–197, 1963.

72. Henson, P.M.: Mechanisms of mediator release from inflammatory cells. *In* Weissmann, G.: (ed.): *Mediators of Inflammation*, 9–50, Plenum Press, New York and London, 1974.

73. Henson, P.M. and Cochrane, C.G.: Acute immune complex disease in rabbits. The role of complement and of a leukocyte-mediated release of vasoactive amines from platelets. *J. Exp. Med. 133*: 554–571, 1971.

74. Henson, J.B., Gorham, J.R., Padgett, G.A., Wash, P., and Davis, W.C.: Pathogenesis of the glomerular lesions in Aleutian disease of mink. Immunofluorescent studies. *Arch. Path. 87*: 21–28, 1969.

75. Henson, J.B., Gorham, J.R., and Tanaka, Y.: Renal glomerular ultrastructure in mink affected by Aleutian disease. *Lab. Invest. 17*: 123–139, 1967.

76. Henson, J.B., Gorham, J.R., Tanaka, Y., and Padgett, G.A.: The sequential development of ultrastructural lesions in the glomeruli of mink with experimental Aleutian disease. *Lab. Invest. 19*: 153–168, 1968.

77. Heymann, W., Hackel, D.B., Harwood, S., Wilson, S.G.F., and Hunter, J.L.P.: Production of nephrotic syndrome in rats by Freund's adjuvant and rat kidney suspensions. *Proc. Soc. Exp. Biol. Med. 100*: 660–664, 1959.

78. Hicks, J.D. and Burnet, F.M.: Renal lesions in the "auto-immune" mouse strains NZB and F1 NZB/NZW. *J. Path. Bact. 91*: 467–477, 1966.

79. Hovig, T., Jørgensen, L., Rowsell, H.C., and Mustard, J.F.: The structure of thrombus-like deposits formed in extracorporeal shunts. *Amer. J. Path. 59*: 75–99, 1970.

80. Howie, J.B. and Helyer, B.J.: The immunology and pathology of NZB mice. *Adv. Immunol. 9*: 215–266, 1968.

81. Huber, H., Polley, M.J., Linscott, W.D., Fudenberg, H.H., and Müller-Eberhard, J.H.: Human monocytes: Distinct receptor sites for the third component of complement and for immunoglobulin G. *Science 162*: 1281–1283, 1968.

82. Jones, D.B.: Inflammation and repair of the glomerulus. *Amer. J. Path. 27*: 991–1009, 1951.

83. Jones, D.B.: Glomerulonephritis. *Amer. J. Path. 29*: 33–51, 1953.

84. Jørgensen, L., Rowsell, H.C., Hovig, T., and Mustard, J.F.: Resolution and organization of platelet-rich mural thrombi in carotid arteries of swine. *Amer. J. Path. 51*: 681–719, 1967.

85. Kay, C.F.: The mechanism by which experimental nephritis is produced in rabbits injected with nephrotoxic duck serum. *J. Exp. Med. 72*: 559–572, 1940.

86. Kelly, V.E. and Cavallo, T.: An ultrastructural study of the glomerular slit diaphragm in New Zealand Black/White mice. *Lab. Invest. 35*: 213–220, 1976.

87. Kinding, D., Spargo, B.H., and Kirsten, W.H.: Glomerular response in Aleutian disease of mink. *Lab. Invest. 16*: 436–447, 1967.

88. Klassen, J., Sugisaki, T., Milgrom, F., and McCluskey, R.T.: Studies on multiple renal lesions in Heymann nephritis. *Lab. Invest. 25*: 577–585, 1971.

89. Kniker, W.T. and Cochrane, C.G.: Pathogenic factors in vascular lesions of experimental serum sickness. *J. Exp. Med. 122*: 83–98, 1965.

90. Kniker, W.T. and Cochrane, C.G.: The localization of circulating immune complexes in experimental serum sickness. The role of vasoactive amines and hydrodynamic forces. *J. Exp. Med. 127*: 119–136, 1968.

91. Kobayashi, Y., Shigematsu, H., and Tada, T.: Nephritogenic properties of nephrotoxic guinea pig antibodies. I. Glomerulonephritis induced by guinea pig IgG_1 antibody in rats. *Virchows Arch. Abt. B 14*: 259–271, 1973.

92. Kobayashi, Y., Shigematsu, H., and Tada, T.: Nephritogenic properties of nephrotoxic guinea pig antibodies. II. Glomerular lesions induced by $F(ab')_2$ fragments of nephrotoxic IgG_1 antibody in rats. *Virchows Arch. Abt. B 15*: 35–44, 1973.

93. Kondo, Y. and Shigematsu, H.: Cellular aspects of rabbit Masugi nephritis. I. Cell kinetics in recoverable glomerulonephritis. *Virchows Arch. Abt. B 10*: 40–50, 1972.

94. Kondo, Y., Shigematsu, H., and Kobayashi, Y.: Cellular aspects of rabbit Masugi nephritis. II. Progressive glomerular injuries with crescent formation. *Lab. Invest. 27*: 620–631, 1972.

95. Kondo, Y., Shigematsu, H., and Okabayashi, Y.: Cellular aspects of rabbit Masugi nephritis. III. Mesangial changes. *Lab. Invest. 34*: 363–371, 1976.

96. Kuriyama, T.: Chronic glomerulonephritis induced by prolonged immunization in the rabbit. *Lab. Invest. 28*: 224–235, 1973.

97. Laguens, R. and Segal, A.: Experimental autologous immune-complex nephritis: An electron microscope and immunohistochemical study. *Exp. Mol. Path. 11*: 89–98 1969.

98. Lambert, P.H. and Dixon, F.J.: Pathogenesis of the glomerulonephritis of NZB/W mice. *J. Exp. Med. 127*: 507–522, 1968.

99. Lazarus, G.S., Brown, R.S., Daniels, J.R., and Fulimer, H.M.: Human granulocyte collagenase. *Science 159*: 1483–1485, 1968.

100. Lazarus, G.S., Daniels, J.R., Lian, J., and Burleigh, M.C.: Role of granulocyte collagenase in collagen degradation. *Amer. J. Path. 68*: 565–576, 1972.

101. Leber, P.D. and McCluskey, R.T.: Immune complex diseases. *In* Zweifach, B.W., Grant, L., and McCluskey, R.T. (eds.): *The Inflammatory Process*, 2nd ed., Vol. III., 401–441, Academic Press, New York, San Francisco, and London, 1974.

102. Lerner, R.A. and Dixon, F.J.: Transfer of ovine experimental allergic glomerulonephritis (EAG) with serum. *J. Exp. Med. 124*: 431–442, 1966.

103. Lindberg, L.H. and Rosenberg, L.T.: Nephrotoxic serum nephritis in mice with a genetic deficiency in complement. *J. Immunol. 100*: 34–38, 1968.

104. Lubaroff, D.M. and Waksman, B.H.: Bone marrow as source of cells in reactions of cellular hypersensitivity. I. Passive transfer of tuberculin sensitivity in syngeneic system. *J. Exp. Med. 128*: 1425–1435, 1968.

105. Lubaroff, D.M. and Waksman, B.H.: Bone marrow as source of cells in reactions of cellular hypersensitivity. II. Identification of allogeneic or hybrid cells by immunofluorescence in passively transferred tuberculin reactions. *J. Exp. Med. 128*: 1437–1449, 1968.

106. Manaligod, J.R., Krakower, C.A., and Greenspon, S.A.: Glomerular changes induced by extrarenal foci of inflammation and by polymorphonuclear cell lysates. *Amer. J. Path. 56*: 533–551, 1969.

107. Mannik, M. and Arend, W.P.: Fate of preformed immune complexes in rabbits and rhesus monkeys. *J. Exp. Med. 134*: 19s–31s, 1971.

108. Masugi, M.: Über das Wesen der spezifischen Veränderungen der Niere und der Leber durch das Nephrotoxin bzw. das Hepatotoxin. Zugleich ein Beitrag zur Pathogenese der Glomerulonephritis und der eklamptischen Lebererkrankung. *Beitr. Path. Anat. 91*: 82–112, 1933.

109. Masugi, M.: Über die experimentelle Glomerulonephritis durch das spezifische Antinierenserum. Ein Beitrag zur Pathogenese der diffusen Glomerulonephritis. *Beitr. Path. Anat. 92*: 429–466, 1934.

110. Masugi, M., Sato, Y., Murasawa, S., und Tomizuka, Y.: Über die experimentelle Glomerulonephritis durch das spezifische antinierenserum. *Trans. Jap. Path. Soc. 22*: 614–628, 1932.

111. Matsuoka, M., Sakuragawa, N., and Shimaoka, M.: Studies on fibrinolytic activities in normal human leucocytes. *Acta Med. Biol. (Niigata) 16*: 91–104, 1969.

112. Mauer, S.M., Sutherland, D.ER., Howard, R.J., Fish, A.J., Najarian, J.S., and Michael, A.F.: The glomerular mesangium. III. Acute immune mesangial injury: A new model of glomerulonephritis. *J. Exp. Med. 137*: 553–570, 1973.

113. McCluskey, R.T. and Benacerraf, B.: Localization of colloidal substances in vascular endothelium. A mechanism of tissue damage. II. Experimental serum sickness with acute glomerulonephritis induced passively in mice by antigen-antibody complexes in antigen excess. *Amer. J. Path. 35*: 275–283, 1959.

114. McCluskey, R.T., Benacerraf, B., Potter, J.L., and Miller, F.: The pathologic effects of intravenously administered soluble antigen-antibody complexes. I. Passive serum sickness in mice. *J. Exp. Med. 111*: 181–194, 1960.

115. McCluskey, R.T. and Vassalli, P.: Experimental glomerular diseases. *In* Rouiller, C. and Muller, A.F. (eds.): *The Kidney. Morphology, Biochemistry, Physiology,* Vol. II, 83–198, Academic Press, New York and London, 1969.

116. McGiven, A.R. and Hicks, J.D.: The development of renal lesions in NZB/NZW mice. Immunohistological studies. *Brit. J. Exp. Path. 48*: 302–204, 1967.

117. McGiven, A.R. and Lynraven, G.S.: Glomerular lesions in NZB/NZW mice. Electron microscopic study of development. *Arch. Path. 85*: 250–261, 1968.

118. McIvor, K.L. and Weiser, R.S.: Mechanisms of target cell destruction by alloimmune peritoneal macrophages. II. Release of a specific cytotoxin from interacting cells. *Immunol. 20*: 315–322, 1971.

119. McKay, D.G.: Participation of component of the blood coagulation system in the inflammatory response. *Amer. J. Path. 67*: 181–204, 1972.

120. McKay, D.G., Philips, L.L., Kaplan, H., and Henson, J.B.: Chronic intravascular coagulation in Aleutian disease of mink. *Amer. J. Path. 50*: 899–912, 1967.

121. Mellors, R.C.: Autoimmune disease in NZB/BL mice. I. Pathology and pathogenesis of a model system of spontaneous glomerulonephritis. *J. Exp. Med. 122*: 25–40, 1965.

122. Mellors, R.C.: Autoimmune and immunoproliferative diseases of NZB/B1 mice and hybrids. *Intern. Rev. Exp. Path. 5*: 217–252, 1966.

123. Mellors, R.C., Aoki, T., and Huebner, R.J.: Further implication of murine leukemia-like virus in the disorders of NZB mice. *J. Exp. Med. 133*: 1045–1062, 1969.

124. Mellors, R.C., Shirai, T., Aoki, T., Huebner, R.J., and Krawczynski, K.: Wild-type Gross leukemia virus and the pathogenesis of the glomerulonephritis of New Zealand mice. *J. Exp. Med. 133*: 113–132, 1971.

125. Miller, F. und Bohle, A.: Electronenmikroskopische Untersuchungen am Glomerulum bei der Masugi-Nephritis der Ratte. *Virchows Arch. Path. Anat. Histol. 330*: 483–497, 1957.

126. Moppert, J. und Fresen, K.O.: Experimentelle Glomerulonephritis und Glomerulonephrose bei der Maus nach wiederholten Ovalbumin-injectionen. Eine licht-, fluorescenz-, und electronenoptische Untersuchung. *Virchows Arch. Path. Anat. Histol. 342*: 304–318, 1967.

127. Morita, T., Kihara, I., Oite, T., and Yamamoto, T.: Participation of blood born cells in rat Masugi nephritis. *Acta Path. Jap. 26*: 409–422, 1976.

128. Movat, H.Z., McGregor, D.D., and Steiner, J.W.: Studies of nephrotoxic nephritis. II. The fine structure of the glomerulus in acute nephrotoxic nephritis of dogs. *Amer. J. Clin. Path. 36*: 306–321, 1961.

129. Movat, H.Z., Mustard, J.F., Taichman, N.S., and Uriuhara, T.: Platelet aggregation and release of ADP, serotonin, and histamine associated with phagocytosis of antigen-antibody complexes. *Proc. Soc. Exp. Biol. Med. 120*: 232–237, 1965.

130. Müller-Eberhard, H.J.: The serum complement system. *In* Miescher, P.A. and Müller-Eberhard, H.J. (eds.): *Textbook of Immunopathology,* 2nd ed., Vol. I, 45–73, Grune & Straton, New York, San Francisco, and London, 1976.

131. Mustard, J.F. and Packham, M.A.: The reaction of the blood to injury. *In* Movat, H.Z. (ed.): *Inflammation, Immunity and Hypersensitivity,* 527–607, Harper & Row Publishers, New York, Evanston, San Franciso, and London, 1971.

132. Myhre-Jensen, O.: Localization of fibrinolytic activity in the kidney and urinary tract of rats and rabbits. *Lab. Invest. 25*: 403–411, 1971.

133. Nairn, R.C., McGiven, A.R., Ironside, P.N.J., and Norins, L.C.: Plasma proteins in the glomerular lesions of NZB/NZW mice. *Brit. J. Exp. Path. 47*: 99–103, 1966.

134. Nakabayashi, M.: Immunochemical properties of rabbit antibodies in membranous glomerulonephritis. *Acta Path. Jap. 24*: 63–77, 1974.

135. Nelson, D.S.: Immune adherence. *Adv. Immunol. 3*: 97–180, 1963.

136. Nelson, D.S.: *Macrophages and Immunity,* North-Holland Publishing Co., Amsterdam and London, 1969.

137. Nelson, R.A.: The complement system. *In* Zweifach, B.W., Grant, L., and McCluskey, R.T. (eds.): *The inflammatory Process,* 2nd ed., Vol. III, 37–84, Academic Press, New York, San Francisco, and London, 1974.

138. Ohnuki, T.: Crescentic glomerulonephritis induced by homologous or heterologous glomerular basement membrane antigen in the goat. *Acta Path. Jap. 25*: 319–331, 1975.

139. Okabayashi, A.: Induction of a disease resembling systemic lupus erythematosus in later stage of prolonged sensitization in rabbits. *Acta Path. Jap. 14*: 345–371, 1964.

140. Okabayashi, A.: Nephritides and dysimmunization. With special reference to the significance of lytic process in immunologically induced experimental glomerulonephritis. *Jap. J. Nephrol. 12*: 1–17, 1970.

141. Okabayashi, A., Kondo, Y., and Shigematsu, H.: Cellular and histopathologic consequences of immunologically induced experimental glomerulonephritis. *Curr. Topics Path. 61*: 1–43, 1976.

142. Okuda, R., Kaplan, M.H., Cuppage, F.E., and Heymann, W.: Deposition of autologous gamma globulin in kidneys of rats with nephrotic renal disease of various etiologies. *J. Lab. Clin. Med. 66*: 204–215, 1965.

143. Okumura, K.: Induction of a disease resembling systemic lupus erythematosus in C57BL/6J mice by prolonged immunization with egg albumin. *Acta Path. Jap. 23*: 695–704, 1973.

144. Okumura, K., Kondo, Y., and Tada, T.: Studies on passive serum sickness. I. The glomerular fine structure of serum sickness nephritis induced by preformed antigen-antibody complexes in the mouse. *Lab. Invest. 24*: 383–391, 1971.

145. Ortega, L.G. and Mellors, R.C.: Analytical pathology. IV. The role of localized antibodies in the pathogenesis of nephrotoxic nephritis in the rat. *J. Exp. Med. 104*: 151–170, 1956.

146. Pan, I.C., Tsai, K.S., Grinyer, I., and Karstad, L.: Glomerulonephritis in Aleutian disease of mink: Ultrastructural studies. *J. Path. 102*: 33–40, 1970.

147. Pan, I.C., Tsai, K.S., and Karstad, L.: Glomerulonephritis in Aleutian disease of mink: Histological and immunofluorescence studies. *J. Path. 101*: 119–127, 1970.

148. Paronetto, F. and Koffler, D.: Autoimmune proliferative glomerulonephritis in monkeys. *Amer. J. Path. 50*: 887–894, 1967.

149. Piel, C.F., Dong, L., Modern, F.W.S., Goodman, J.R., and Moore, R.: The glomerulus in experimental renal disease in rats as observed by light and electron microscopy. *J. Exp. Med. 102*: 573–580, 1955.

150. Pincus, T., Haberkern, R., and Christian, C.L.: Experimental chronic glomerulitis. *J. Exp. Med. 127*: 819–832, 1968.

151. Porter, D.D. and Larsen, A.E.: Aleutian disease of mink: Infectious virus-antibody complexes in the serum. *Proc. Soc. Exp. Biol. Med. 126*: 680–682, 1967.

152. Porter, D.D., Larsen, A.E., and Porter, H.G.: The pathogenesis of Aleutian disease of mink. I. In vivo viral replication and the host antibody response to viral antigen. *J. Exp. Med. 130*: 575–593, 1969.

153. Rich, A.R.: Hypersensitivity in diseases; With especial reference to periarteritis nodosa, rheumatic fever, disseminated lupus erythematosus and rheumatoid arthritis. *Harvey Lect. 42 (1946-47)*: 106–147, 1947.

154. Rich, A.R. and Gregory, J.E.: The experimental demonstration that periarteritis nodosa is a manifestation of hypersensitivity. *Bull. Johns Hopkins Hosp. 72*: 65–82, 1943.

155. Riddle, J.M. and Barnhart, M.I.: Ultrastructural study of fibrin dissolution via emigrated polymorphonuclear neutrophils. *Amer. J. Path. 45*: 805–823, 1964.

156. Rennke, H.G. and Venkatachalam, M.A.: Glomerular permeability: *In Vitro* tracer studies with polyanionic and polycationic ferritins. *Kid. Intern. 11*: 44–53, 1976.

157. Robertson, D.M. and More, R.H.: Structure of glomerular axial region in normal and nephritic rabbits. *Arch. Path. 72*: 331–342, 1961.

158. Rother, K., Rother, U., Vassalli, P., and McCluskey, R.T.: Nephrotoxic serum nephritis in C'6-deficient rabbits. I. Study of the second phase of the disease. *J. Immunol. 98*: 965–971, 1967.

159. Sakaguchi, H., Suzuki, Y., and Yamaguchi, T.: Electron microscopic study of Masugi nephritis. I. Glomerular change. *Acta Path. Jap. 7*: 53–66, 1957.

160. Sano, M.: Participation of monocytes in glomerulonephritis in acute serum sickness of rabbit. *Acta Path. Jap. 26*: 423–433, 1976.

161. Sarre, H. und Wirtz, H.: Geschwindigkeit und Ort der "Nephrotoxin"-bindung bei der experimentellen Glomerulonephritis. *Klin. Wscher. 18*: 1548–1550, 1939.

162. Seegal, B.C., Hsu, K.C., and Andres, G.A.: Specific nephrotoxic nephritis: Old facts and present concepts. *IIIrd Intern. Symp. Immunopath.* 208–219, 1963.

163. Seegal, B.C., Hsu, K.C., Rothenberg, M.S., and Chapeu, M.L.: Studies of the mechanism of experimental nephritis with fluorescein-labeled antibody. II. Localization and persistence of injected rabbit or duck anti-rat-kidney serum during the course of nephritis in rats. *Amer. J. Path. 41:* 183–203, 1962.

164. Shibata, S., Sakaguchi, H., and Nagasawa, T.: Induction of chronic progressive glomerulonephritis with immunofluorescent 'mesangial pattern' in rats. *Nephron 16:* 241–255, 1976.

165. Shigematsu, H.: Glomerular events during the initial phase of rat Masugi nephritis. *Virchows Arch. Abt. B 5:* 187–200, 1970.

166. Shigematsu, H. and Kobayashi, Y.: The development and fate of the immune deposits in the glomerulus during the secondary phase of rat Masugi nephritis. *Virchows Arch. Abt. B 8:* 83–95, 1971.

167. Shigematsu, H. and Kobayashi, Y.: The distortion and disorganization of the glomerulus in progressive Masugi nephritis in the rat. *Virchows Arch. Abt. B 14:* 313–328, 1973.

168. Shigematsu, H. and Kobayashi, Y.: Accelerated serum sickness in the rabbit. II. Glomerular ultrastructural lesions in transient proliferative and progressive disorganizing glomerulonephritis. *Virchows Arch. Path. Anat. Histol. 369:* 269–282, 1976.

169. Shigematsu, H., Sano, M., Suguro, T., and Kobayashi, Y.: Accelerated serum sickness in the rabbit. III. Histopathological study of the development of tissue injuries of the heart. *Acta Path. Jap. 26:* 325–339, 1976.

170. Shimizu, F., Abe, F., Ito, K., and Kawamura, S.: On the age-associated presence of immunoglobulin and complement in the renal glomeruli of mice. *Contr. Nephrol. 6:* 79–93, 1977.

171. Shirai, T. and Mellors, R.C.: Natural thymocytotoxic autoantibody and reactive antigen in New Zealand Black and other mice. *Proc. Nat. Acad. Sci. 68:* 1412–1415, 1971.

172. Shirasawa, K. and Chandler, A.B.: Phagocytosis of platelets by leukocytes in artificial thrombi and in platelet aggregates induced by adenosine diphosphate. *Amer. J. Path. 63:* 215–224, 1971.

173. Simpson, I.J., Amos, N., Evans, D.J., Thompson, N.M., and Peters, D.K.: Guinea pig nephrotoxic nephritis. I. The role of complement and polymorphonuclear leukocytes and the effect of antibody subclass and fragments in the heterologous phase. *Clin. Exp. Immunol. 19:* 499–511, 1975.

174. Siqueira, M. and Nelson, R.A.: Platelet agglutination by immune complexes and its possible role in hypersensitivity. *J. Immunol. 86:* 516–525, 1961.

175. Snyderman, R. and Mergenhagen, S.E.: Chemotaxis of macrophages. *In* Nelson, D.S. (ed.): *Immunobiology of the Macrophages,* 323–348, Academic Press, New York, San Francisco, and London, 1976.

176. Sorkin, E., Borel, J.F., and Stecher, V.J.: Chemotaxis of mononuclear and polymorphonuclear phagocytes. *In* van Furth, R. (ed.): *Mononuclear Phagocytes,* 397–418, Blackwell Scientific Publications, Oxford and Edinburgh, 1970.

177. Steblay, R.W.: Glomerulonephritis induced in sheep by injections of heterologous glomerular basement membrane and Freund's complete adjuvant. *J. Exp. Med. 116:* 253–272, 1962.

178. Steblay, R.W.: Glomerulonephritis induced in monkeys by injections of heterologous glomerular basement membrane and Freund's adjuvant. *Nature 197:* 1173–1176, 1963.

179. Steblay, R.W. and Rudofsky, U.: In vitro and in vivo properties of autoantibodies eluted from kidneys of sheep with autoimmune glomerulonephritis. *Nature 218:* 1269–1271, 1968.

180. Steinman, R.H. and Cohn, Z.A.: The metabolism and physiology of the mononuclear phagocytes. *In* Zweifach, B.W., Grant, L., and McCluskey, R.T. (eds.): *The Inflammatory Process,* 2nd ed., Vol. I., 450–510, Academic Press, New York, San Francisco, and London, 1974.

181. Stilmant, M.M., Couser, W.G., and Cotran, R.S.: Experimental glomerulonephritis in the mouse associated with mesangial deposition of autologous ferritin immune complexes. *Lab. Invest. 32:* 746–756, 1975.

182. Sugisaki, T., Klassen, J., Andres, G.A., Milgrom, F., and McCluskey, R.T.: Passive transfer of Heymann nephritis with serum. *Kid. Intern. 3:* 66–73, 1973.

183. Suzuki, Y., Churg, J., Grishman, E., Mautner, W., and Dachs, S.: The mesangium of the renal glomerulus. Electron microscopic studies of pathologic alterations. *Amer. J. Path. 43:* 555–578, 1963.

184. Thomas, L.: Possible role of leucocyte granules in the Shwartzman and Arthus reactions. *Proc. Soc. Exp. Biol. Med. 115*: 235–240, 1964.

185. Thompson, N.M., Naish, P.F., Simpson, I.J., and Peters, D.K.: The role of C3 in the autologous phase of nephrotoxic nephritis. *Clin. Exp. Immunol. 24*: 464–473, 1976.

186. Turk, J.L.: *Delayed Hypersensitivity*. 2nd ed., North-Holland Publishing Co., Amsterdam and Oxford, 1975.

187. Unanue, E.R. and Dixon, F.J.: Experimental glomerulonephritis. IV. Participation of complement in nephrotoxic nephritis. *J. Exp. Med. 119*: 965–982, 1964.

188. Unanue, E.R. and Dixon, F.J.: Experimental glomerulonephritis. V. Studies on the interaction of nephrotoxic antibodies with tissues of the rat. *J. Exp. Med. 121*: 697–714, 1965.

189. Unanue, E.R. and Dixon, F.J.: Experimental glomerulonephritis. VI. The autologous phase of nephrotoxic serum nephritis. *J. Exp. Med. 121*: 715–725, 1965.

190. Unanue, E.R. and Dixon, F.J.: Experimental glomerulonephritis: Immunological events and pathogenetic mechanisms. *Adv. Immunol. 6*: 1–90, 1967.

191. Unanue, E.R. and Dixon, F.J.: Experimental allergic glomerulonephritis induced in the rabbit with heterologous renal antigens. *J. Exp. Med. 125*: 149–162, 1967.

192. Unanue, E.R. and Dixon, F.J.: Experimental allergic glomerulonephritis induced in the rabbit with homologous renal antigens. *J. Exp. Med. 125*: 163–176, 1967.

193. Unanue, E.R., Mardiney, M.R., and Dixon, F.J.: Nephrotoxic serum nephritis in complement intact and deficient mice. *J. Immunol. 98*: 609–617, 1967.

194. Unkeless, J.C., Gordon, S., and Reich, E.: Secretion of plasminogen activator by stimulated macrophages. *J. Exp. Med. 139*: 834–850, 1974.

195. Vassalli, P. and McCluskey, R.T.: The pathogenic role of the coagulation process in rabbit Masugi nephritis. *Amer. J. Path. 45*: 653–677, 1964.

196. Vassalli, P. and McCluskey, R.T.: The coagulation process and glomerular disease. *Amer. J. Med. 39*: 179–183, 1965.

197. Vassalli, P., Simon, G., and Rouiller, C.: Electron microscopic study of glomerular lesions resulting from intravascular fibrin formation. *Amer. J. Path. 43*: 579–617, 1963.

198. Vogt, A. and Kochem, H.G.: Immediate and delayed nephrotoxic nephritis in rats. The role of complement fixation. *Amer. J. Path. 39*: 379–392, 1961.

199. Volkman, A. and Gowans, J.L.: The production of macrophages in the rat. *Brit. J. Exp. Path. 46*: 50–61, 1965.

200. Volkman, A. and Gowans, J.L.: The origin of macrophages from bone marrow in the rat. *Brit. J. Exp. Path. 46*: 62–70, 1965.

201. Ward, P.A.: A plasmin-split fragment of C' as a new chemotactic factor. *J. Exp. Med. 126*: 189–206, 1967.

202. Ward, P.A., Cochrane, C.G., and Müller-Eberhard, H.J.: Further studies on the chemotactic factor of complement and its formation in vivo. *Immunology 11*: 141–153, 1966.

203. Ward, P.A. and Newman, L.T.: A neutrophil chemotactic facotr from human C'5. *J. Immunol. 102*: 93–99, 1969.

204. Warren, B.A. and Khan, S.: The ultrastructure of the lysis of fibrin by endothelium in vitro. *Brit. J. Exp. Path. 55*: 138–148, 1974.

205. Watanabe, T. and Tanaka, K.: The role of coagulation and fibrinolysis in the development of rabbit Masugi nephritis. *Acta Path. Jap. 26*: 147–165, 1976.

206. Weissmann, G., Zurier, R.B., and Hoffstein, S.: Leukocytic proteases and the immunologic release of lysosomal enzymes. *Amer. J. Path. 68*: 539–560, 1972.

207. Werb, Z. and Gordon, S.: Secretion of a specific collagenase by stimulated macrophages. *J. Exp. Med. 142*: 346–360, 1975.

208. Werb, Z. and Gordon, S.: Elastase secretion by stimulated macrophages. Characterization and regulation. *J. Exp. Med. 142*: 361–377, 1975.

209. Werdelin, O. and McCluskey, R.T.: The nature and the specificity of mononuclear cells in experimental autoimmune inflammations and the mechanisms leading to their accumulation. *J. Exp. Med. 133*: 1242–1263, 1971.

210. Wilson, C.B. and Dixon, F.J.: Antigen quantitation in experimental immune complex glomerulonephritis. I. Acute serum sickness. *J. Immunol. 105*: 279–290, 1970.

211. Wilson, C.B. and Dixon, F.J.: Quantitation of acute and chronic serum sickness in the rabbit. *J. Exp. Med. 134*: 7s-18s, 1971.
212. Yoshiki, T., Mellors, R.C., Strand, M., and August, J.T.: The viral envelope glycoprotein of murine leukemia virus and the pathogenesis of immune complex glomerulonephritis of New Zealand mice. *J. Exp. Med. 140*: 1011–1027, 1974.
213. Zucker, M.B.: Platelets. *In* Zweifach, B.W., Grant, L., and McCluskey, R.T. (eds.): *The Inflammatory Process*, 2nd ed., Vol. I, 511–543, Academic Press, New York, San Francisco, and London, 1974.

Chapter **6**

Nephrotoxic Serum Nephritis and Some Other Immunologically Induced Experimental Models: A Coherent View

Atsushi OKABAYASHI, Yoichiro KONDO, and Tomio TADA

I. Introduction

With the establishment of nephrotoxic serum or Masugi nephritis and other immunologically induced experimental models, abundant issues concerning morphologic and immunologic events in experimental glomerulonephritis have been successively described. Advances in the studies of immunologically induced experimental glomerulonephritis have been reviewed: Experimental Glomerulonephritis: Immunological Events and Pathogenetic Mechanisms (Unanue and Dixon, 1967) [66], Experimental Glomerular Diseases (McCluskey and Vassalli, 1969) [35], Immunopathology of the Renal Glomerulus: Immune Complex Deposit and Antibasement Membrane Disease (Germuth and Rodriguez, 1973) [16], Cellular and Histopathologic Consequences of Immunologically Induced Experimental Glomerulonephritis (Okabayashi et al., 1976) [49], and others. Undoubtedly the experimental results provide invaluable implications on the search for the immunopathology of human glomerular diseases.

In the experimental models induced by immunologic means, the glomerular alterations vary depending upon the amount and property of immune reactants which are produced either in situ or deposited in the form of immune complexes. This in turn indicates that the glomerular pathology is causatively related to the host immune response. In fact, for example, the aspect of prolonged antigenic stimulation leads one to imagine that crucial questions concerning glomerulonephritis can be settled by studying the behavior of the immune system.

In this chapter, while surveying some known models of experimental glomerulonephritis, the immunopathologic implications of these experimental studies will be discussed briefly.

II. Some Models of Immunologically Induced Experimental Glomerulonephritis

In the preceding chapter (Chapter 5) we have studied the fine structure of Masugi and some other experimental nephritides. For the present study it is proposed to outline certain important pathogenic aspects of experimental glomerulonephritis and then, to see the essential features in the animal models. Here almost the same experimental models as in Chapter 5 will be selected. They are: Masugi nephritis in rats and rabbits (Model 1),

Steblay nephritis in sheep and goats (Model 2), Heymann nephritis in rats (Model 3), serum sickness in rabbits (Model 4), prolonged antigenic stimulation in rabbits and C57BL mice (Model 5), Aleutian disease of mink (Model 6), New Zealand mouse disease (Model 7), and immunologically mediated glomerulitis of horses (Model 8).

1. Glomerulonephritis following injection of heterologous antikidney sera (nephrotoxic sera) in rats and rabbits — Masugi nephritis

Masugi for the first time presented unequivocal evidence of experimental production of glomerulonephritis by immunologic means, i.e., by using heterologous nephrotoxic sera [31–33].   In this experimental model, immediate glomerulonephritis is induced in animals with the injection of mammalian nephrotoxic antibodies (NTAbs) whereas there is a latent period before the onset of glomerular changes when fowl NTAbs are employed.   The latter case was a puzzling issue for Masugi and other investigators at that time.   Kay clearly settled this by showing that the latent period corresponded with the induction phase of the host antibody response [23].   At present, it has been interpreted that there are two se-

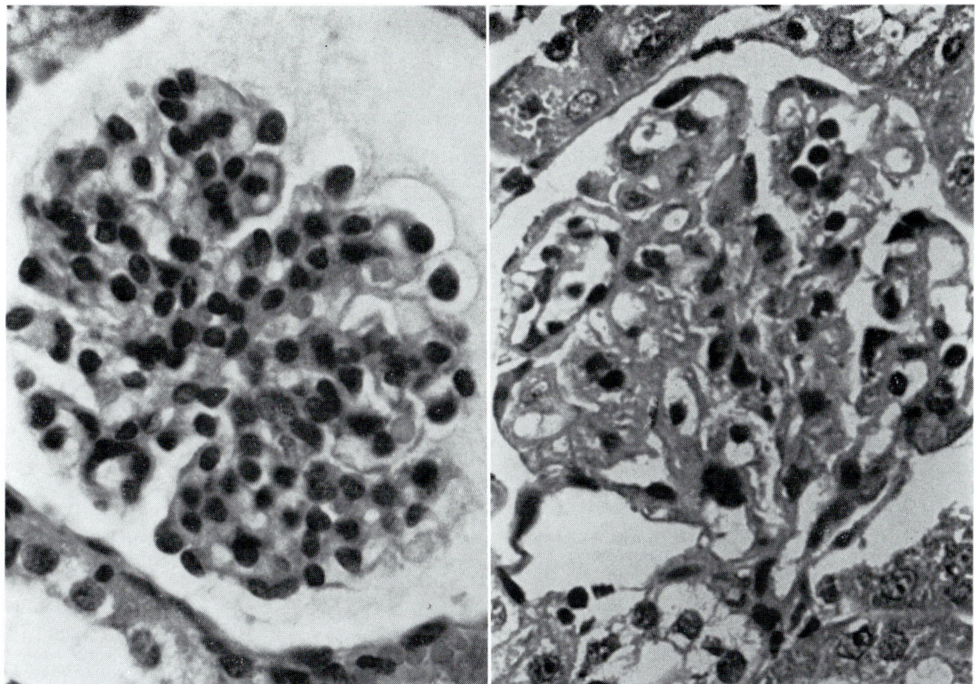

Figs. 6-1 and 6-2 Degenerative conversion of Masugi, or anti-rabbit-kidney duck serum, nephritis of the rabbit.
Fig. 6-1 *(left)* Masugi nephritis induced in a native, control rabbit. The nephritis is proliferative. Seven days after the onset of albuminuria. H & E stain,   ×660. Rabbit E40 (Masugi nephritis).
Fig. 6-2 *(right)* Masugi nephritis induced in a rabbit having had prolonged immunization with egg white for 140 days. The nephritis is degenerative or wire-looping. Eight days after the onset of albuminuria. H & E stain, ×660. At biopsy on the 138th experimental day no remarkable glomerular changes had been found. Rabbit E15 (egg white sensitization plus Masugi nephritis). (From Okabayashi, A.: *Jap. J. Nephrol. 9*: 29–32, 1967)
These two rabbits received an injection of the same dose (8 ml) of the same nephrotoxic serum. Interestingly a recent reexamination confirms that in this rabbit E15 there had been established the wasting and imbalance in the immune system (see Model 5).

quential immunologic events, consisting of immediate fixation of the heterologous NTAb to the glomerulus (the first or heterologous phase) and its in situ interaction with host antibody (the second or autologous phase) [13, 66].   Because the major antigenic constituents are included in the glomerular basement membrane (GBM), the distribution of the NTAb and of the host antibody in the glomerulus is identical, exhibiting a distinctive continuous, linear pattern in immunofluorescence [13, 66].   Broadly speaking fowl NTAbs are incapable of inducing glomerular injury in the first phase because they are unable to activate the complement system via the classical pathway [66] and differ in some biologic properties from mammalian antibodies [13].   In contrast, mammalian NTAbs with high nephrotoxicity commonly cause a biphasic glomerular injury.

The glomerular changes induced are therefore variable depending upon many factors such as species of recipient animals, source and amount of NTAb, or intensity of host immune response.   For instance rabbit Masugi nephritis is usually characterized by florid inflammatory changes but rarely enters the chronic phase unless the rabbit has received repeated injections of NTAb.   Rat Masugi nephritis, however, frequently becomes chronic despite rather mild inflammatory changes taking place during the acute phase.   The spectrum of histologic and ultrastructural changes developing in rat or rabbit Masugi nephritis is described in the foregoing chapters.

In brief, an enhanced host immune response leads principally to the occurrence of severe, often disorganized glomerular injury.   Moreover, if there exists a wasting in the immune response, the glomerular pathology might be significantly modified.   In fact we have proved that at the later stage of prolonged antigenic stimulation, the rabbits that received duck NTAbs showed peculiar degenerative glomerulonephritis, rather than the usual proliferative change seen in native, control rabbits [41, 45] (Figs. 6-1 and 6-2).

Although nephrotoxic serum nephritis has been studied mainly in rats and rabbits, it has also been reported in dogs, mice, monkeys, and sheep [13, 66] (see also Chapter 5).

2. Glomerulonephritis following injection of heterologous glomerular basement membrane plus Freund's complete adjuvant in sheep and goats — Steblay nephritis

Steblay produced severe crescentic glomerulonephritis in sheep with injections of heterologous GBM antigens and Freund's complete adjuvant (FCA) [60].   The immunologic mechanism of Steblay's sheep nephritis has been shown to be of the antiGBM-type since the glomerular distribution pattern of host antibodies is linear in immunofluorescence. In addition, it has been found that antibodies capable of reacting with autologous GBM are elutable from the diseased kidneys [61] and that they are also detectable in the serum of the nephritic animal undergoing bilateral nephrectomy [30].   Interestingly crescentic, rapidly progressive glomerulonephritis is seen in the sheep [60] or goat [49, 67] while in other animal species, glomerular changes are generally far milder.   In this connection McCluskey says that similar, although less severe, glomerulonephritis has been produced in monkeys, rabbits, and rats by injections of homologous or heterologous glomerular basement membrane preparations [36].   In any case, this model is very important as the first example to demonstrate the occurrence of autologous antiGBM nephritis.

Although the basic pathogenesis has been determined, the mode of immune response in this model of so-called autoallergic disease still remains unknown.

3. Glomerulonephritis following injection of homologous kidney plus Freund's complete adjuvant in rats — Heymann nephritis

Heymann and associates originally reported the experimental production of glomerulonephritis in the rat by using homologous kidney emulsion and FCA [21]. This rat nephritis is characterized by membranous thickening of the GBM with negligible inflammatory response. Granular deposits of host immunoglobulins could be found diffusely along the GBM in immunofluorescence, corresponding to dense deposits in electron microscopy. These features resemble membranous glomerulonephritis and indicate the immune complex pathogenesis. Edgington et al. disclosed that antigenic constituents were derived from brush border of the proximal tubular epithelium [10]. It has thus been realized that the nephritogenic complexes consisting of brush border antigen(s) and antibodies are circulating in the blood of the immunized rat. The amount of the circulating complexes are believed to be minimal because of the considerable difficulty in passive transfer of the disease by means of sera from the nephritic rat [62].

4. Serum sickness in rabbits

Serum sickness is an unwelcome, sometimes serious complication taking place after the therapeutic application of a large dose of antisera. In 1943 Rich and Gregory demonstrated that a variety of hypersensitivity diseases including acute glomerulonephritis were produced in rabbits that received large intravenous injection(s) of horse serum [58]. Germuth [15], and Dixon and associates [8] clarified immunologic mechanisms leading to the initiation of serum sickness diseases (Fig. 6-3). It was shown that the antigen (usually purified plasma protein, e.g., bovine serum albumin) was rapidly eliminated from

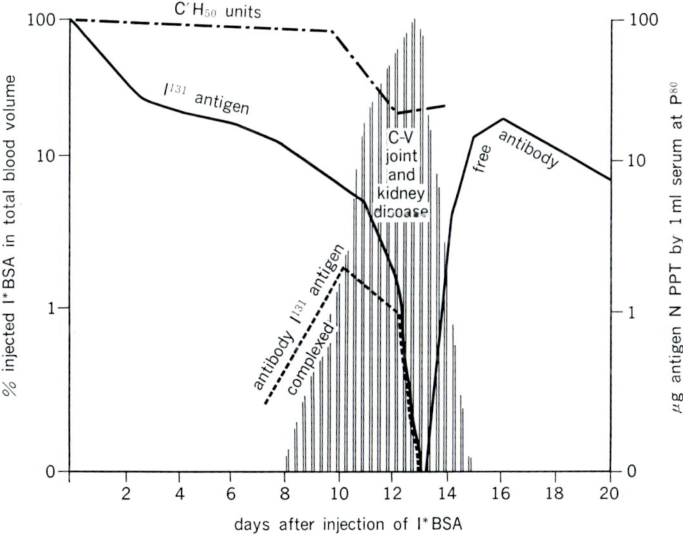

Fig. 6-3 Sequence of events following injection of 250 mg I*BSA/kg body weight in rabbits. Elimination of ¹³¹I antigen indicated by solid line relating to log scale at left. Amount of free antibody in the circulation relates to log scale at right. Antigen-antibody complexes plotted as percent of total I*BSA injected. Level of complement indicated as percent of normal. Incidence of cardiovascular, joint and kidney disease indicated by shaded area, reaching 100 percent on day 13. (From Dixon, F.J.: *In* Samter, M. (ed.) *Immunological Diseases,* 161–171, Little, Brown, and Company, Boston, 1965)

the circulation following the formation of host antibodies [8, 15]. During this immune phase of antigen elimination, soluble antigen and antibody complexes were produced in the circulation in an antigen excess environment. By immunofluorescence the complexes were found deposited at the site of the lesions of serum sickness [8]. These experimental results have contributed greatly in carifying the pathogenesis of many hypersensitivity diseases in man. Influencing factors related to immune complex diseases have been thoroughly reviewed recently [5]. The organs and tissues involved in experimental serum sickness are the kindeys, lungs, arteries, and heart (see [9, 51]).

Passive serum sickness is also a convenient experimental model for examining differences in inflammatory tissue manifestations in connection with those of the nature of immune complexes [27, 53].

Chronic serum sickness or immune complex nephritis probably develops on the basis of mechanisms which are similar to those revealed in acute serum sickness. However, chronic serum sickness nephritis is not uniform in histologic features owing to variations of the immune complexes produced. It has been indicated that the size and chemical nature of the complexes are important in determining the deposition site and, accordingly, the characteristics of the disease process [28]. The heterogeneity of produced antibodies governing the property of the complexes is apparently correlated with that of immune responses which can be further ascribed to alterations of the immune system as will be discussed later.

5. Prolonged antigenic stimulation in rabbits and C57BL mice

It is of considerable interest to know what happens in the host associated with the failure in the elaborate systemic defense mechanism performed by the immune system. Presumably such a critical situation could be created experimentally in animals by enforced overwork of the immune system, e.g., by repeated immunizations with an appreciable but not tolerogenic amount of antigens. Okabayashi and collaborators, since 1940, have carried out a series of experiments in the rabbit or C57BL/6J mouse, to clarify the overall sequence of events taking place in the immune system of the host by means of prolonged antigenic stimulation by using foreign protein or bacterial antigens [43–49, 51, 52, 54]. With such repeated immunizations, the animals showed an enhanced immunocyte proliferation in the immune system organs, together with accelerated hematopoiesis in the bone marrow. The observations indicated that the sensitized host responses were eatablihed by

---

Figs. 6-4 – 6-7 Immune system in prolonged antigenic stimulation with foreign protein: the prior activation (the extensive induction of immunocytes) and consequent exhaustion (progressive reduction or loss of the immunocytes).

Fig. 6-4 Hyperplasia of the spleen: increase in the lymphocytes (T cells) of periarterial lymphoid sheaths, formation of germinal follicles, leukocyte accumulation in the marginal zones, and immunoblastic and plasma cellular proliferation in the cords of red pulp. H & E stain, ×170. Autopsy at 72 experimental days. Rabbit T543 (egg albumin plus Freund's incomplete adjuvant-sensitization).

Fig. 6-5 Atrophy or exhaustion of the spleen. Autopsy at 378 experimental days. H & E stain, ×170. Rabbit R341 (egg white-sensitization).

Fig. 6-6 Hyperplasia of a popliteal lymph node: increase in the lymphocytes (T cells) of thymusdependent or deep cortical areas, formation of germinal follicles, and immunoblastic and plasma cellular proliferation in the medullary cords. H & E stain, ×67. Autopsy at 72 experimental days. Rabbit T543 (egg albumin plus Freund's incomplete adjuvant-sensitization). (From Okabayashi, A.: *In* Okabayashi, A. (ed.) *Immunopathology and Disease*, 165–223, Bunkodo, Tokyo, 1979)

Fig. 6-7 Atrophy or exhaustion of a popliteal lymph node. H-E stain, ×330. Autopsy at 271 experimental days. Rabbit S575 (egg white-sensitization). (From Kondo, Y.: *Acta Path. Jap. 17*: 252–258, 1967)

Figs. 6-4 – 6-7 Immune System in Polonged Antigenic Stimulation

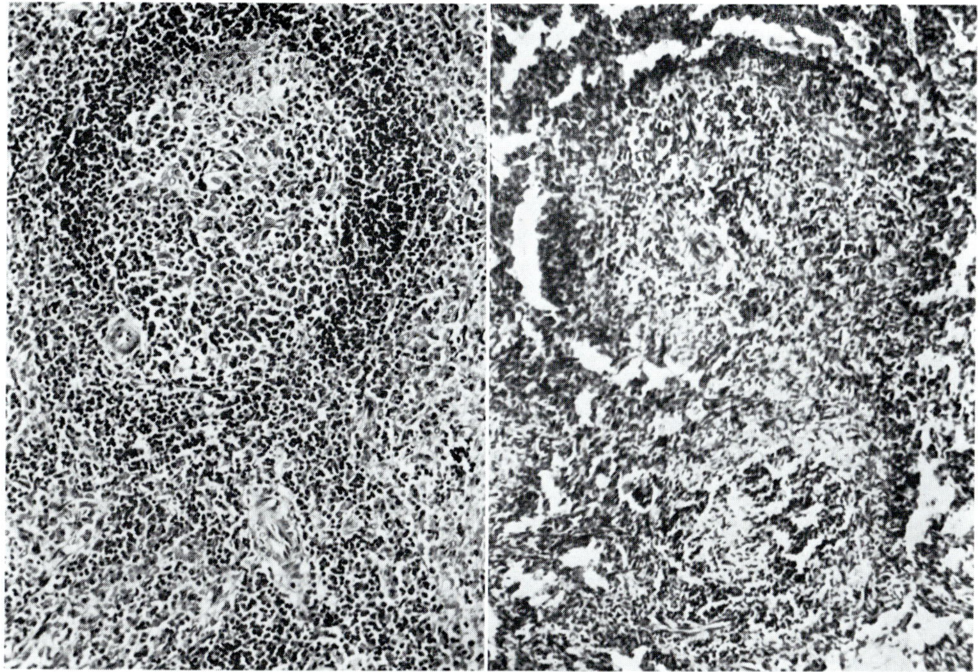

Fig. 6-4 Spleen in the early stage.

Fig. 6-5 Spleen in the late stage.

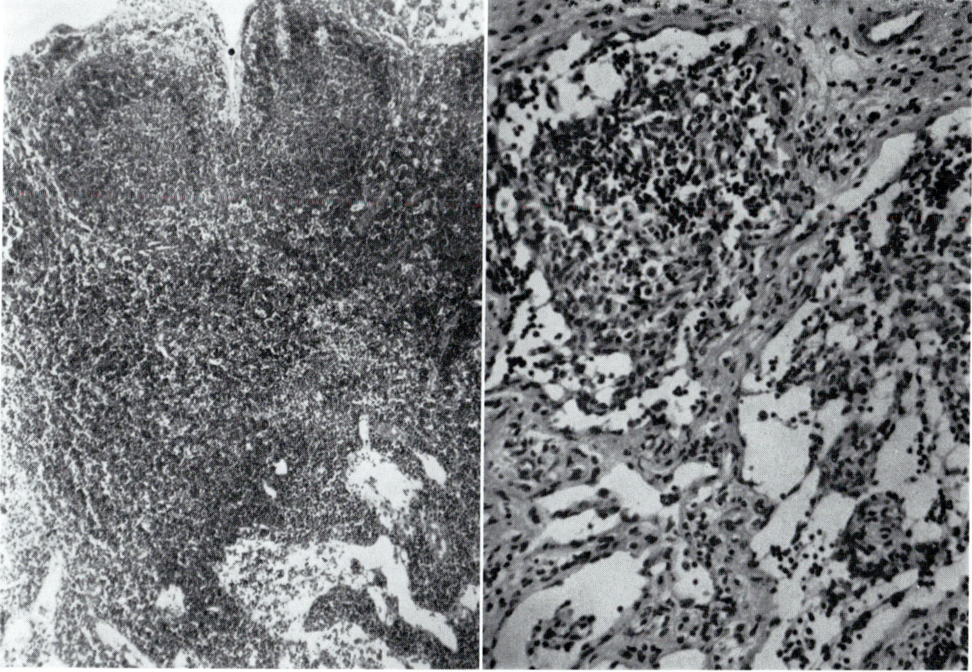

Fig. 6-6 Lymph node in the early stage.

Fig. 6-7 Lymph node in the late stage.

cooperative action of the immune system or myelo- and lymphoid organs, referred to as systemic immune reaction [43].

Even though it is adequate to endure continuous antigenic invasion and maintain the homeostasis, the reactivity of the immune system may not be permanent. Following continued antigen administration, the systemic immune reaction developed to the highest level during the middle stage (80–100 experimental days in rabbits) but gradually became less reactive [25, 43]. The early reactivity and consequent exhaustion were therefore thought to be the basic course of the systemic immune reaction. A wasting in the systemic immune reaction thus ensued in the terminal stage as evidenced by progressive exhaustion of lymphocytic and plasma cellular responses (Figs. 6-4 – 6-7). The bone marrow likewise showed prominent hypoplasia with or without fibrosis. During the fluctuating course of prolonged antigenic stimulation in animals (rabbits and C57BL/6J mice) there occurred a variety of diseases of the blood and tissues at various levels in sequence (Fig. 6-8) [46, 47]. It was noted that exaggerated immunocyte proliferation in the lymphoid organs with polyclonal hyperimmunoglobulinemia, as well as a systemic (or myeloid) blood cell-forming disorder resulting in myelofibrosis syndrome or a systemic (or hepatolienal) blood cell-

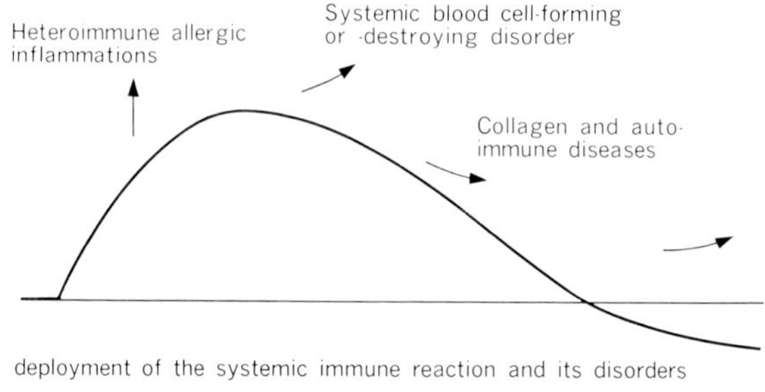

Fig. 6-8   The prior activation and consequent exhaustion. (From Okabayashi, A.:
In Oshima, Y. et al. (eds.) *Clinical Allergology*, 67–77, Asakura Shoten, Tokyo, 1967)

Fig. 6-9   Localization of autologous immunoglobulin in the sarcolemma and striations of cardiac myofibers. Direct immunoflorescence of frozen section of the heart with FITC-labeled goat antirabbit IgG, ×660. Autopsy at 97 experimental days. Rabbit U111 (the rabbit had been thymectomized during young adulthood before immunization with monthly injections of 0.5 mg of dinitrophenylated bovine immunoglobulin plus Freund's complete adjuvant). (Courtesy of Drs. T. Tada and M. Taniguchi. See also [50])

Fig. 6-10   Localization of autologous immunoglobulin in the glomerulus. Direct immunofluorescence of frozen section of the kidney with FITC-labeled goat anti-rabbit IgG, ×400. Experimental glomerulonephritis with changes similar to wire loop lesions induced by the intraperitoneal inoculation of emulsion of the own unilateral kidney in a rabbit given prolonged antigenic stimulation with egg white plus Freund's incomplete adjuvant for 162 days. Autopsy at 176 experimental days. Neither hen's egg albumin nor antibody against egg albumin was detected in this glomerulonephritis. In this rabbit, moreover, the circulating antikidney antibody was demonstrated: the glomerular basement membrane of normal rabbit kidney was positively stained (frozen section treated with the serum and FITC-labeled goat antirabbit IgG). Rabbit S425. (From Tanaka, N. et al.: *Jap. J. Exp. Med. 34*: 53–57, 1964)

Fig. 6-11   Glomerular as well as tubular nuclei show distinct specific fluorescence. Frozen kidney section of normal mouse treated with ×10 diluted serum of a mouse at 200 experimental days and then stained with FITC-labeled rabbit antimouse IgG, ×660. Autopsy at 200 experimental days showed experimental systemic lupus accentuated by nephritis with characteristic organized deposits in the mesangium under conditions of wasting and imbalance in the immune system. C57BL mouse CB38 (egg albumin-sensitization). (From Okumura, K.: *Acta Path. Jap. 23*: 695–704, 1973)

Fig. 6-12   Experimental in vitro-prepared LE cell: leukocyte with two LE bodies. Preparation consisted of crossed rabbit serum and human leukocytes. Wright stain, ×1,700 Autopsy at 118 experimental days showed systemic degenerative alterations of the connective tissue accentuated by endocarditis degenerative in nature. (From Okabayashi, A: *Acta Path Jap. 14*: 345–371, 1964)

Figs. 6-9 – 6-12   Autoantibodies Induced during the Later Stage of Prolonged Antigenic Stimulation

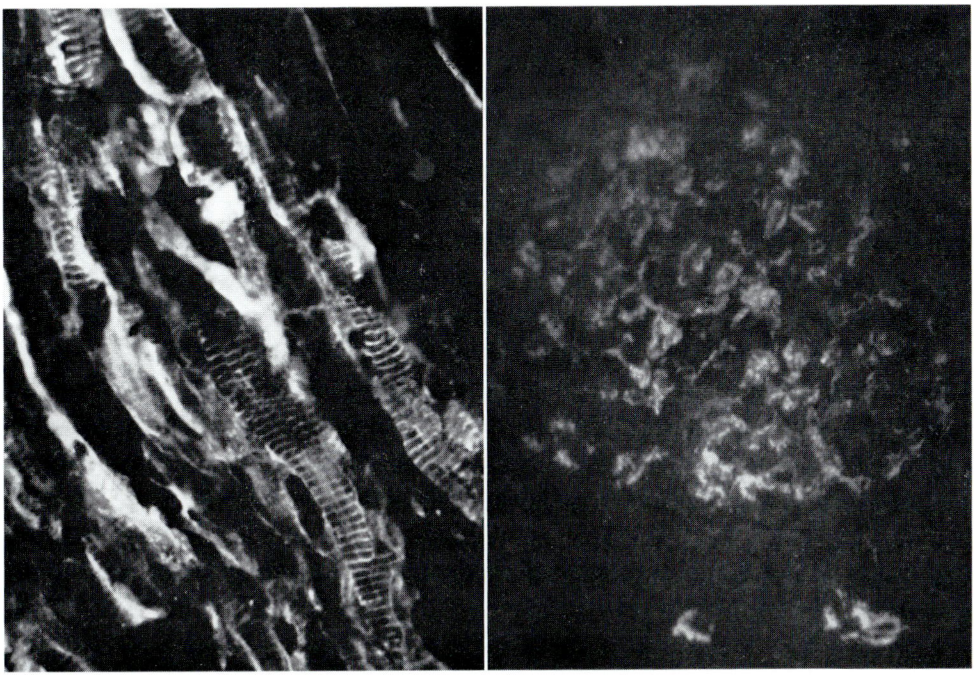

Fig. 6-9   Heart muscle.   Fig. 6-10   Glomerulus.

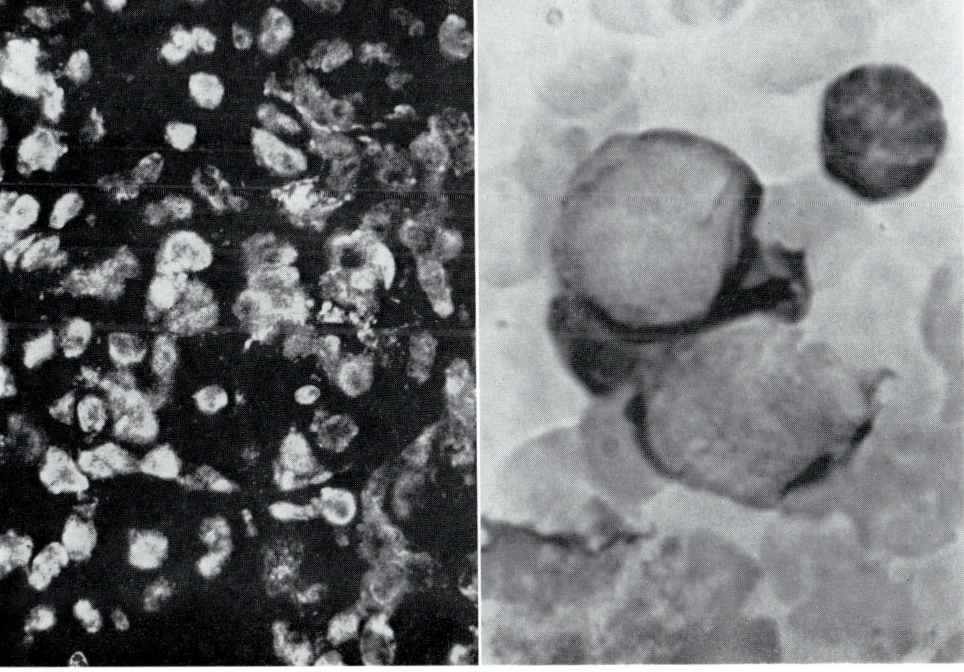

Fig. 6-11   Cellular nuclei (glomerulus).   Fig. 6-12   Leukocyte.

Prolonged Antigenic Stimulation and the Blood

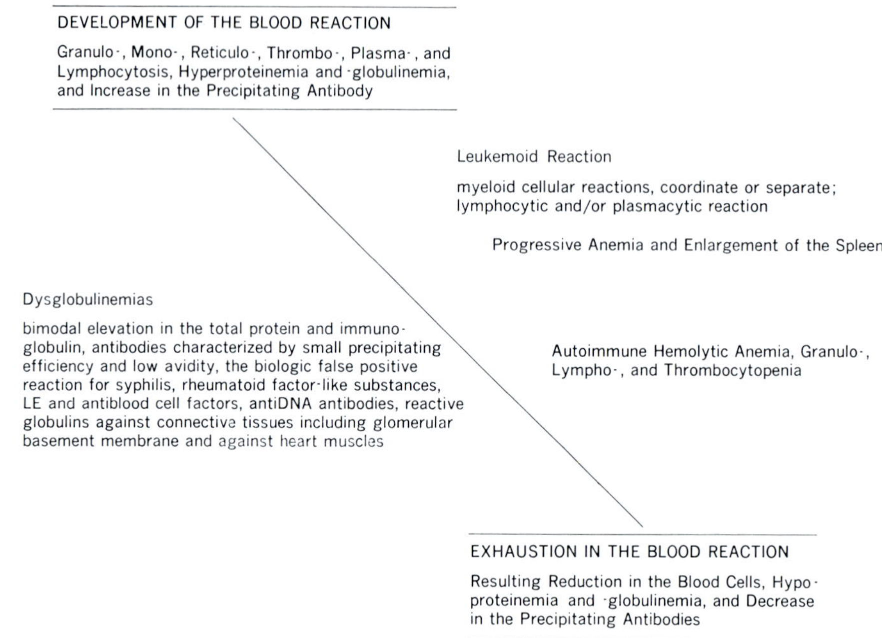

Fig. 6-13 Dysglobulinemias induced during the later stage of prolonged antigenic stimulation. (From Okabayashi, A.: *In* Oshima, Y. et al. (eds.) *Clinical Allergology*, 67–77, Asakura Shoten, Tokyo, 1967. Partly modified, see [50])

destroying disorder resulting in Banti's syndrome, were brought about during the middle stage of stimulation most conspicuously in experimental rabbits. In studies along similar lines, Kitamura and collaborators also demonstrated changes of the blood and tissues including crescentic glomerulonephritis, carditis of the rheumatic type, etc. in rabbits [24].

Following the augmentation of the systemic immune reaction, hypersensitivity diseases occurred in organs with typical features of acute inflammation. Especially renal glomeruli were frequently involved in severe proliferative inflammation. The alterations were basic-

Figs. 6-14 – 6-17 Unbalanced exaggerated proliferations in the wasting immune system developed during the later stage of prolonged antigenic stimulation.

Fig. 6-14 An unbalanced exaggerated proliferation of lymphocytes (T cells) in the thymus-dependent or deep cortical areas and follicular atrophy, largely under conditions of wasting, in a mesenteric lymph node. Autopsy at 242 experimental days. H & E stain, ×67. Transient monoclonal gammopathy and amyloidosis. Rabbit T521 (egg albumin plus Freund's incomplete adjuvant-sensitization).

Fig. 6-15 Marked depletion of lymphocytes (T cells) in the thymus-dependent or deep cortical areas and follicular hyperplasia in a popliteal lymph node. Biopsy at 23 weeks. H & E stain, ×67. Autopsy at 241 experimental days revealed a membranous glomerulonephritis under conditions of wasting and imbalance in the immune system. Rabbit T515 (egg albumin plus Freund's incomplete adjuvant-sensitization).

Fig. 6-16 Follicular immunoblastic dysplasia in a mesenteric lymph node. Note the nodular and diffuse extension deeply into medulla of the node. Autopsy at 200 experimental days. H & E stain, ×67. Experimental systemic lupus accentuated by nephritis under conditions of wasting and imbalance in the immune system. C57BL mouse CB39 (egg albumin-sensitization). (From Okabayashi, A.: *Rinsho Men-eki 5*: 683–692, 1973)

Fig. 6-17 Follicular or nodular immunoblastic and plasma cellular hyperplasia in the atrophying thymus. Autopsy at 200 experimental days. H & E stain, ×87. Experimental systemic lupus accentuated by nephritis under conditions of wasting and imbalance in the immune system. C57BL mouse CB39 (egg albumin-sensitization). (From Okabayashi, A.: *Rinsho Men-eki 5*: 683–692, 1973)

Figs. 6-14 – 6-17 Pathology in the Immune System during the Later Stage of Prolonged Antigenic Stimulation

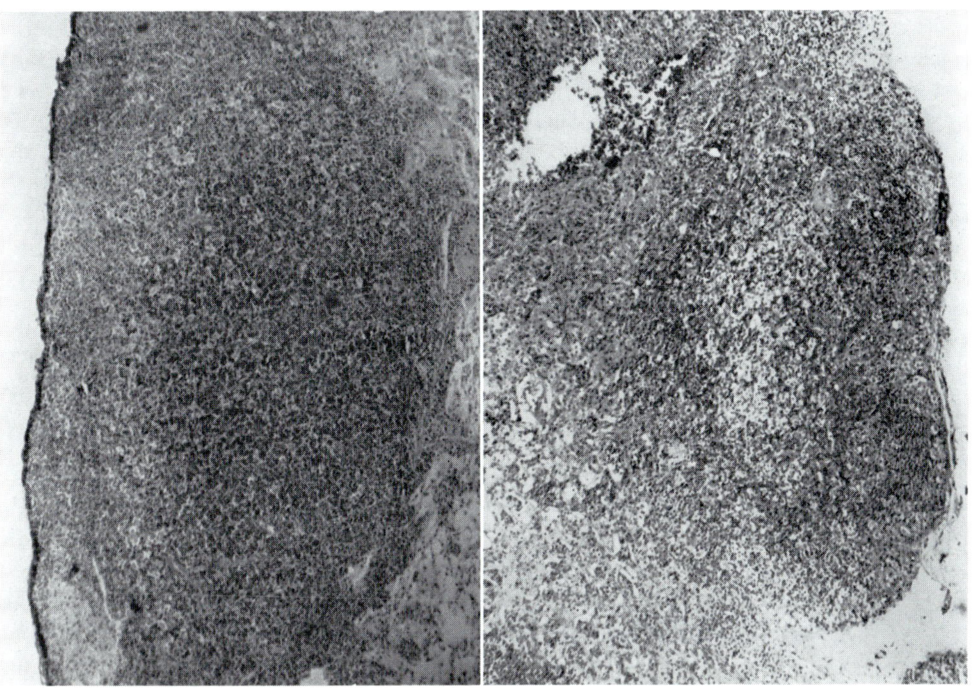

Fig. 6-14 Lymph node.   Fig. 6-15 Lymph node.

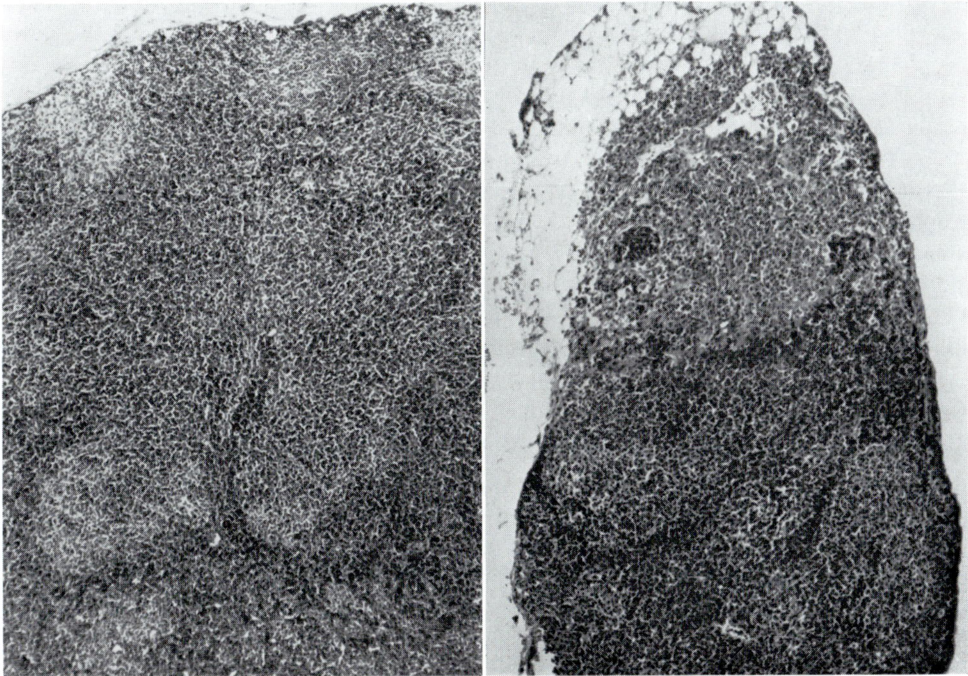

Fig. 6-16 Lymph node.   Fig. 6-17 Thymus.

ally similar to those found in experimental acute serum sickness and were probably caused by local deposition of immune complexes. Okabayashi has emphasized that before entering into the overt anergic or exhausted terminal phase, certain immunologic disorders develop in the later stage of prolonged antigenic stimulation which are significantly different from those observed during the early stages [47, 48]. Remarkably, alterations of the organs and tissues now became degenerative in nature. The glomerular change was often characterized by numerous subepithelial deposits of immune complexes without notable inflammatory responses like that in human membranous glomerulonephritis [28]. The mechanism involved in this degenerative conversion of the inflammatory process is still puzzling. In studying immunochemical properties of immune complexes, however, it was found that rabbits with this membranous nephropathy produced low avidity antibodies directed against injected antigen [40], suggesting that an alteration of the host immune response was crucial in the degenerative conversion of tissue manifestations. In the immune system, a progressive depletion of lymphocytes in the thymus-dependent areas (T cells) appeared to coincide with follicular immunoblastic (B cell) dysplasia — the imbalance in the wasting immune system [48].

It is remarkable that under conditions of the imbalance in the wasting immune system there appeared not only the degenerative conversion of the inflammatory process but also the development of autoimmunization. The spontaneous appearance of autoantibodies to nuclear and erythrocyte antigens has been confirmed in only certain strains of mice or some other animals but not in rabbits or C57BL/6J mice before the advanced aging stage (see, for example, [54]). In the later stage of prolonged antigenic stimulation, some cases of experimental rabbits or C57BL/6J mice produced a variety of autoantibodies (Figs. 6-9 – 6-13) and virtually developed a multisystem disease, inflammatory and/or degenerative in nature, resembling human systemic lupus. Glomerulonephritis experimentally induced in these animals has hallmarks of human lupus nephritis, rather than of common immune complex nephritis [44, 54] (see also Chapter 5). Interestingly, it was here that wasting and imbalance in the immune system was most conspicuous.

In fact, a confusing situation, i.e., a frank imbalance between the T and B lymphocyte populations, was observed in the later stage of prolonged antigenic stimulation [44, 47, 51]. Fig. 6-14 shows an exceptional, peculiar finding in a lymph node. There is an unbalanced exaggerated proliferation of lymphocytes in the thymus-dependent areas and a marked atrophy of lymphoid follicles. Most of the imbalances evolved both in rabbits and in C57BL/6J mice were however characterized by progressive depletion of lymphocytes in the thymus-dependent areas (T cells) coinciding with the follicular hyper- and dysplasia — the wasting and imbalance in the immune system (Figs. 6-15 and 6-16). In lymphoid follicles there appeared exaggerated immunoblastic or plasma cellular (B cell) proliferation, frequently monotonous in character. The follicular dysplasia sometimes showed a broad distribution, extending deeply into the medulla of the lymph node (Fig. 6-16). Similar follicular or nodular immunoblastic and plasma cellular (B cell) hyperplasia was also noted in the atrophying thymus (Fig. 6-17). It was shown that this wasting and imbalance in the immune system paralleled the degenerative conversion and autoimmunization in animals. In an experiment utilizing C57BL/6J mice [26], a decrease in the T (Thy-1 positive) cell populations was actually confirmed by histologic as well as cytologic examinations (Fig. 6-18).

In summary, later in the course of prolonged antigenic stimulation it was revealed that characteristic dysglobulinemias (Fig. 6-9 – 6-13) and two associated intimately related tissue manifestations developed — (1) degenerative conversion of the inflammatory re-

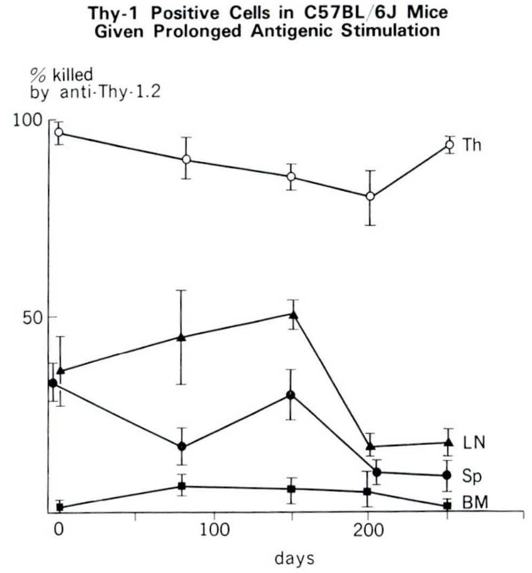

Fig. 6-18 Time course analysis of T cell number in the C57BL/6J mice given prolonged immunization with egg albumin.
The number of T cells (Thy-1 positive cells) was examined by the cytotoxic dye exclusion test using antiThy-1.2 and guinea pig complement. Lymphocytes from the thymus (Th), lymph nodes (LN), spleen (Sp), and bone marrow (BM) were investigated. The number of T cells in each organ was increased until about 150 days of experiment and hereafter the prominent decrease was observed as indicated. (Courtesy of Dr. T. Takemori. See also [26])

sponses including the induction of membranous glomerulonephritis-like disease and (2) autoimmunization accentuated by the induction of lupuslike nephritis. Beside these glomerular and blood changes there existed an abnormality of immune response, i.e., the wasting and imbalance in the immune system (Fig. 6-15 – 6-17). Conceivably the primary seat of the glomerular diseases of immune origin is to be found in the immune system and its alterations.

6. Aleutian disease of mink

Systemic angiitis and progressive, often fatal glomerulonephritis develop in mink that have Aleutian gene aa. This mink disease is presumed to be caused by local deposition of immune complexes which are produced in association with infection of Aleutian disease virus [5, 42]. In addition, antibodies directed against single or double stranded DNA have been detected in the sera of diseased mink [5]. At present, therefore, it is uncertain which of these two mechanisms, i.e., viral immune complexes or DNA-antiDNA complexes are pathogenetically more important. In the renal glomerulus, trace amounts of viral antigens could be detected occasionally [5] in contrast to abundant lumpy deposits of host antibodies and complement [56]. Progressive deposition of eosinophilic material, most likely immune deposits, result in diffuse obliteration of the glomerular tufts to produce renal insufficiency.

Henson et al. investigated sequential changes in the immune system [19, 20]. Progressive proliferation of plasma cells was noted from the early stage, accounting for marked elevation of the serum immunoglobulin titer. Later, however, the immune system became atrophic correlated with decrease in the lymphocyte population while plasma cells were still recognized diffusely. Alterations in the thymus have not been described. Porter et al. reported the transition from an electrophoretically heterogenous hyperglobulinemia to a homogeneous myeloma-like hyperglobulinemia in mink affected with Aleutian disease [55].

7. New Zealand (NZ) mouse disease

Naturally occurring systemic disorders in NZB mice and their hybrids have been known as a representative animal model of autoimmune diseases, notably of human SLE. With age, the NZB mice have autoimmune hemolytic anemia, antinuclear antibodies, and progressive nephropathy. The mice are highly susceptible to infection with murine leukemia virus and show a marked immune response against viral antigens. Obviously the mouse autoimmune disease develops on the basis of genetic abnormalities, though the mode of the inheritance has not yet been elucidated conclusively. It is also unknown whether or not viral infection plays a crucial role for the induction of the autoimmunity.

At the age of several months, many of the animals may develop definite glomerulonephritis with lumpy deposition of immunoglobulins, complement, and other plasma proteins [22]. In $(NZB \times NZW)$ F_1 hybrids, especially in females, the incidence and severity of glomerulonephritis are even more prominent. Segmental proliferation of glomerular cells is first seen between 5 and 6 months of age [22], which is later modified by some degenerative lesions with necrosis of the tufts and crescent formation.

Concerning the pathogenesis of the glomerulonephritis, two possibilities have been proposed; Lambert and Dixon stated that nephritogenic immune complexes were largely composed of DNA and antiDNA antibodies [29]. Alternatively Mellors and associates have emphasized the pathogenetic importance of viral antigen-antibody complexes [37, 68]. These conflicting results indicate the multiplicity of the underlying mechanisms of the mouse nephropathy.

Prominent hyperplastic changes in the immune system are another hallmark of the NZB mice. In the spleen and lymph nodes hyperplasia and/or enlargement of lymphoid follicles with a germinal center formation may be an initiating sign of the lymphoproliferative disorder [22]. Follicular accumulation of lymphocytes can be observed in the medulla of the thymus. With age marked proliferation of plasma cells occurs in the immune system which may be correlated with the appearance of autoimmune phenomena [22]. Beyond the frank hyperplasia in the immune system, various lymphomas develop in appreciable numbers of animals, including thymoma, plasmacytoma, and reticulum cell sarcoma.

Despite the accumulation of multiple publications dealing with NZB mice and their hybrids, no comprehensive concept has been established accounting for the occurrence of abnormalities in the immune response. However, there is circumstantial evidence to indicate that T cell function may be in some way concerned with the unusual immune response. For example thymectomy did not suppress but frequently enhanced the development of these diseases in mice [22]; it was also reported that natural thymocytotoxic antibodies were circulating in the blood of the NZB mice [59]. These results suggest that in the NZB mice, there exists a dysfunction of Tcells in controlling the antibody formation performed by B cells.

8. Immunologically mediated glomerulitis of horses

Recently, it has been revealed by Banks and Henson [3] that horses developed not only immune complex-induced glomerulitis (glomerular inflammation) but also spontaneous antiglomerular basement membrane (antiGBM) disease. They determined the occurrence of immunologically mediated glomerulitis in the horse related [2] or not related [3] equine infectious anemia (EIA) viral infection. Interestingly, in the latter it has been observed that horses sometimes developed spontaneous antiGBM antibody production [3]. AntiGBM antibodies were furthermore confirmed by them in the eluate of the isolated glomeruli of one of three horses with linear fluorescent deposits in the glomeruli.

III. Concluding Remarks (Immunologic Bases and a Unifying Concept)

Masugi nephritis and some other immunologically induced experimental models have been described in previous chapters and sketched in this communication. It is remarkable that glomerulonephritis varied considerably from an abrupt and acute to an insidious and chronic process. It was also noted that there could appeare (1) phagocyte accumulating and recoverable, proliferative glomerulonephritis, (2) disorganizing (histolytic), rapidly progressive glomerulonephritis resulting in scarring, (3) a membranous glomerulonephritis characterized by numerous subepithelial deposits of immune complexes, and (4) lupuslike nephritis with deposits exhibiting a peculiar organized structure (see Chapter 5) and wire loop lesions. Following advances in experimental investigations performed during the past decades (as described above), fundamental immunologic processes in the glomerular changes have been now realized and these can be categorized into three basic patterns (Fig. 6-19).

First of all renal glomeruli can be damaged by a direct action of antibodies directed against their own constituents, e.g., by antiGBM antibodies as clearly shown in the first phase of rat Masugi nephritis induced by rabbit NTAbs. Obviously glomerulonephritis produced in this way is not actually present in human beings; however a pathogenetically similar situation is seen associated with production of autologous antiGBM antibodies as experimentally evidenced by Steblay [60]. Goodpasture's syndrome is a representative human case of this type of nephritis. In all of these experimental and human examples of antiGBM nephritis, diffuse linear localization of antibodies may be seen along the GBM by immunofluorescent examination. An appreciable number of other human cases are sup-

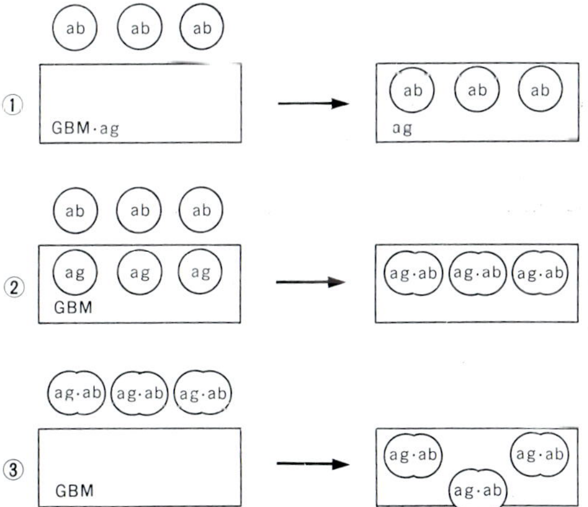

Fig. 6-19 Three possible immunologic processes occurring around the glomerular basement membrane (GBM). (1) Interaction between endogenous GBM antigens (ag) and circulating heterologous or autologous anti-GBM antibodies. (2) Interaction between antigens previously fixed on the GBM (ag) and circulating antibodies (ab). (3) Deposition of circulating antigen-antibody complexes (ag · ab) which have no specific affinities to the glomerular constituent. (From Okabayashi, A. et al.: *Current Topics Path. 61*: 1–43, 1976)

posed to be included in this category as far as the possibility is evaluated by immunofluorescence [8]. Similar glomerular distribution of host antibodies is often observed in renal allografts thereby implicating a production of antiGBM antibodies during the rejection reaction [57].

As seen in Model 8, it has recently been observed that horses sometimes develop naturally occurring antiGBM disease with linear fluorescent deposits in their glomeruli.

Second, immunologic glomerular injury may also be brought about by an interaction between antigens previously fixed in the glomerulus and circulating antibodies. This is indeed the case in the second phase of Masugi nephritis whereby the prefixed nephrotoxic antibodies react with host antibodies later produced, resulting in either initiation or exacerbation of glomerulonephritis. Apart from such a distinctive but rare instance, it is not unlikely that some glomerular diseases are induced by the above mentioned pathway, since antigens or other macromolecules are often shown to be entrapped by renal glomeruli. Unfortunately, until the present, this possibility has been proved only in a complex experiment [34] but not definitely in many other conditions.

The third mechanism concerns deposition of circulating antigen-antibody complexes which have no specific affinities to the glomerulus. The deposition of immune complexes conceivably occurs related to peculiar physiologic and anatomic organization of the glomerulus. It has been indicated that the deposition is not a simple but highly complicated process influenced by many factors [5]. Presumably glomerular diseases in humans along with those occurring spontaneously in animals are, for the most part, of the immune complex-type.

As mentioned before, because of broad diversities in the composition of immune complexes, histologic and immunohistochemical findings in immune complex-associated glomerulonephritis are quite variable. The immune deposits basically exhibit a granular distribution in immunofluorescence, distinct from the linear pattern shown in antiGBM nephritis. The deposits may occur at any sites of a glomerulus involving the tufts diffusely or locally related to the difference in conditions.

Although the basic pathogenesis has been clarified, there are still several important questions to be answered with respect to the pathology of immunologically induced glomerulonephritis, especially those including the mediation of the inflammatory process and behavior of the host immune response.

Concerning the latter issue, our attention has come to focus on the problem of "nephritis and the dysimmunization" through studies on the experimental models elaborated by Masugi and other investigators. Dysimmunization referred at first to an abnormality in the immune response taking place during the later stage of prolonged antigenic stimulation (Model 5) [46]. As demonstrated above it has been proved that, under this condition, there emerged wasting and imbalance in the immune system being associated with degenerative conversion and autoimmunization (Fig. 6-20). To be sure, each experimental model sketched above is characteristic and peculiar. However, it should not be overlooked that the animal models, especially Models 5-7 having a prolonged pattern of disease, have subtle ties and that their basic pathogenic mechanisms seem to be comparable. The dysimmunization or related conditions in these animal models seem to be characterized by dysimmunoglobulinemias and the progressive depletion of lymphocytes in the thymus-dependent areas coincides with follicular immunoblastic dysplasia. It is noted that the imbalance between the T and B cell populations in the immune system manifests itself grossly under the condition of wasting. The immunologic wasting seems to result from aging (Models 6 and 7) or from prolonged antigenic stimulation (Model 5).

We could see no escape from assuming that the experimental induction of collagen and

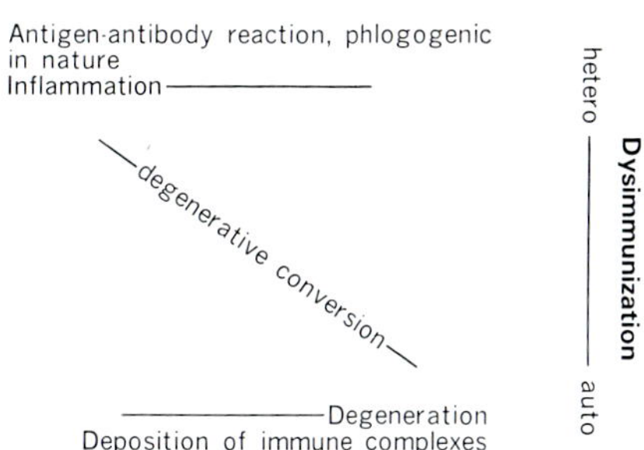

Fig. 6-20 Degenerative conversion and autoimmunization in the later stage of prolonged antigenic stimulation. (From Okabayashi, A.: *In* Okabayashi, A. (ed.) *Immunopathology and Disease*, 165–223, Bunkodo, Tokyo, 1979. Partly modified)

autoimmune diseases may be related to the wasting and imbalance in the immune system. This concept has been troubling us because of the evidence that was different from the usual aspect of emergence of autoimmunity. As, for example, Fudenberg (1974) [12] points out, it has long been thought that autoimmunity results merely from inappropriate hyperactivity of immune mechanisms.

Fortunately, a new light has been thrown on the fundamental nature of dys- and autoimmunization through recent studies by Tada in our laboratory, whose point of view and related ones on the dual regulatory role of T cells (T lymphocytes) will be summarized as follows:

It has recently been well documented that the antibody response is initiated via collaborative interactions between T and B cells [4, 7, 39, 65]. The term 'helper' was conferred to the cell type which assists in the antibody synthesis by B cells. It is obvious that in many instances the amount and quality of antibody response are direct functions of the activity of helper T cells. Both antigen-specific and antigen-nonspecific helper effects have been demonstrated. As the autoreactive B cells do exist in normal animals, the production of autoantibodies would be influenced on one hand by the stimulation of helper T cells with continuous activation by antigen.

Recent reports by several investigators (reviewed by Gershon, 1975 [18]), however, indicate another very important regulatory activity of T cells, namely the 'suppressor' T cell function. This was first observed as the ability of T cells to suppress specific antibody response to sheep erythrocytes, haptenated ascaris antigen and pneumococcal polysaccharide (Gershon and Kondo, 1971 [17]; Tada and Okumura, 1971 [63]; Baker et al., 1971 [1]), and later substantiated by a number of experiments using different antigens and animal species. The role of suppressor T cells in genetically determined unresponsiveness to certain antigens and even self components has been demonstrated. Thus the antibody responses by B cells were regulated by two balanced cell types under physiologic conditions, the helper and suppressor T cells. A number of maneuvers which eliminated suppressor T cells were found to augment antibody response, and under certain conditions to facilitate autoimmune and allergic manifestations in mice and chickens. Furthermore, the impairment of the suppressor T cell has recently been described in SLE patients.

The recent immunogenetic studies have focused the attention on the phenotypic expressions on helper and supperssor T cells, and yielded a fruitful outcome in defining these cell types. Suppressor T cells are generally sensitive to treatments with x-irradiation, cyclophosphamide and adult thymectomy, whereas helper T cells are usually resistant to these treatments. They have different phenotypic exprssions on their cell surface, which

11. Ehrlich, P.: Die Schutzstoffe des Blutes. *Verh. Ges. dtsch. Naturf. Ärzte 73*: 250–275, 1901.

12. Fudenberg, H.H.: Are autoimmune diseases immunologic deficiency states? *In* Good, R.A. and Fisher, D.W. (eds.): *Immunobiology*, 7th printing, 175–183, Sinauer Associates, Inc., Sunderland, 1974.

13. Fujimoto, T., Okada, M., Kondo, Y., and Tada, T.: The nature of Masugi nephritis. Histo- and immunopathological studies. *Acta Path. Jap. 14*: 275–310, 1964.

14. Fujimoto, T. and Kitamura, T.: Pathology of lupus nephritis with special reference to the immunological bases of glomerular changes. *Tohoku J. Exp. Med. 122*: 355–374, 1977.

15. Germuth, F.G., Jr.: A comparative histologic and immunologic study in rabbits of induced hypersensitivity of the serum sickness type. *J. Exp. Med. 97*: 257–282, 1953.

16. Germuth, F.G., Jr. and Rodriguez, E.: *Immunopathology of the renal glomerulus; Immune complex deposit and antibasement membrane disease.* Little, Brown and Company, Boston, 1973.

17. Gershon, R.K. and Kondo, K.: Infectious immunological tolerance. *Immunology 21*: 903–914, 1971.

18. Gershon, R.K.: A disquisition on suppressor T cells. *Transplant. Rev. 36*: 170–185, 1975.

19. Henson, J.B., Leader, R.W., Gorham, J.R., and Padgett, G.A.: The sequential development of lesions in spontaneous Aleutian disease of mink. *Path. Vet. 3*: 289–314, 1966.

20. Henson, J.B., Gorham, J.R., Padgett, G.A., Wash, P., and Davis, W.C.: Pathogenesis of the glomerular lesions in Aleutian disease of mink. Immunofluorescent studies. *A.M.A. Arch. Path. 87*: 21–28, 1969.

21. Heymann, W., Hackel, D.B., Harwood, S., Wilson, S.G.F., and Hunter, J.L.P.: Production of nephrotic syndrome in rats by Freund's adjuvant and rat kidney suspensions. *Proc. Soc. Exp. Biol. Med. 100*: 660–664, 1959.

22. Howie, J.B. and Simpson, L.O.: The immunopathology of the NZB mice and their hybrids. *In* Miescher, P.A. and Müller-Eberhard, H.J. (eds.): *Textbook of Immunopathology*, 2nd ed., 247–278, Grune & Stratton, New York, 1976.

23. Kay, C.F.: The mechanism by which experimental nephritis is produced in rabbits injected with nephrotoxic duck serum. *J. Exp. Med. 72*: 559–572, 1940.

24. Kitamura, S. and Koizumi, F.: Experimental studies on the Aschoff body by prolonged sensitization. *In* Otaka, Y. (ed.): *Immunopathology of Rheumatic Fever and Rheumatoid Arthritis*, 129–138, Igaku-Shoin, Tokyo, 1976.

25. Kondo, Y.: Lymph node and antigenic stimulation; Experimental studies. *Acta Path. Jap. 17*: 252–258, 1967.

26. Kondo, Y. and Tada, T.: T cell system and immune response (in Japanese). *Tr. Soc. Path. Jap. 64*: Suppl. 61–66, 1975.

27. Koyama, A., Niwa, Y., Shigematsu, H., Taniguchi, M., and Tada, T.: Studies on passive serum sickness. II. Factors determining the localization of antigen-antibody complexes in the murine renal glomerulus. *Lab. Invest. 38*: 253–262, 1978.

28. Kuriyama, T., Chronic glomerulonephritis induced by prolonged immunization in the rabbit. *Lab. Invest. 28*: 224–235, 1973.

29. Lambert, P.H. and Dixon, F.J.: Pathogenesis of the glomerulonephritis of NZB/W mice. *J. Exp. Med. 127*: 507–522, 1968.

30. Lerner, R. and Dixon, F.J.: Transfer of ovine experimental allergic glomerulonephritis (EAG) with serum. *J. Exp. Med. 124*: 431–442, 1966.

31. Masugi, M. und Tomizuka, Y.: Über die specifischen zytotoxischen Veränderungen der Niere und der Leber durch das spezifische Antiserum (Nephrotoxin und Hepatotoxin). Zugleich ein Beitrag zur Pathogenese der Glomerulonephritis. *Tr. Jap. Path. Soc. 21*: 329–341, 1931.

32. Masugi, M., Sato, Y., Murasawa, S., und Tomizuka, Y.: Über die experimentelle Glomerulonephritis durch das spezifische Antinierenserum. *Tr. Jap. Path. Soc. 22*: 614–628, 1932.

33. Masugi, M.: Referat. Die Allergie und ihre pathologische Bedeutung. *Tr. Soc. Path. Jap. 29*: 603–631, 1939.

34. Mauer, S.M., Sutherland, D.E.R., Howard, R.J., Fish, A.J., Najarian, J.S., and Michael, A.F.: The glomerular mesangium. III. Acute immune mesangial injury: A new model of glomerulonephritis. *J. Exp. Med. 137*: 553–570, 1973.

35. McCluskey, R.T. and Vassalli, P.: Experimental glomerular diseases. *In* Rouiller, C. and Muller, A.F. (eds.): *The Kidney; Morphology, Biochemistry, Physiology II*: 83–198, Academic Press, New York and London, 1969.

36. McCluskey, R.T.: Immunologic mechanisms in renal disease. *In* Heptinstall, R.H.: *Pathology of the Kidney*, 2nd ed., 273–317, Little, Brown and Company, Boston, 1974.

37. Mellors, R.C., Shirai, T., Aoki, T., Huebner, R.J. and Krawczynski, K.: Wild-type Gross leukemia virus and the pathogenesis of the glomerulonephritis of New Zealand mice. *J. Exp. Med. 133*: 113–132, 1971.

38. Metcalf, D.: Reticular tumors in mice subjected to prolonged antigenic stimulation. *Brit. J. Cancer 15*: 769–779, 1961.

39. Miller, J.F.A.P. and Mitchell, G.F.: Thymus and antigen-reactive cells. *Transplant. Rev. 1*: 3–42, 1969.

40. Nakabayashi, M.: Immunochemical properties of rabbit antibodies in membranous glomerulonephritis. *Acta Path. Jap. 24*: 63–77, 1974.

41. Nogiwa, H.: Histopathological studies of Masugi nephritis in rabbits by prolonged sensitization with egg white (in Japanese). *J. Chiba Med. Soc. 35*: 1850–1861, 1959.

42. Norton, W.L.: Aleutian mink and New Zealand mice: Models of viral induced connective tissue disease. *Rheumatol. 3*: 194–223, 1970.

43. Okabayashi, A.: *Immunity and Allergy; A septic aspect of infection* (in Japanese). Nagai Shoten, Osaka, 1950.

44. Okabayashi, A.: Induction of a disease resembling systemic lupus erythematosus in later stage of prolonged sensitization. *Acta Path. Jap. 14*: 345–371, 1964.

45. Okabayashi, A.: Degenerative conversion of glomerulitis in the later stage of prolonged sensitization; Experimental studies. *Jap. J. Nephrol. 9*: 29–32, 1967.

46. Okabayashi, A.: Dysimmunization and the concept of sensitization disease. *In* Oshima, Y. et al. (eds.): *Clinical Allergology*, 67–77, Asakura Shoten, Tokyo, 1967.

47. Okabayashi, A.: Pathogenesis of autoimmunity; Experimental induction of a systemic lupus-like disease in the later stage of prolonged antigenic stimulation and its pathogenetic suggestion (in Japanese). *Rinsho Men-eki 5*: 683–692, 1973.

48. Okabayashi, A.: Degenerative conversion of the inflammatory responses; A new concept of collagen diseases (in Japanese). *Infection · Inflammation · Immunity 6*: 149–156, 1976.

49. Okabayashi, A., Kondo, Y., and Shigematsu, H.: Cellular and histopathologic consequences of immunologically induced experimental glomerulonephritis. *In* Grundmann, E. (ed.): *Glomerulonephritis (Current Topics in Pathology 61)*, 1–43, Springer-Verlag, Berlin, 1976.

50. Okabayashi, A., Kondo, Y., and Tomioka, H.: The role of antiheart antibodies in experimental induction of myocardial lesions of the rheumatic type. *In* Otaka, Y. (ed.): *Immunopathology of Rheumatic Fever and Rheumatoid Arthritis*, 106–128, Igaku Shoin, Tokyo, 1976.

51. Okabayashi, A.: Concepts of immunologic disorder (in Japanese). *In* Okabayashi, A. (ed.): *Immunopathology and Disease*, 165–223, Bunkodo, Tokyo, 1979.

52. Okada, M.: Kidneys in prolonged sensitization; An experimental histopathological study (in Japanese). *J. Chiba Med. Soc. 38*: 396–416, 1963.

53. Okumura, K., Kondo, Y., and Tada, T.: Studies on passive serum sickness. I. The glomerular fine structure of serum sickness nephritis induced by preformed antigen-antibody complexes in the mouse. *Lab. Invest. 24*: 283–391, 1971.

54. Okumura, K.: Induction of a disease resembling systemic lupus erythematosus in C57BL/6J mice by prolonged immunization with egg albumin. *Acta Path. Jap. 23*: 695–704, 1973.

55. Porter, D.D., Dixon, F.J., and Larsen, A.E.: The development of a myeloma-like condition in mink with Aleutian disease. *Blood 25*: 736–742, 1965.

56. Porter, D.D., Larsen, A.E., and Porter, H.G.: The pathogenesis of Aleutian disease of mink. I. In vitro viral replication and the host antibody response to viral antigen. *J. Exp. Med. 130*: 575–593, 1969.

57. Porter, K.A., Andres, G.A., Calder, M.W., Dossector, J.B., Hsu, K.C., Rendall, J.M., Seegal, B.C., and Starzl, T.E.: Human renal transplants. II. Immunofluorescent and immunoferritin studies. *Lab. Invest. 18*: 159–171, 1968.

58. Rich, A.R. and Gregory, J.E.: The experimental demonstration that periarteritis nodosa is a manifestation of hypersensitivity. *Bull. Johns Hopkins Hosp. 72*: 65–82, 1943.

59. Shirai, T. and Mellors, R.C.: Natural thymocytotoxic autoantibody and reactive antigen in New Zealand Black and other mice. *Proc. Nat. Acad. Sci. 68*: 1412–1415, 1971.

60. Steblay, R.W.: Glomerulonephritis induced in sheep by injections of heterologous glomerular basement membrane and Freund's complete adjuvant. *J. Exp. Med. 116*: 253–272, 1962.

61. Steblay, R.W. and Rudofsky, U.: In vitro and in vivo properties of autoantibodies eluted from kidneys of sheep with autoimmune glomerulonephritis. *Nature 218*: 1269–1271, 1968.

62. Sugisaki, T., Klassen, J., Andres, G.A. Milgrom, F., and McCluskey, R.T.: Passive transfer of Heymann nephritis with serum. *Kidney International 3*: 66–73, 1973.

63. Tada, T. and Okumura, K.: Regulation of homocytotropic antibody formation in the rat. V. Cell cooperation in the anti-hapten homocytotropic antibody response. *J. Immunol. 107*: 1137–1145, 1971.

64. Tanaka, N., Nishimura, T., Tada, T., and Okabayashi, A.: Autoimmune phenomenon occurred in the course of prolonged sensitization of heterologous protein. *Jap. J. Exp. Med. 34*: 53–57, 1964.

65. Taylor, R.B.: Cellular cooperation in the antibody response of mice to two serum albumins: Specific function of thymus cells. *Transplant. Rev. 1*: 114–149, 1969.

66. Unanue, E.R. and Dixon, F.J.: Experimental glomerulonephritis: Immunological events and pathogenetic mechanisms. *Adv. Immunol. 6*: 1–90, 1967.

67. Williams, R. and Steblay, R.W.: Glomerulonephritis induced in goats by injection of human glomerular basement membrane and Freund's adjuvant. *Fed. Proc. 24*: 243–243, 1965.

68. Yoshiki, T., Mellors, R.C., Strand, M., and August, J.T.: The viral envelope glycoprotein of leukemia virus and the pathogenesis of immune complex glomerulonephritis of New Zealand mice. *J. Exp. Med. 140*: 1011–1027, 1974.

Chapter **7**

Renal Tissue Antigens and Antikidney Antibodies in the Serum and Urine of Patients with Glomerular, or Tubular and Interstitial Renal Diseases

MASAFUMI WAKASHIN and YOKO WAKASHIN

I. Introduction

It has been well known that the immunological renal injury can be caused by two immune processes, first by the injection of heterologous antibodies reacting with antigens in the kidney, namely nephrotoxic serum nephritis, and, second, by the circulating antigen-antibody immune complexes which accumulate in the glomeruli as in the case of serum sickness. Historically two important researches have been conducted on immunological renal injury. Lindeman (1900) succeeded in demonstrating the nephrotoxicity of heterologous anti-kidney sera after the injection of antiserum against rabbit kidneys raised in guinea pigs. von Pirque (1911) reported a clinical case of nephropathy in serum sickness following the injection of foreign proteins.

In the series of experimental nephrotoxic serum nephritis, Masugi nephritis has been well known as a classic model of experimental nephritis for the study of renal injuries induced with heterologous nephrotoxic serum. Further, pathological studies on nephrotoxic nephritis have been conducted extensively and numerous experimental researches have been undertaken in order to define the immunopathological mechanisms. Kay [27] showed the importance of the host's response against injected nephrotoxic serum. He postulated that heterologous nephrotoxic serum would fix into the kidney without any remarkable injury and that the following antiheterologous gamma globulin response was the main explanation for the injury. Various nephrotoxic serum nephritides have usually been divided into two phases which are dependent upon different pathogenetic mechanisms. The heterologous phase which promptly occurs in the animals after the antibody against kidney constituents has been injected, is due to the interaction of the heterologous nephrotoxic antibodies with glomerular antigens. The autologous phase usually appears several days after the injection, and is dependent on the host immune response to heterologous gamma globulin. This concept with regard to mechanisms of the heterologous nephrotoxic serum nephritis has recently been developed to include also the mechanisms of autoantibody nephropathy and immune complex nephropathy.

Glomerulonephritis might be caused by the immunization with homologous, or with heterologous kidney antigens such as glomerular basement membrane (GBM), renal tubular epithelium (RTE) and tubular basement membrane (TBM), all being cross-reactive with renal tissues of the host. Development of autoantibodies to own kidney constituents would play an important role in the initiation of the renal injury. Much evidence suggesting this mechanism has been provided.

About 30 years after Masugi, Dixon and his coworkers demonstrated antiGBM antibody in the kidney and sera of patients with human glomerulonephritis [32, 38, 39, 40, 59]. They also reported that soluble GBM antigen obtained from normal rabbit urine caused renal injuries to the injected rabbits [33].   Further, in 1971, Steblay [52] described a new cortical tubular disease and presence of autoantibodies to TBM in the serum and also their presence along the cortical TBM of the diseased animals.   Therefore we will describe here the renal injuries caused by auto- and hetero-antibodies to kidney constituents.

In 1911, von Pirque first reported the relationship between the host immune response to foreign protein after therapeutic injection and the development of serum sickness. Following the report, the immunopathogenesis of immune complex (IC) induced glomerulonephritis has been extensively studied.   During the 1950's, IC nephritis was clearly identified by Germuth [12] who demonstrated the substantial features and immune mechanisms of IC induced nephropathy, showing the fact that a sufficient amount of circulating foreigh protein stimulated the host antibody formation, and development of IC which was composed of antigen and the host antibody was seen in the circulation and the IC accumulated in glomerular capillary walls and initiated the renal injury.   As an experimental classic model of IC-induced tissue injury, acute (one-shot) serum sickness has been well understood.   As to the renal lesion, a precise investigation using immunochemical and immunohistological techniques was carried out by Dixon et al. [9].   They described the fate of large amounts of radioiodinated protein such as bovine serum albumin (BSA) in the circulation, the appearance of free circulating antiBSA antibody and also the characterization of the glomerular deposits of IC by immunofluorescence.

At the same time, chronic serum sickness has been extensively studied, mostly in the following way.   Rabbits were daily given an injection of foreign protein, which resulted in the development of chronic glomerulonephritis for the period of two or three months after the initial injection.   The renal lesions are similar in many respects to human glomerulonephritis.   As a peculiar type of IC nephropathy, Edgington and his coworkers described an autologous immune complex nephropathy [11] which was induced with the immune complexes composed of renal tubular epithelial antigen and autoantibody to the antigen.   The histological manifestations were similar to chronic serum sickness nephritis in rabbits.   In the circulation of the animals, autoantibody against the host renal tubular epithelium was raised and the glomerular deposits contained the antigen and host antibody.

In human renal diseases, it also appears that various forms of renal injury might be induced by autoantibodies against different kidney constituents, just as in experimental animals.   Concerning the pathogenetic role of renal antigens, autoantibody associated renal diseases should be divided into three types: the first one is GBM antigen related glomerulonephritis in which autoantibodies against GBM antigen play a main role as in Goodpasture's syndrome and in certain cases of nephrotic syndrome, especially focal sclerosing and membranoproliferative varieties.   The second is TBM antigen associated interstitial nephropathy in which autoantibodies against TBM would become involved in mechanisms of the development of the main manifestations of renal injury.   The third is RTE antigen related nephropathy, namely autologous immune complexes nephropathy, in which depositis along the GBM contain autoantibodies to RTE and RTE antigen.

Based upon a series of clinical surveys on the relationship between the form of renal injury and the incidence of autoantibodies against renal antigens, the following report consists of three sections: the first dealing with GBM antigen and antiGBM antibodies induced nephropathy, the second with TBM antigen and tubulointerstitial nephropathy, and the third with RTE antigen and RTE antigen-antibody complex induced membranous nephropathy.

II. GBM Antigen in Human Glomerular Diseases

Kidney homogenate was used in Masugi nephritis, and in the homogenate, kidney antigens were presumed to play a role in the production of heterologous antibodies. Subsequently it was postulated that the antiserum against the antigen was nephrotoxic being capable of producing glomerulonephritis, with striking similarities to the diseases in man. Heymann and his coworkers [16] confirmed that the antigen existed in the renal cortex but not in the medulla. This antigen might be GBM antigen. As this antigen had not been well purified from other renal tissue constituents, renal diseases in experimental animals might exhibit various patterns of alterations. In addition the antigenic character of the glomerular antigen had not been fully explained. GBM was first isolated from the kidney by Krakower and Greenspon [29] and the antigen was eluted. Thereby the method of isolating the GBM from the kidney was established. The nephritogenic character of the antigen eluted from the GBM as well as the chemical components are now well investigated by several authors, with histopathological analyses of the GBM of normal and nephritic animals.

The main antigen of the glomeruli is in its basement membrane. The structure of the GBM, possessing specific antigenic sites, is similar to that of vascular and epithelial basement membranes, stomal reticulum and also collagen fibers. The glomerular basement membrane is rich in hydroxyproline and has an amino acid composition similar to collagen. The amino acid composition of the GBM is composed of about 14% proline and hydroxyproline and 20% glycine, with the amount of hydroxylysine being much greater than that in vertebrate collagen. The carbohydrate contained in GBM is about 10% in weight of the GBM, in the form of glucose, mannose, galactose, fucose, hexosamines and sialic acids [28]. The carbohydrate of the GBM appears to have two moieties, one being disaccharide which originated from the collagenous region of the molecule, and the other a sugar component derived from the non-collagenous region.

Histochemically the GBM reacts strongly with the periodic acid-Schiff stain indicating a high carboxyhydrate content, in contrast to the weak reactions exhibited by collagen. Ultrastracturally, the GBM consists of three amorphous layers of varying density — two laminae lucidae and one laminae densa, with no evidence of structural periodicity like that observed in collagen fibers.

The precise localization of the glomerular antigen has been determined with immunochemical techniques by several authors [5, 6, 14, 19, 48]. The GBM appears to contain two types of antigens, i.e., those common to vascular basement membranes and those to reticulum fibers of other organs. But the GBM has been shown to still have distinct antigenicity from tubular cell cytoplasm and other renal basement membrane antigens.

More recently, the purification accuracy of GBM was improved by using immunochemical and physicochemical methods. So, to study the GBM antigen, one must first isolate the original antigen in pure form, that is, free of cellular components and other tissue proteins. As mentioned above, the crude GBM might include several antigens common to other tissue origin antigens such as vascular basement membranes and tubular cell cytoplasm. Some antigens of the GBM included in the TBM sometimes cause a confusion. That is why we presume that, among certain common substances which may contain both tubular basement membrane and glomerular basement membrane, original antigens, i.e., pure TBM and GBM antigens might exist.

By tryptic digestion, and other immunochemical and physicochemical methods, the original GBM antigen can be separated from those common substances and other components. The antigen we thus obtained had a molecular weight of about 40,000 and could induce a specific antibody upon immunization of rabbits which was reactive only to GBM but not to TBM and RTE antigen.   We detected that this GBM antigen was excreted into the urine of patients in various cases of glomerulonephritis.   Not only in Goodpasture's syndrome but also in certain cases of nephrotic syndrome, especially of focal sclerosing and membranoproliferative changes, GBM antigen was excreted into the urine in a quantity much higher than that in other cases of glomerulonephritis, and antiGBM antibody was also detected in patients' sera as well as in the kidney.   With this in mind, the following section will be divided into three parts: the first one is concerned with the purification and characterization of normal human GBM, the second with patients' urinary GBM and the third deals with antiGBM antibody in patients' kidney and sera.

1. Materials and methods

a. GBM antigen preparation

Normal human kidneys from cadaver subjects without any renal diseases were immediately washed and perfused with cold isotonic saline.   Cortices were sliced approximately 5 mm in thickness and were forced through a 100 mesh stainless steel sieve.   The glomerular suspension was further purified from other tissue components by a second passage through a 180 mesh sieve, the glomeruli remaining on the sieve.   The glomeruli suspended in cold isotonic saline were centrifuged at 400 g for 15 min and the supernatant was discarded.   The glomeruli were washed and centrifuged several times until the supernatant became clear.   The final precipitate was suspended in isotonic saline and then disrupted by supersonic vibration and centrifuged at 700 g for 10 min.   The pellets including GBM were also washed and centrifuged several times.   The final precipitate was suspended in a buffer of 0.1 M Tris-HCl, 0.02 M $CaCl_2$.   Then this GBM fraction was digested by trypsin and solubilized GBM fraction was obtained.   The activity of the trypsin was stopped with soybean trypsin inhibitor which was added excessively.   This trypsinized materials were centrifuged at 16,000 r.p.m. for 60 min and at 24,000 r.p.m. for 60 min. The final supernatant was obtained as a digested GBM fraction.   From this digested GBM fraction we purified a GBM antigen by immunochemical and physicochemical analysis.

b. Further purification of GBM antigen

The crude solubilized GBM antigen was electrophoretically fractionated in agar (Fig. 7-1).   The protein content of each block was determined according to the Folin-Ciocalteu method and 4 protein peaks were detected: one in the alpha fraction, 2 in the beta fraction and last one in the gamma fraction.   Both blocks in the beta zone containing GBM antigen were pooled and concentrated.   Next, the antigen was purified by DEAE cellulose column chromatography (Fig. 7-2).   DEAE cellulose, equilibrated with 0.0175 M sodium phosphate buffer, pH 7.4, was packed into a column 20×1 cm.   The sample, obtained by agar block electrophoresis, was dialysed against the same buffer, and eluted by step wise elution of NaCl (0, 0.1, 0.3, and 7.0 M).   A sharp elution peak containing pure GBM antigen was obtained at 0.3 M NaCl concentration.   This sample was next eluted from a Sephadex G-200 column.   Two major protein peaks were detected, with the second peak of low molecular weight including GBM antigen.   This peak was also analyzed in SDS-polyacryl amid gel electrophoresis.

c. Preparation of rabbit antiserum to normal human GBM

Crude solubilized GBM antigen incorporated with Freund's complete adjuvant was

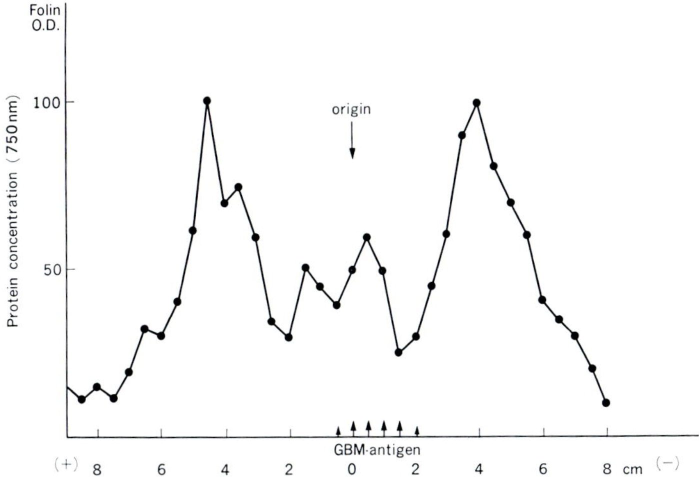

Fig. 7-1   Electrophoretic patterns of trypsinized GBM antigen. Protein concentration of each fractions were measured by the method of Folin. Separation carried out in 0.85% agar, barbital buffer, pH 8.6 ionic strength=0.1. The region containing GBM antigen is shown by arrows.

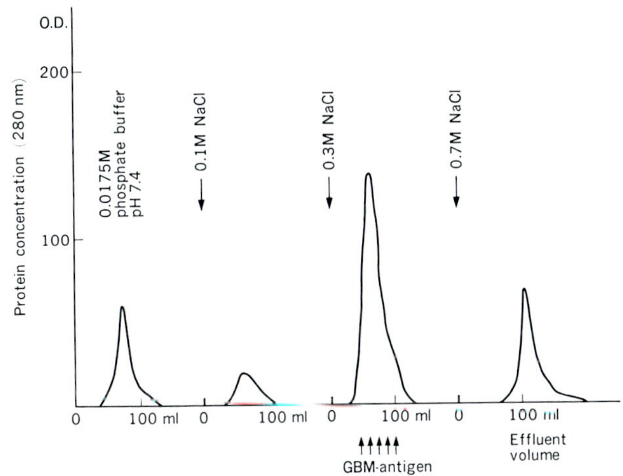

Fig. 7-2   Chromatogram on DEAE cellulose column of GBM antigen. Column size: 1.5× 20 cm. A discontenuous gradient of sodium chloride was used, starting at 0.0175 M phosphate buffer pH 7.4. GBM antigen was eluted in 0.3 M NaCl peak.

injected into the footpads and back muscle of rabbits 3 times at biweekly intervals.   The antiserum thus obtained was absorbed with normal human whole serum, renal epithelial antigen, TBM antigen, and soybean trypsin inhibitor.   The IgG fraction of the rabbit serum was prepared by 50% ammonium sulfate precipitation followed by DEAE cellulose column chromatography with 0.01 M sodium phosphate buffer, pH 8.0.   The specificity of the antiserum confirmed immunoelectrophoresis and by immunofluorescence.

d. Preparation of urine specimens

Urine specimens were obtained from 37 adult patients with various renal diseases. Urine specimens were dialysed against cold isotonic saline and then were concentrated by negative pressure dialysis.   The concentrated urine specimens were centrifuged at 20,000 r.p.m. for 30 min at 4–8 °C and tested against antihuman GBM antibody.   Molecular sieving of patients' urine with Sephadex G-200 was performed with borate buffered saline. Existence of GBM antigen in each fraction was examined by immunodiffusion with antihuman GBM.

e. Measurement of GBM antigen in urine

The concentration of GBM antigen in the urine samples was measured according to an indirect single radial radioimmunodiffusion method, in which rabbit antihuman GBM and radioactive iodinated goat antirabbit IgG were used.   As standard antigen we used the purified GBM antigen eluted from DEAE cellulose column chromatography.   The protein concentration was determined according to the Folin-Ciocalteu method.   The diameters of the radioactive rings were measured and GBM concentration in urine was determined from this standard curve.   We designated that 1 unit of the GBM in urine corresponded to 1 μg prot/ml of purified GBM antigen.

2. Immunochemical characters of normal human GBM

Purified GBM antigen was shown to have mobility in the beta zone by electrophoresis. In this zone, other renal tissue origin antigens such as tubular basement membrane and tubular epithelial antigen were not detected (Fig. 7-1).   This GBM antigen revealed a moderate ionic strength of pH 7.4, which was analyzed in DEAE cellulose column (Fig. 7-2).   Further, the antigen showed a molecular weight which is lower than that of normal human serum albumin according to molecular sieving such as Sephadex G-200 column chromatography.   SDS-polyacryl amide gel electrophoresis then showed that the GBM antigen molecular weight was about 40,000 (Fig. 7-3).   Furthermore, the purified GBM antigen raised specific antibody to human GBM, when immunizing rabbits with Freund's complete adjuvant.   This specific antiserum to human GBM reacted only with purified GBM antigen in a gel plate but did not react with other renal tissue origin antigens and human serum components.   This antiserum also reacted specifically with normal human GBM of frozen kidney section by immunofluorescent technique.   The fluorescence was detected linearly along the GBM but not detected on the other kidney components (Fig. 7-4).

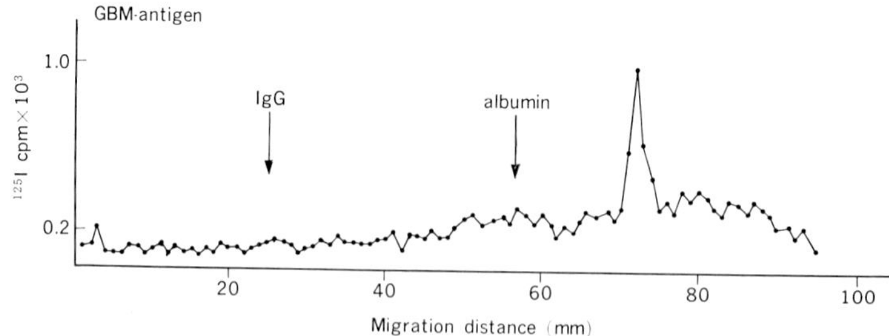

Fig. 7-3 SDS polyacrylamide gel electrophoresis of a ^{125}I-labeled GBM antigen. Gels with an acrylamide concentration of 7.5% were used. After completion of the electrophoretic separation the gel was divided into segments of 1 mm width and counted for radioactivity in a gammer-well type scintillation counter.

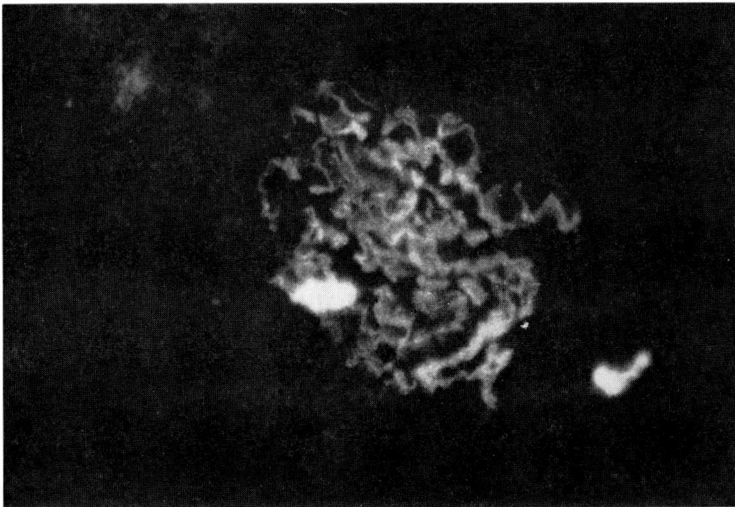

Fig. 7-4 Immunofluorescence showing linear pattern along the glomerular basement membrane. Normal human kidney treated with fluorescein-labeled rabbit antihuman GBM.

3. GBM antigen in urine of patients of glomerular diseases

GBM antigen is excreted into the urine of various renal diseases in a soluble form. The GBM in urine reacts specifically with our antiserum to human GBM at the beta zone of the plate as well as to purified GBM antigen on immunoelectrophoresis. The molecular weight of the GBM in urine was revealed to be relatively lower than that of human serum albumin. On a Sephadex G-200 column, concentrated patient urine showed four protein peaks; in the fourth peak the GBM antigen was detected with human serum albumin (Fig. 7-5) and in sucrose density gradient elution, the GBM was eluted following human serum

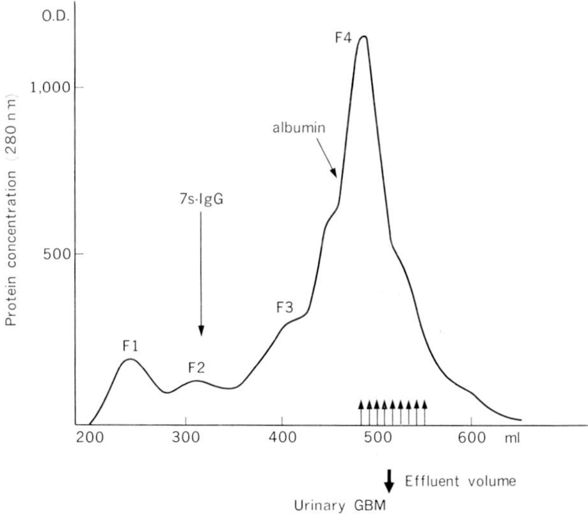

Fig. 7-5 Chromatography on Sephadex G-200 of concentrated urine samples from a patient. Elution speed: 16 ml/hr. Column size: 3×180 cm. Four peaks of urine protein were observed. GBM antigen was eluted only from the fourth peak with human albumin, as shown with arrows.

albumin (Fig. 7-6) indicating that this urine GBM antigen was a molecular weight less than that of human serum albumin.   This antigen also produced specific antibody in rabbits immunized with patient urine specimens.   The antigenicity of the GBM in urine was compared with that of purified GBM by a double immunodiffusion method.   In an agarose plate, the urine specimens from two patients showed an identical immunological reaction. However, the trypsinized GBM formed a spur over these urine specimens (Fig. 7-7).

To summarize these observations, the GBM antigen in urine is antigenically distinct from renal tubular epithelial antigen, renal tubular basement membrane antigen, as well as other normal serum components.   The size of the molecule is somewhat smaller than that of human serum albumin and the same as trypsinized human GBM, and can therefore be reabsorbed through the kidney epithelial cells.   The fact that the GBM antigen has displayed a partial identity to the purified GBM antigen intimates that the GBM antigen in urine would share one determinant with the trypsinized GBM antigen and that it would

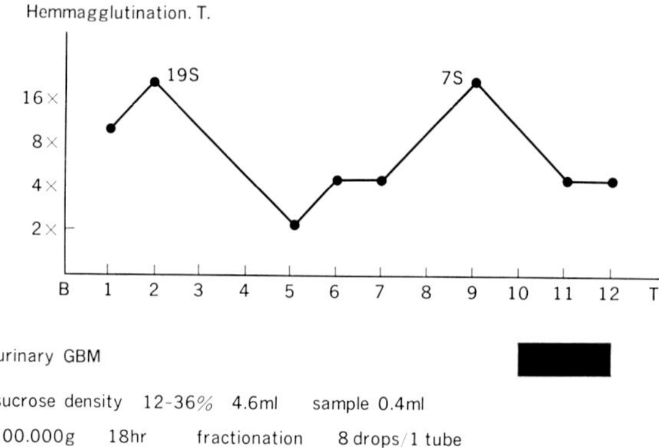

Fig. 7-6   The sucrose density (12–36%) ultracentrifugation patterns (av. 100,000 kg, 18 hrs) of urinary protein. Purified rabbit 19s and 7s gammer globulin served as markers. GBM in urine is seen at the top side from 7s markers.

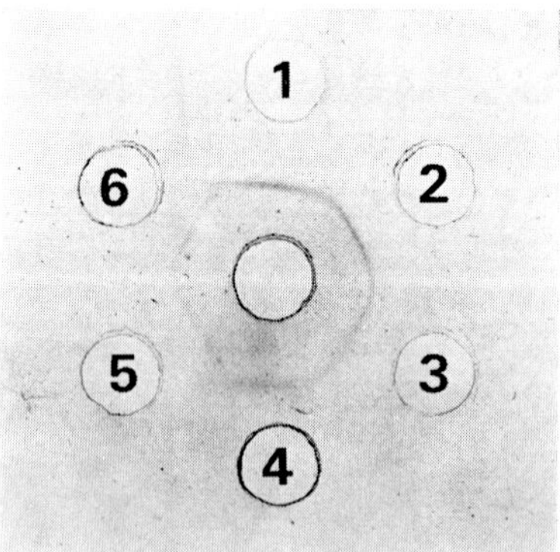

Fig. 7-7   Ouchterlony plate showing antigenic character of GBM in urine and purified GBM antigen. The central well was filled with an antiserum against normal human GBM. The No. 1 well contained crude trypsinized GBM antiggen, the No. 2 well was placed with GBM fractions from block electrophoresis, No. 3 was placed with the fraction eluted from Sephadex G-200, and No. 4 was placed with finally purified GBM antigen. The No. 5 well was placed with the crude preparation of one patient's urine, and No. 6 was placed with purified urinary GBM eluted from a Sephadex G-200 column.

have one deficient antigenic determinant.   The GBM antigen in urine is probably a molecule which is a degrading product of the glomerular basement membrane in a soluble form in vivo, distinct from the form in which the GBM antigen is solubilized with trypsin in vitro.

The GBM antigen was detected in 26 out of 37 cases of glomerular diseases: 1 chronic glomerulonephritis, 14 nephrotic syndrome, 5 chronic renal insufficiency, and 6 lupus nephropathy.   The concentration of the GBM antigen varied in each case, in which most of the nephrotic syndrome and lupus nephropathy cases showed very high concentrations. Only one case of chronic glomerulonephritis and 2 cases of renal insufficiency showed measurable amounts of GBM antigen (Fig. 7-8).

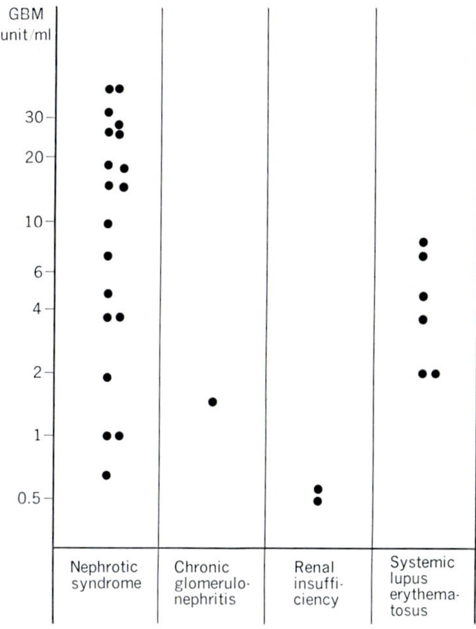

Fig. 7-8   GBM concentration in urine and various renal diseases.

This indicates that GBM antigen may be frequently detected in patients with systemic lupus nephropathy, nephrotic syndrome and renal insufficiency.   Particularly in nephrotic syndrome, cases of a high concentration level may be often seen.   As to its relationship to renal function, urinary GBM concentration was not correlated with the glomerular filtration rate (sodium thiosulfate clearance) and the excretion of GBM antigen was not controlled by the renal function.   Histologically, we divide glomerular diseases into five groups as classified by Burch [7]: minimal change, proliferative change, membranous change, membranoproliferative change and sclerosing change.   In the case of minimal change, GBM antigen was not detectable at all, but in proliferative change it was frequently detected, although its concentration value was usually low (Fig. 7-9).   However, in membranous and membranoproliferative change, most cases excreted GBM antigen over 10 units/ml.   These findings lead to the obvious suggestion that damaged GBM has at least some partial effect on the excretion of GBM antigen.   In membranous change, immune deposits fixed to the GBM probably release some chemical mediators which might partially

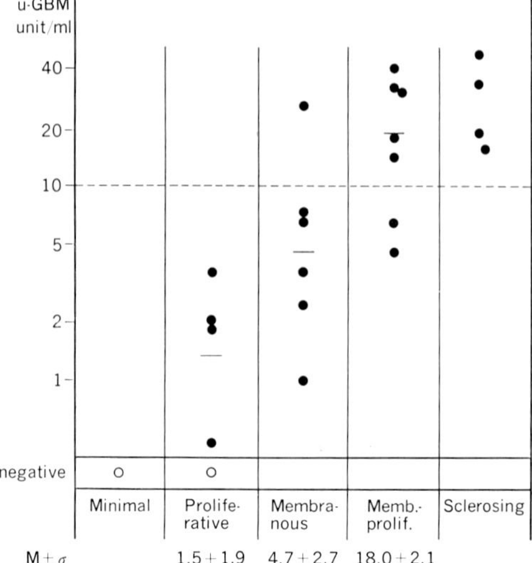

Fig. 7-9   Relationship of GBM concentration in urine to histological findings of nephrotic syndrome.

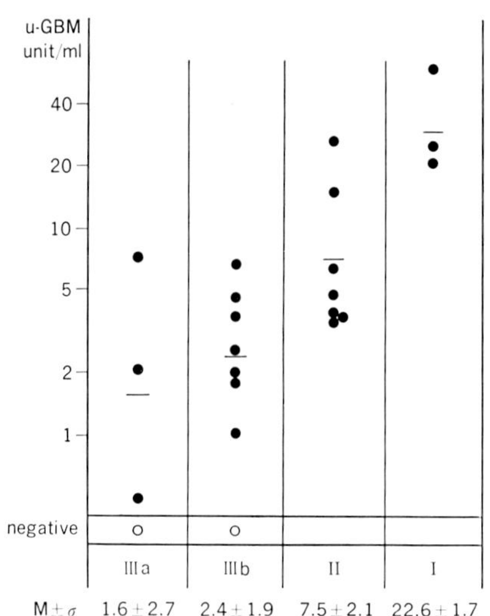

Fig. 7-10   Relationship of GBM concentration in urine to steroid hormone treatment.

solubilize the GBM, causing the GBM antigen to excrete into the urine of patients.   The group of membranoproliferative change included the cases associated with antiGBM antibody and the cases excreted very high amounts of GBM into urine.   In these cases some factors would influence the autoantibody formation to the host GBM antigen in the kidney; then the antiGBM antibody would damage its own GBM and from the damaged GBM, antigen would be continuously discharged into the urine.   Therefore the clinical features would not have improved completely, and the effectiveness of steroid hormone therapy, for example, would be inhibited (Fig. 7-10).   The results of quantitative estimation of GBM antigen in urine will be correlated with the prediction of histological diagnosis as well as the response to steroid therapy. The probably significance of this is that large amounts of GBM antigen in urine indicate the degree of severity of the glomerular lesions.

4. AntiGBM antibody in glomerular diseases

Various experiments have been conducted on the nephritogenicity of the GBM antigen towards animals. Shibata and his coworkers [49] found that glycopeptide associated with GBM would have nephritogenic activity in rats. Lerner and Dixon [33] also demonstrated that GBM antigen in urine induced glomerulonephritis in rabbits. They also demonstrated that, while observing antiGBM antibody associated glomerulonephritis of rabbits, GBM antigen in urine had increased and altered its physical characteristics in response. Their report suggested that the GBM antigen in urine may have become an autoimmunogen to the glomerulonephritis. In human nephritis, antiGBM antibody has been demonstrated in glomerulonephritic kidneys [39]. We have also detected anti GBM antibody in sera and kidney of 4 cases with high amounts of GBM antigen in urine, 2 cases with membranoproliferative change and 2 cases with sclerosing change. The clinical course of all 4 cases was progressive and advanced. These patients resisted all therapeutic means and subsequently succumbed to the diseases after 2–3 years.

By direct immunofluorescence, typical linear depositions of IgG along the GBM were demonstrated in their kidneys. From these kidneys elution of antiGBM antibody was performed by lowering the pH value [32]. The cortical portion of the kidneys was dissected and glomeruli and glomerular basement membranes were obtained as described previously. From the GBM, IgG was eluted by glycin-HCl buffer, pH 2.4. The eluted IgG reacted with the GBM of a normal human kidney section by an indirect immunofluorescent technique (Fig. 7-11).

The findings resembled very much the so-called Goodpasture's syndrome. It is well known that Goodpasture's syndrome is induced with autoantibody to the host's GBM antigen [32, 39]. After typical lung disorders, autoantibody to GBM is raised and typical kidney diseases are established. The renal manifestation is followed by the glomerular lesion in which cellular proliferation and crescent formation are detected (Fig. 7-12) and in immunofluorescence, typically linear depositions of host immunoglobulin and complement components are seen. The linearly deposited IgG eluted from the kidney reacts specifically with purified GBM antigen by agarose double immunodiffusion. In the sera, antiGBM antibody is also detected, and in the urine a high amount of GBM antigen is seen.

These results seem to provide some confirmation that the GBM antigen in urine may change into an autoimmunogen because the extensively excreted amounts of GBM antigen, the molecular size being the same as albumin, can be easily reabsorbed in the proximal tubular cells in the kidney. The host antibody proliferated and invaded the GBM as the target organ, following which the degrading GBM antigen would be noted in the patients' urine again, thereby indicating that the clinical course would be progressive and advanced.

5. Summary

A soluble glomerular basement membrane (GBM) antigen was detected in the urine of patients with various glomerular diseases including chronic glomerulonephritis, nephrotic syndrome, chronic renal insufficiency, and lupus nephropathy. The urinary GBM antigen (u-GBM) was immunochemically distinct from other renal antigens and other serum components, but it was crossreactive with trypsinized human GBM antigen. The molecular size of urinary GBM was approximately the same as human serum albumin

studies [2] have demonstrated that the immune responses of strains II and XIII guinea pig to various antigens are controlled by immune response (Ir) genes which are linked to a major histocompatibility complex of the guinea pigs.   AntiTBM antibody production and severity of the disease were predominant in animals having the XIII gene, and therefore were linked to the strain XIII major histocompatibility.

In other animals, the pathogenesis of the autoantibody formation to TBM with the development of the interstitial nephropathy has not yet been clarified.   In our laboratory, antiTBM nephritis was induced in goats immunized with highly purified human TBM in complete Freund's adjuvant three times at 2-week intervals.   The TBM antigen was solubilized with proteolytic enzyme and further purified by physicochemical and immunochemical methods.   The antigen had a molecular weight of about 30,000 and could develop a specific antibody upon immunization of goats, an antibody which is only reactive to human and goat TBM but not GBM antigen.   The antibody was produced only at a low titer during the first 2 months, but it suddenly increased at 4 months after immunization even without further antigenic stimulation.   The histological findings of renal biopsy at this stage revealed an occurrence of severe interstitial nephritis which was similar to the findings in the rats described previously [52] (Fig. 7-13).   Host immunoglobulin was demonstrated along the TBM and Bowman's capsular membrane but not along the GBM by direct immunofluorescence.   Subsequently, soluble TBM antigen of the goats was excreted in urine.

A similar antiTBM antibody nephritis was successfully induced in goats which had been immunized with TBM antigen separated from unilaterally nephrectomized own kidney in a soluble form in Freund's complete adjuvant two times at 2-week intervals.   In this experiment, antiTBM antibody was also raised at a moderate titer and lasted for 6 months. AntiGBM antibody was not raised.   At 3 months after the first injection severe inflammatory changes in the interstitium were demonstrated and mild changes in glomeruli were also seen.   The renal cortical lesion as a primary disease showed interstitial cellular infiltration of mononuclear leucocytes, periglomerular fibrosis and focal tubular destruction.

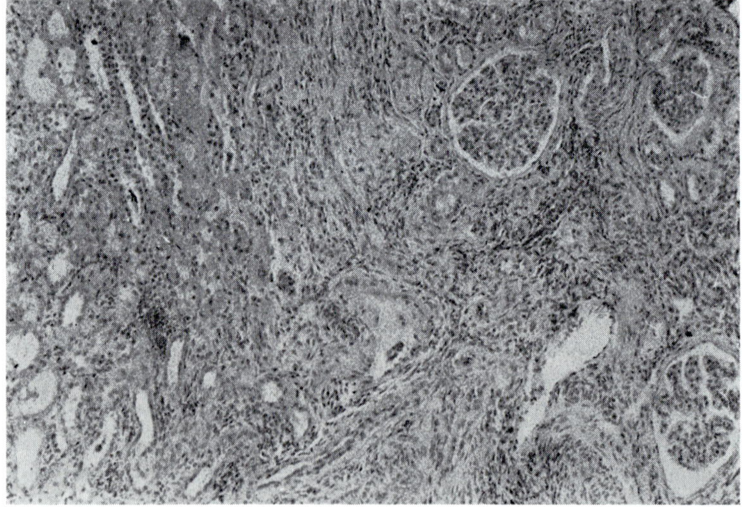

Fig. 7-13 Light microscopic findings of a goat interstitial nephropathy. Severe interstitial nephropathy with focal intensive infiltration of mononuclear cells and spindle shaped cells among fibrou tissues. Tubular atrophy, vacuolation and remarkable changes of TBM are also seen. H & E stain. (Courtesy of Dr. I. Takei)

Irregular thickening and double contour or reduplication of the TBM, and the destruction of tubular epithelial cells were noted. Remarkable compressions of glomerular tuft were seen in certain areas, which indicated an increase of the inner pressure of Bowman's capsular space caused by tubular obstruction. Linear staining along the TBM and Bowman's capsular membrane and positive fine granular staining in the mesangial area corresponding to electron microscopic findings were seen by immunofluorescence.

The above described goats excreted a large amount of host TBM antigen into urine which was reactive with the goat antihuman TBM antibody, or the host autoantiTBM antibody. The immunization of TBM antigen which is crossreactive with host TBM raised autoantibody against host TBM and the antibody caused the tubular injury. Then lysis of TBM antigen from the diseased TBM would occur and the excreted TBM antigen into the urine might be reabsorbed through the tubular cells into the circulating blood and led to stimulate immune response to TBM antigen and form immune complexes composed of TBM antigen and antiTBM antibody (Fig. 7-24).

Now, the important question concerning antiTBM-tubulointerstitial nephritis is whether or not it occurs in man. Antibodies against TBM have occasionally been detected in antiGBM associated glomerulonephritis including Goodpastures' syndrome and renal transplantation. However, primary antiTBM associated interstitial nephritis was very rare. Morel-Maroger [41] and his coworkers have reported antiTBM induced nephritis in rapidly progressive poststreptococcal glomerulonephritis in one 40-year-old man. Linear staining for IgG and beta-1-C was observed along the TBM but not the GBM, and the serum reacted with normal TBM. Severe tubular damage and interstitial fibrosis were noted. Possibly, the initial acute glomerulonephritis somehow led to stimulate the antiTBM response. Tung and Black [54] reported that a renal biopsy specimen of a 2-year-old boy with nephrotic syndrome revealed heavy granular deposits of IgG, C3, IgM and IgA along the GBM and most of the TBM by immunofluorescence. AntiTBM antibody in this case was detectable in the patient's serum 6 months after the onset of the nephrotic syndrome; 6 months later, the patient developed Fanconi's syndrome. The circulating antiTBM antibody reacted with the TBM and Bowman's capsule and was eliminated by absorption with purified TBM antigen, but not with purified GBM antigen.

AntiTBM antibody was also observed by Borden and his coworkers [4] in a patient treated with methicillin in whom interstitial nephritis with mononuclear cell infiltration and focal tubular damage as well as severe renal failure had developed. The immunofluorescence studies of the renal biopsy material showed linear deposits of IgG, C3 and methicillin antigen assumed to be dimethoxyphenyl penicilloyl (DPO), a breakdown product of methicillin, along the TBM but not the GBM. These facts suggested that the DPO-TBM "hapten protein conjugate" stimulated the production of antiTBM antibody reactive with the carrier portion of the protein-hapten conjugate.

In addition, Bergstein and Litman [3] demonstrated interstitial nephritis induced with antiTBM antibody. Renal biopsy from a six-year-old boy revealed linear staining of IgG and C3. The patient's serum reacted of with the TBM of a normal kidney frozen section in a linear pattern. This staining was abolished by absorption of the serum with purified TBM, but not diminished by absorption with purified GBM. Light microscopic studies showed chronic interstitial nephritis. Most of the glomeruli were hyalinized, with the remainder being relatively unaffected, although periglomerular fibrosis was present around some glomeruli. Tubular destruction and atrophy, and marked fibrosis were noted in the interstitium. Recently, our laboratory identified antiTBM associated nephropathy in patients with rheumatoid arthritis who had been treated with gold therapy. Renal biopsy of a patient with nephrotic syndrome revealed coarse granular deposits of IgG and beta-

1-C along the GBM and linear deposits along the TBM by immunofluorescence.   The patients serum and kidney eluate obtained from the renal biopsy specimen was fixed specifically along the TBM.   Furthermore, a precipitin line was identified between the kidney eluate and the purified soluble TBM antigen by radioimmunodiffusion.   Renal biopsy studies of another patient showed minimal changes in glomeruli, although moderate tubular degeneration was noted in the interstitium.   Immunofluorescent studies revealed linear staining of the TBM with IgG and beta-1-C and slight mesangial deposits in the glomeruli. In three other rheumatoid arthritis patients and one with phenacetin toxicity, the serum reacted with the TBM of normal cryostat sections in linear patterns by indirect immunofluorescence.   These observations suggested the possibility that antiTBM antibody had a primary role in the pathogenesis of the patients' interstitial nephritis.

Therefore, this work was divided into three parts: the first one is characterization of normal human TBM, the second is TBM antigen in patient's urine, and the third is antiTBM antibody in patient's kidneys and/or sera.

1. Materials and methods

a. Purification of the TBM

The normal human kidney obtained at autopsy was perfused with isotonic cold saline. The kidney cortices were diced and passed through a rough mesh and then filtered through #100, 150 and 200 mesh stainless steel screens.   The fiber-rich materials which remained on the stainless #100 mesh were centrifuged at 4°C for 30 min at 1500 g on a Ficoll discontinuous gradient (10–60%).   After centrifugation the layer of the most fiber-rich portion was obtained (Fig. 7-14).   The materials were also sonicated for 3 min to exclude the fragments of renal tubular epithelium fixed to fibers.   Crude soluble TBM antigen was obtained by digestion of the material with trypsin.

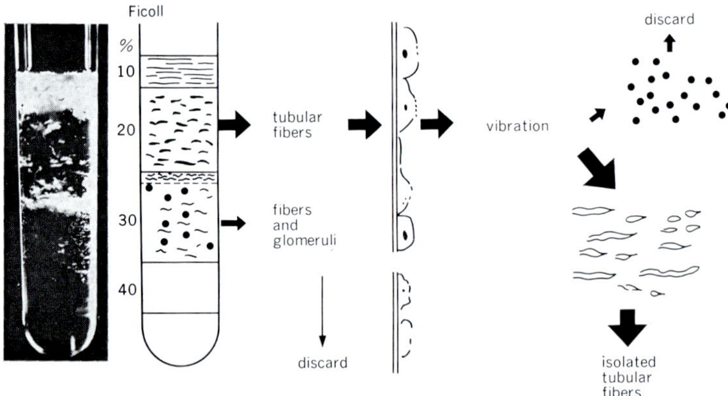

Fig. 7-14   Isolation procedure of tubular basement membrane.

b. Further purification of the TBM antigen

The digestive soluble TBM antigen was centrifuged at 30,000 g for 30 min.   The supernatant was collected and concentrated by negative pressure.   The sample was separated by zone electrophoresis on 0.85% agar at 4°C in barbital-NaOH buffer, pH 8.6, ionic strength 0.1, under an electric potential of 12 V cm^{-1} for 36 hours at 4°C (1.0 × 10 × 24 cm in agar).   The gel was cut into segments 5 mm wide and the proteins were ex-

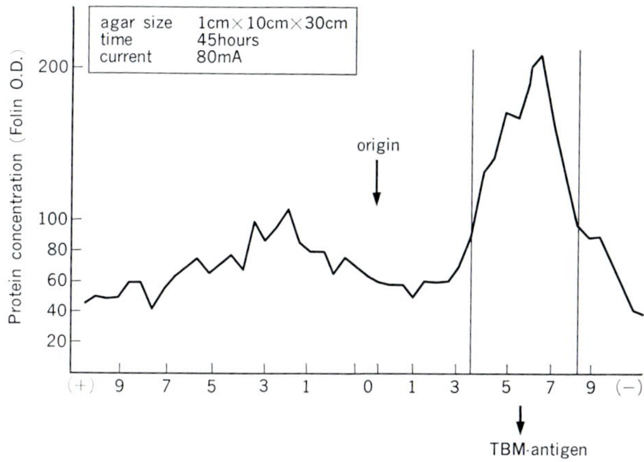

Fig. 7-15 Electrophoretic patterns of trypsinized TBM antigen. The regions containing TBM
antigen are shown by arrows.

tracted by repeated freezing and thawing. Three protein peaks were obtained in the
alpha, beta and gamma portions (Fig. 7-15). Each extract was tested by using the specific
antibody (see below) against the soluble TBM antigen. The fractions which had migrated
to the gamma portion reacted with the antiserum. The material recovered from the gamma portion was further fractionated by DEAE cellulose (DE 52 Whatman; W & R. Boston
Ltd., Springfield Mill, England) column chromatography. The column (20×0.8 cm)
was equilibrated with 0.005 M phosphate buffer, pH 8.0. Before application, the sample
was dialysed extensively against the starting buffer. The applied protein was eluted at
pH 8.0 with a salt gradient from 0 to 1 M NaCl. Effluent fractions reacting with the
specific antiserum were concentrated and applied to a column of Sephadex G-200 (Phar-
macia Fine Chemicals AB, Upsala, Sweden). The fractions eluted from gel filtration were
also tested for the presence of the TBM antigen and the relevant fractions were pooled and
concentrated.

For further examination, the following immunological procedure was performed to
examine the purity and the molecular weight of the antigen. The sodium dedocyl sulfate
polyacrylamide gel electrophoresis (SDS-PAGE) was carried out with an indirect precipitation method using radioiodinated TBM antigen, specific antiserum to TBM rabbit IgG,
and goat IgG against rabbit IgG [36, 55]. The concentrated peak from Sephadex G-200
was radioiodinated using the chloramin-T method with a carrier-free Na^{125}I. Reaction
mixtures were incubated at room temperature for 30 min and overnight at 0°C. After
adding an excess of goat IgG against rabbit IgG, the precipitate was pelleted at 1500 g
for 30 min at 4°C, washed three times with 0.01 M phosphate buffered saline, pH 7.4,
and dissolved with a small amount of PBS, pH 7.2, containing 2% sodium dedocyl sulfate,
0.14 M 2-mercaptoethanol, 50% glycerol and 0.002% bromophenol blue. The samples
were electrophoresed in polyacrylamide gels at 8 mA/gel for 5 hours. The acrylamide
gels were frozen, cut in 1 mm wide sections, and counted in a scintillation spectrophoto-
meter.

c. Preparation of antisera

Crude solubilized TBM antigen was immunized to rabbits with Freund's complete
adjuvant, 3 times at 2-week intervals. The antiserum was absorbed with normal human
whole serum, renal epithelial antigen, purified GBM antigen, and soybean trypsin inhibitor. The specific antiserum was prepared from the IgG fraction of rabbit serum, and the

specificity was confirmed by immunofluorescence.   The fractions from zone electrophoresis and the eluted peak from DEAE column chromatography were also injected into rabbits. These antisera were also tested for their specificity to human TBM by immunofluorescent techniques, gel diffusion methods, and immunoelectrophoresis.

d. Preparation of urine concentrates and patients' sera

Fresh urine collections were obtained from 35 patients and 11 healthy subjects.   Fifteen patients were affected with renal tubular disease, with two cases of Wilson's disease, one case of chronic cadmium poisoning, one of renal tubular acidosis, one of phenacetin induced tubular necrosis, three of acute rejection of renal transplantation, and eight of gold therapy associated tubular disorders with rheumatoid arthritis.   Another 19 patients contained nine with nephrotic syndrome, four of systemic lupus erythematosus and six of chronic glomerulonephritis.   The urine samples were kept at 4°C with the addition of a concentration of 0.1% sodium azide.   For the concentration of the urine specimens, ultrafiltration through Visking tubings (8/32 inch) was used.   The sera from these patients were obtained at the same time when urine specimens were collected.

e. Protein estimation

Quantitative determination of soluble TBM-antigens in the concentrated urine specimens was measured by the indirect single radial immunodiffusion method of Mancini and his coworkers [37] using an antirabbit IgG-goat serum.   Quantitation of the purified renal antigen was used as the standard of this antigen.   The protein concentration of the purified renal antigen was measured by the Folin Ciocalteu method described by Lowry and associates [35].   The concentrations of antigens were obtained by plotting the squares of the diameters on a standard curve.   We designated that 1 U/ml of urinary TBM antigen corresponds to 1 μg/ml of the standard TBM antigen, as previously described in the GBM section in this paper.   Quantitation of albumin in urine specimens was also made by single radial immunodiffusion method.

f. Detection of circulating antiTBM antibodies

Indirect immunofluorescence was performed on frozen normal kidney sections in order to examine the presence of circulating antiTBM antibody of the sera from patients.   The patients in these experiments were suspected of having tubulointerstitial nephritis according to the renal histological findings and the patterns of urinary protein with the SDS-PAGE examination.

Additionally, immunological procedures were carried out for confirmation of the presence of the circulating antiTBM antibody.   Indirect radioimmunodiffusion on agarose was performed between purified TBM antigen and patients' sera using specific antihuman-IgG labeled with Na^{131}I.

g. Elution studies from kidney biopsy specimens

Four-micron frozen sections of needle biopsy specimens were fixed to slide glass and incubated at 4°C with glycine-HCl buffer, pH 2.4, and with agitation with a vibrator. The acid buffer was then neutralized with 0.1 M NaOH, dialysed against 0.01 M PBS, pH 7.2, and concentrated.   Very small amounts of immunoglobulins were obtained and available to use for indirect immunofluorescence and indirect radioimmunodiffusion.

2. Immunochemical characters of normal human TBM antigen

Electrophoresis revealed that purified TBM antigen had the mobility of the gamma range (Fig. 7-15).   This electrophoretic pattern of soluble TBM antigen was reproducible from one experiment to another with several consecutive preparations and only the peak of this gamma portion has reacted with specific antiserum against TBM.   On DEAE column

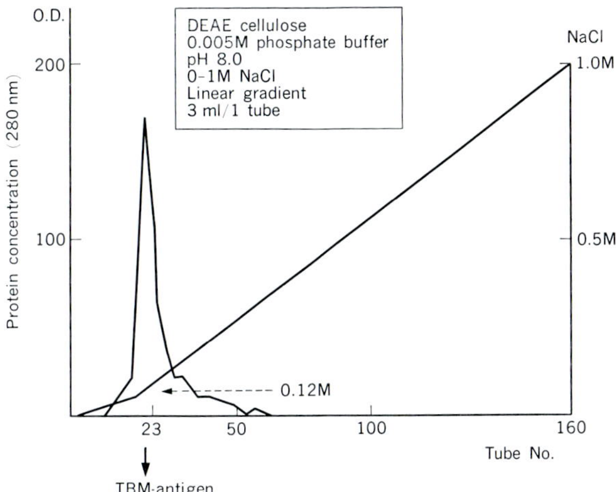

Fig. 7-16 Elution patterns from DEAE cellulose column chromatography of TBM antigen. A linear gradient of sodium chloride was used, starting at 0.005 M phosphate buffer. TBM antigen was eluted in a single peak of 0.12 M peak.

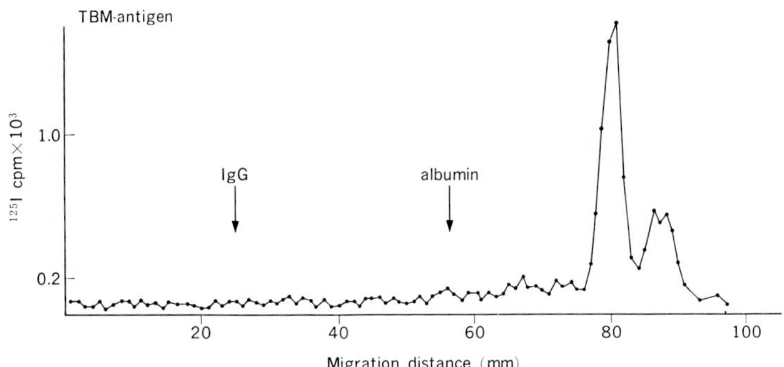

Fig. 7-17 SDS polyacrylamide gel electrophoresis of a ^{125}I-labeled TBM antigen. Gels with an acrylamide concentration of 7.5% were used. After completion of the electrophoretic separation the gel was divided into segments of 1 mm width and counted for radioactivity in a gammer well type scintillation counter.

chromatography TBM antigen was eluted in a single peak at 0.12 M NaCl with a continuous gradient method (Fig. 7-16).   The molecular size of the antigen was smaller than that of human albumin by gel filtration on Sephadex G-200.   Furthermore, the antigen had a molecular weight of about 30,000 with SDS-PAGE (Fig. 7-17), which approximately coincides with the gel filtration pattern.

The purified TBM antigen produced specific antibody in rabbits.   The specific antiserum reacted only with purified TBM antigen (Fig. 7-18) and not with other renal tissue antigens (GBM antigen or RTE antigen) even without any absorption study.   By immunofluorescence, the antiserum also reacted with Bowman's capsular basement membrane and the TBM but not with the other kidney constituents (Fig. 7-19).

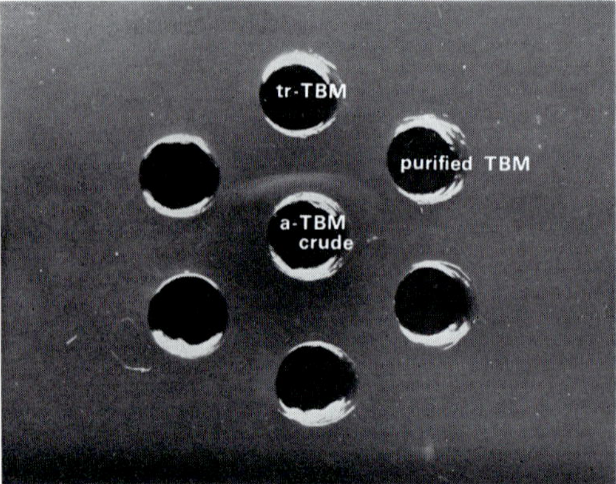

Fig. 7-18 Ouchterlony plate showing the specificity of an antiserum against TBM. The central well was filled with an antiserum against TBM (rabbit serum). The top well contained trypsinized TBM antigen, the upper right well contained finally purified TBM antigen, the lower right well contained purified GBM antigen, and upper left well contained purified RTE antigen. The antiserum reacted only with TBM antigen.

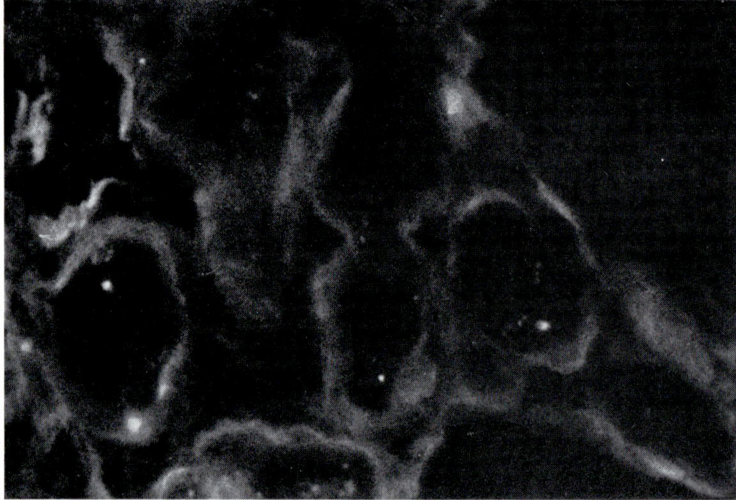

Fig. 7-19 Indirect immunofluorescence staining of normal human kidney with a specific antibody aganist human TBM. Note the bright selective staining of the tubular basement membrane. GBM and tubular cells are completely negative.

3. TBM antigen in urine of patients

The TBM antigen was observed in urine of various renal patients in a soluble form. The excreted TBM antigen reacted with the specific antibody against TBM antigen and was identified in the gamma portion by immunoelectrophoresis. The TBM antigen in urine had a molecular weight smaller than that of human IgG by gel filtration (Fig. 7-20). The elution pattern of the excreted TBM on DEAE cellulose column showed the same pattern on that of purified TBM under the same condition, that is, the urinary TBM antigen was eluted with a salt gradient at 0.12 M NaCl. The antigenicity of the TBM antigen in urine was the same as that of prepared TBM antigen against the specific antiserum in

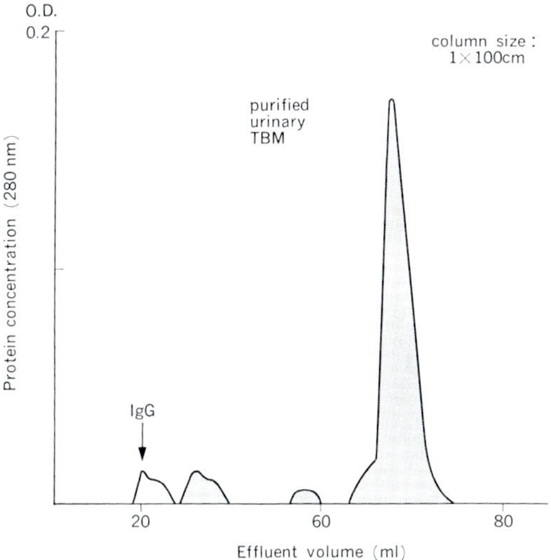

Fig. 7-20 Chromatography on Sephadex G-200 of partially purified TBM from a patient's urine sample. Three peaks were observed after the peak of human IgG. (Courtesy of Dr. K. Iesato)

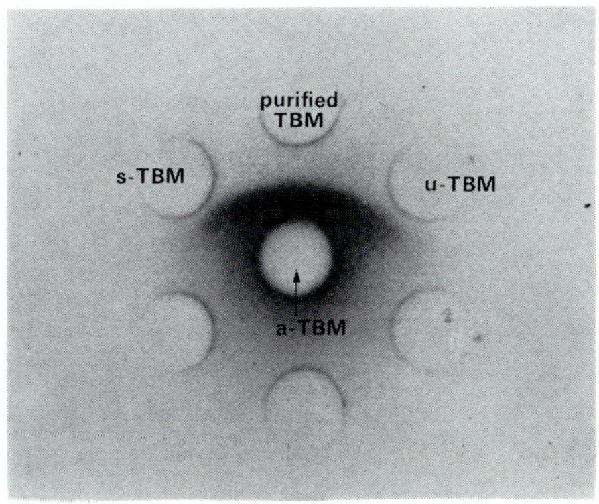

Fig. 7-21 Ouchterlony plate showing the antigenic character of TBM in urine and serum, and purified TBM antigen. The central well was filled with the specific antiserum against TBM. The well of u-TBM contained TBM antigen from urine samples and the well of s-TBM contained TBM from a patient's serum. (Courtesy of Dr. K. Iesato)

immunodiffusion (Fig. 7-21). The excreted TBM in urine also produced the antiserum in rabbits, which in turn reacted specifically with normal human TBM by indirect immunofluorescence.

The TBM antigen in urine was detected in 20 out of 36 cases with various renal disorders. We divided these cases into 3 groups according to the difference of renal lesion, namely, tubular damage only, glomerular damage only, and diseases with both tubular and glomerular damage ("mixed type"). The classification was done by histological examinations of patients' biopsied kidney and by functional examination including urinary protein analysis [23]. Urinary TBM antigen was found in 6 cases with glomerular damage, 5 cases with tubular damage, 8 cases with both tubular and glomerular damage, and in one of the normal subjects (Table 7-1). In other words, TBM antigen was frequently excreted in the urine of all groups. However, the frequency was highest in the "mixed type" group.

Table 7-1 Incidence of TBM antigen in urine as detected by a doule diffusion method in agarose using a specific antiserum against TBM.

Classification of damaged region	Number of urines tested (36)	Positive	Per cent
Tubular damage	8	5	62.5
Glomerular damage	10	6	60.0
Tubular and Glomerular damage	11	8	72.7
Normal subject	7	1	14.3

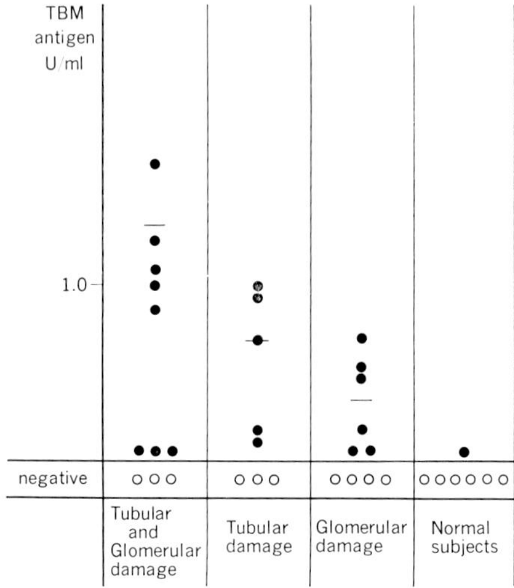

Fig. 7-22 TBM concentration in urine and various renal damages (tubular damage, glomerular damage and tubular and glomerular damage).

In normal subjects the incidence was very low as evidenced by the solitary case detected. The remarkable differences among the 3 groups was also characterized by the excretion amounts of TBM antigen in urine. The high concentration of the excreted antigen was observed in the "mixed type" (Fig. 7-22). Clinical features of the patients in this group disclosed rapidly progressive glomerulonephritis with nephrotic syndrome, gold induced membranous glomerulonephritis, renal tubular acidosis and cadmium poisoning with glomerulonephritis. In three patients having "Minamata disease" with simple tubular lesion, the antigen was but moderately excreted into their urine. Although patients with glomerular lesion only also excreted the antigen into their urine, the concentration was very low. These findings showed that the quantitative determination of TBM antigen in urine was useful for examining the grade of tubular damage, and/or the type of renal injury.

4. Autoantibody to TBM antigen and interstitial nephropathy in human

Antibody to TBM antigen was detected in sera of 3 patients with both interstitial and glomerular changes. These 3 cases included the gold induced membranous nephropathy associated with rheumatoid arthritis, rapidly progressive glomerulonephritis with unknown etiology and renal transplantation. The interstitial changes were characterized by a focal, mononuclear cell infiltration, tubular atrophy and peritubular fibrosis.   The glomerular changes were represented by typical membranous changes.   By immunofluorescence, IgG and beta-1-C were demonstrated strongly along the GBM in a granular pattern, and IgG and beta-1-C were also demonstrated finely and/or linearly along the TBM. Kidney eluates from these patients contain IgG type of immunoglobulin which reacted specifically with normal human TBM by immunofluorescence and also reacted with purified TBM antigen by the methods of radioimmunodiffusion.   The antibody in sera was confirmed by indirect immunofluorescence using normal human kidney as targets and fluorescein conjugated specific antibody to human IgG, and also by radioimmunoelectrophoresis using radio-iodinated purified TBM antigen (Fig. 7-23).   These patients excreted extremely large amounts of TBM antigen from the damaged TBM into their urine.

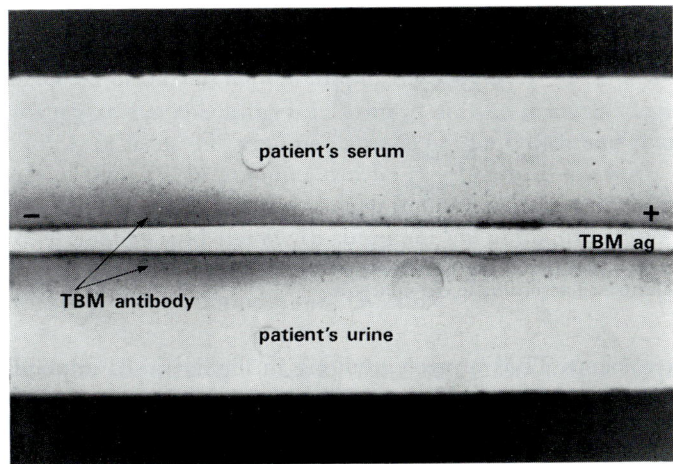

Fig. 7-23   Immunoeletrophoretic patterns of circulating antibody against TBM from a patient. The trough was filled by TBM antigen labeled with Na[131]I. The upper well was filled with patient's serum and the lower was filled with patient's urine. The precipitin lines were faintly noted in gamma region.

These findings showed that eluted immunoglobulin-G from the kidney apparently contained the antibody against its own TBM, and also showed that the eluted antibody and circulating antibody may participate in the both tubular and glomerular changes in the above cases.   It is surprising evidence that immune complex glomerulonephritis was accompanied by antiTBM antibody induced interstitial nephritis in human.   In contrast, in experimental animals, antiTBM-related interstitial nephritis has failed to show any evidence of immune complex glomerulonephritis.

Although the mechanisms of immune complex formations in these cases are not yet clarified, the antigen source may be gradually supplied by its own damaged TBM and the autoantibody formation might also slowly continue.   It may be that when the ratio between amounts of antigen and antibody is adequate for the production of immune complexes, they will induce the glomerular lesion.   It can also be considered that the TBM may be damaged by some other agents and lysed in a soluble form.   The denatured TBM antigen may be reabsorbed into the circulation and may stimulate antibody formation continuously (Fig. 7-24).

In experimental animals, initial antigen stimulations have been performed with the

endogenous, to form antibodies which can react with the host soluble antigen in the circulation to form complexes. When this immune process is accomplished, the host's circulating antigen may stimulate antibody formation to form nephritogenic complexes. In this immune complex glomerulonephritis, non-glomerular antigens such as thyroglobulin [58], tumor associated antigens [8, 34], DNA [30, 50] and/or non-glomerular renal antigen included in the brush border of the proximal tubular cells have been well identified, and they may stimulate the host antibody formation. The finest model of immune complex glomerulonephritis associated with non-glomerular renal antigen was first described by Heymann et al. [17]. Homologous rat whole kidney was repeatedly injected into the peritoneum of rats and the diseased kidney showed fine granular immune deposits along the GBM with typical subepithelial electron dense deposits. Further examinations have been performed by Glassock and Dixon in rats which were immunized with homologous renal tubular epithelial antigen named RTE-alpha 5 [11, 13]. The antigen was eluted from the proximal tubular cells and could form antibody reacting with the cell brush border. This antigen was organ-specific and not widely distributed among the various other tissues according to immunofluorescence. In immune complex glomerulonephritis with RTE-alpha 5, the antigen was demonstrated in glomeruli after partial elution treatment by immunofluorescence. Host immunoglobulin and complement were deposited in glomeruli and within the brush border of the proximal tubule. This type of immune complex nephritis was considered as an autologous immune complex disease which was caused by the immunizing antigen and circulating antibodies capable of reacting with autologous renal tubular antigen.

Recently, membranous nephritis induced with this immune process has been identified in man by Naruse and his associates [42] as well as in our laboratory [56]. Additionally, Shwayder and his coworkers reported a case of a patient with Fanconi syndrome and nephrotic syndrome associated with RTE antigen-antibody complex [51]. In our laboratory the identification of RTE antigen in glomerular immune complexes was presented by immunofluorescence using antiRTE rabbit serum in 5 membranous cases. RTE antigen was also detected in urine specimens of patients as well as of normal subjects. In some cases, 2 components of urinary RTE antigen were detected, one of which had a higher molecular weight than that of human IgG and the other was between IgG and albumin in gel filtration. The macromolecular RTE antigen has been commonly found in normal urine as well as in most patients' urine. Low molecular RTE antigen was demonstrated in the urine of the above 5 cases and also in their sera. This fact suggested that this low molecular RTE antigen might be associated with this nephropathy. In this presentation, we will demonstrate the nephritogenic characterization of RTE antigen and the analysis of excreted urinary RTE antigen of renal disease in juxtaposition with the clinical features.

1. Materials and methods

a. Preparation of RTE antigen

Renal tubular epithelial antigen was prepared by the methods of Edgington and associates [11] with modifications [23]. From autopsied kidney specimens without renal diseases, tubular epithelial cells were obtained with a stainless steel sieve. They were suspended in 0.25 M sucrose with a Potter-Elvejhem homogenizer. The homogenate was centrifuged at 700 g for 10 min, and the sediment was suspended in 2.2 M sucrose. The suspension was centrifuged at 50,000 g for 30 min. The upper nonsedimented portion in the 2.2 M sucrose contained most of the tubular epithelial cell wall. This fraction was then solubilyzed by trypsin.

b. Further preparation of RTE

Appropriate antigen was applied to a column of Sephadex G-200. Fractions corresponding to the third peak containing RTE antigen were pooled and concentrated. The concentrated sample was electrophoretically fractionated in agar. The alpha-region contained RTE antigen and fractions of this region were collected and concentrated. Finally, DEAE cellulose column chromatography was carried out by a linear gradient (Fig. 7-25). The mixing vessel contained 0.175 M phosphate buffer, pH 6.3, and the reservoir vessel 2 M KCl.

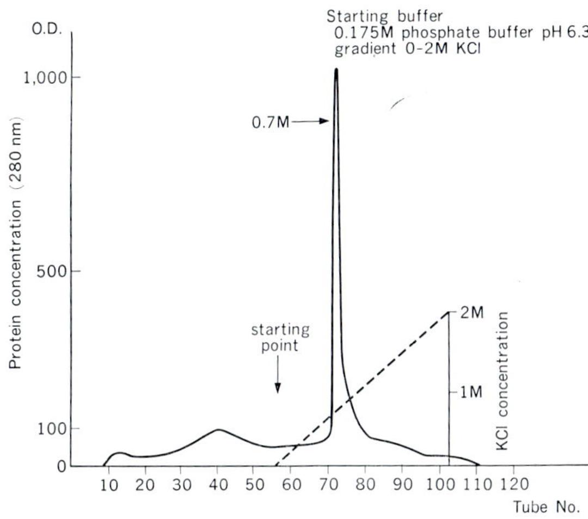

Fig. 7-25 Chromatogram on DEAE cellulose column of RTE antigen. A discontinuous gradient of potassium chloride (0–2 M) was used, starting at 0.175 M phosphate buffer pH 6.3. RTE antigen was eluted in 0.7 M KCl peak.

c. Collection of urine and blood

Forty liters of urine from healthy subjects were collected. The urine samples were kept at 4°C during the collection period. After completion of the collection sodium azide was added to a concentration of 0.1%. The specimens were filtered through No. 2 filter paper (Toyo Roshi Kaisha, Ltd., Tokyo, Japan) while at a constant 4°C. The specimens were then concentrated by ultrafiltration using 8/32-inch boiled Visking dialysis tubing (Union Carbide Corp., Chicago, Illinois). Chromatography on Sephadex G-200 of concentrated proteins from normal subjects was carried out.

Fresh specimens of urine were also obtained from 32 patients with nephrotic syndrome. All the urine specimens were concentrated by ultrafiltration as well. Preparation of RTE antigen in urine specimens of one patient was done by immunochemical and physico-chemical methods by the combined techniques of ammonium sulfate precipitation, Sephadex G-200 column and DEAE cellulose column chromatography. Preparation of RTE antigen in serum was also carried out by the same methods.

d. Preparation of antisera

An antiserum against renal tubular epithelial antigen was prepared in rabbits by repeated immunization in complete Freund's adjuvant. The immunization procedure was repeated at 2-week intervals and the animals were bled 2 weeks after the last injection. The antiserum was absorbed with normal human serum and purified glomerular and tubular basement membrane antigens were examined to determine the antiserum specific for the renal tubular epithelial antigen. The specificity of this antiserum was confirmed by the specific staining of the renal tubular epithelium in indirect immunofluorescence. Antisera against all fractions from Sephadex G-200 column of urine specimens of normal subjects and patients were also prepared by a similar immunization method. An antiserum against the purified RTE antigen was also prepared in rabbit (AntiRTE F III).

e. Immunofluorescent study

By immunofluorescent study the distribution and cross-reactivity of the RTE antigen were examined. Using the antiserum against crude preparation of RTE, purified RTE and urinary RTE, staining procedure of various tissues was done on frozen sections including renal tubular epithelium, esophagus, stomach, duodenum, colon, liver, lung, bronchial epithelium and placenta.

Immunofluorescent study on the biopsied specimens of patients' kidney was performed using the fluorescein conjugated antiserum against the purified RTE, human IgG and beta-1-C.

f. Immunodiffusion method

All urine specimens of 32 patients and purified RTE antigen were tested by immunodiffusion methods using the specific antiserum against purified RTE (Anti-FIII) on detection and characterization of the antigen.

2. Immunochemical characters of purified RTE antigen

Gel filtration of crude RTE preparation on Sephadex G-200 gave five distinct peaks (Fig. 7-26). RTE antigen could be widely detected from the first to the fourth peak by immunodiffusion using antiserum against crude RTE antigen. The antiserum against crude RTE preparation could stain various tissues of normal subjects by indirect immunofluorescent technique. Renal tubular epithelium and duodenum were strongly stained, and bronchial tubular epithelium and colon were also noticeably stained. Esophagus, stomach, liver and lung were not stained (Table 7-2). On the other hand, the antiserum against the third peak on Sephadex G-200 (anti-FIII) could also strongly stain renal tubular epithelium (Fig. 7-27) but not any of the other tissues. All of these antisera did not stain glomerular basement membrane and tubular basement membrane. Therefore, from the third peak, RTE antigen was further purified. By block electrophoresis of the third peak, RTE antigen was detected in the alpha region. The antigen corresponding to the alpha region was eluted from a column of DEAE cellulose in 0.7 M KCl peak (Fig. 7-25). The staining pattern of the antiserum against purified RTE was the same as that of the antiserum against the third peak. Both of the antisera also stained the depositions of the biopsied kidney of membranous nephropathy by direct immunofluorescence.

Table 7-2 Crossreactivity of RTE antigen with various human organs by a method of immunofluorescent techniques using crude antiRTE and antiRTE FIII.

	Crude anti-RTE	Anti-RTE FIII
Renal Tubular Epithelium	+++	+++
Oesophagus	−	−
Stomach	±	−
Duodenum	+++	±
Colon	+	−
Liver	−	−
Lung	−	−
Bronchus Epithelium	+	−
Placenta	−	−

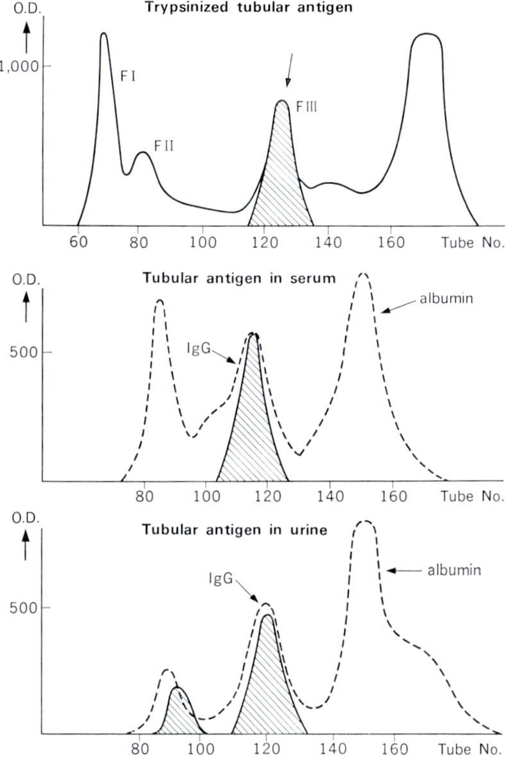

Fig. 7-26   Chromatogram on Sephadex G-200 of trypsinized tubular antigen, tubular antigen in serum, and tubular antigen in urine.

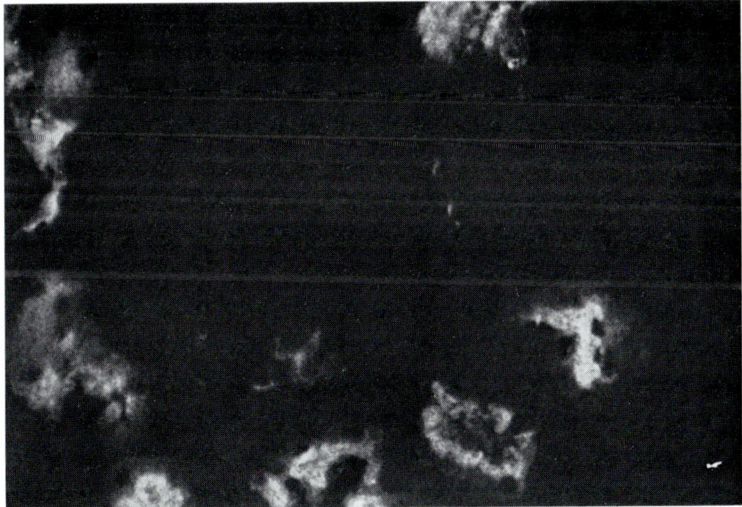

Fig. 7-27   Direct immunofluorescence staining of normal human kidney with a specific antibody against RTE antigen FIII. Marked staining is observed in the luminal layer of proximal tubular epithelium.

3. Immunochemical characters of RTE antigen in urine of normal subjects

RTE antigen was usually found in urine of normal subjects.   Gel filtration of concentrated urine specimens of Sephadex G-200 revealed three protein peaks of which only the first one gave RTE-specific antigenicity [56].   By immunodiffusion methods a single precipitin line was observed between purified RTE antigen and the antiserum against normal urine RTE, and the precipitin line was fused with spur formation to a precipitin line which was seen between the urine specimen and the same antiserum [56].   By immunofluorescence, specific staining was observed on frozen normal human kidney section, using the same antiserum as against normal urine RTE.   Thus antiserum also stained various other tissues such as duodenum, bronchial epithelium, and colon.   The staining characteristics were very similar to those of the antiserum against crude RTE preparation.

4. RTE Antigen in urine of patients

RTE antigen was identified in urine of all 32 patients as examined by immunodiffusion methods.   In 5 of these 32 patients two precipitin lines were seen, with both lines fused to that formed between RTE antigen and specific antiserum against RTE on the same gel diffusion plate, whereas others could form only a single line against the same antiserum [56].   These five cases consisted of two of membranous nephropathy, two of lupus nephropathy and one of nephrotic syndrome associated with cadmium poisoning.   Chromatogram on Sephadex G-200 of a urine sample from one of these five cases revealed 4 protein peaks.   RTE antigen was eluted in the first peak (u-RTE 1) and in the third peak (u-RTE) (Fig. 7-26).   The first peak RTE antigen had similar molecular weight as that of normal subjects and also that of the other 27 patients.   Only these 5 cases had another RTE antigen of a molecular weight lower than that of normal subjects.   By immunofluorescence, the staining characteristics of the antiserum against u-RTE 1 are similar to that of the antiserum against normal urine RTE, while the antiserum against u-RTE 2 is similar to that of the antiserum against purified RTE.

5. Detection and characterization of RTE antigen in serum of patients

RTE antigen was also found in serum of a patient who had two components of urinary RTE antigen.   The antigen in serum was detected in the supernatant when the serum was treated by the methods of ammonium sulfate precipitation at 50% saturated concentration. Chromatogram on Sephadex G-200 of the sample revealed four peaks of which only the third had RTE-specific antigenicity.   On the same column human IgG was eluted in the peak which contained the RTE antigen (Fig. 7-26).   Chromatogram on DEAE cellulose column of the serum disclosed that the antigen was eluted in the peak of 0.15 M KCl which was different from that of purified RTE antigen.   The chromatogram was done by the same immunochemical procedure as the preparation of purified RTE antigen (Fig. 7-28).

6. Detection of RTE antigen in the kidney

The clinical manifestations of the above 5 cases were typical nephrotic syndrome with systemic lupus erythematosus, cadmium poisoning and unknown etiology.   The histo-

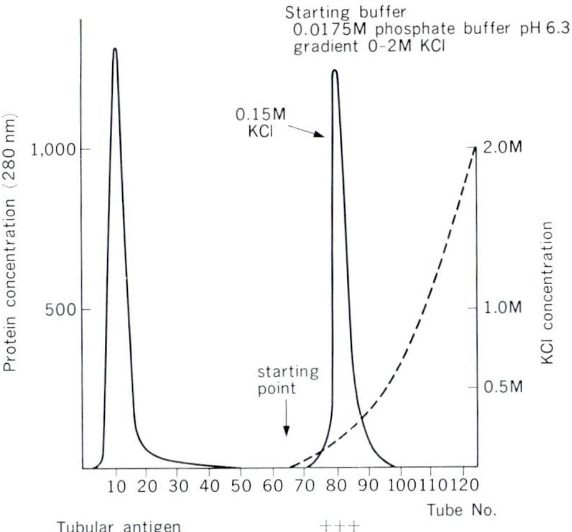

Fig. 7-28 Chromatogram on DEAE cellulose column of TBM antigen from a patient's serum. A discontinuous gradient of potassium chloride (0–2 M) was used, starting at 0.175 M phosphate buffer pH 6.3. Tubular antigen in serum was disclosed in 0.15 M KCl peak.

logical findings of the diseased kidney showed typical membranous change in glomeruli in all cases.   The depositions on GBM were well stained by fluorescein conjugated antisera against human IgG and beta-1-C (Fig. 7-29).   The depositions were also stained by the specific antiserum against purified RTE antigen.   Fluorescence was demonstrated on the tubular epithelial brush border and also along the GBM in a granular pattern (Fig. 7-30). Moreover, the depositions were stained by the antiserum against u-RTE 2 [56].

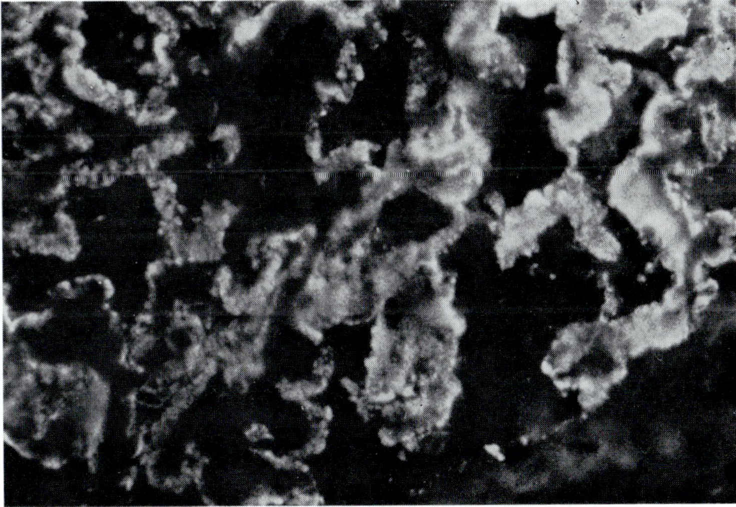

Fig. 7-29 Immunofluorescence staining of biopsied nephrotic patient's kidney. Typical granular deposits of IgG are seen along the GBM.

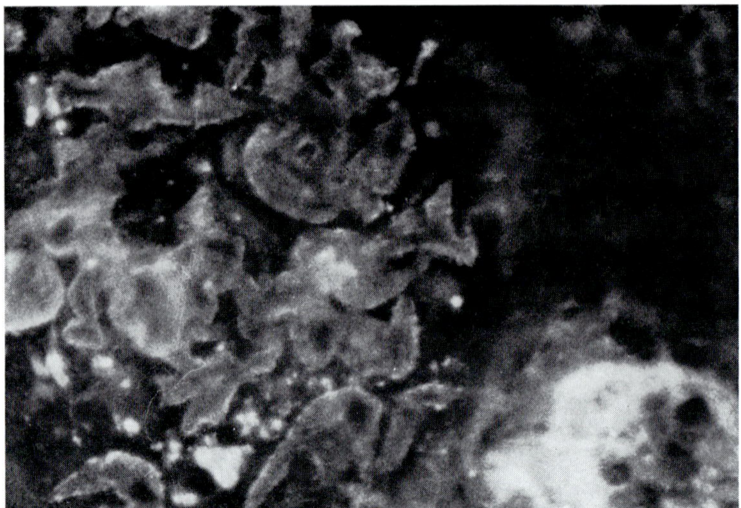

Fig. 7-30   Staining of RET-antigen by indirect immunofluorescent technique showing a thick layer of granular deposits of antigen along the walls of the glomerular loops.

7. Discussion

Another antigen exists in the renal tissue, i.e., RTE and it has been implicated as an etiological agent in renal injury as like GBM and TBM antigen.   The specific antiserum to RTE is only reactive with RTE antigen and not with GBM, TBM or any other organs. The crude RTE preparation is also not crossreactive with GBM and TBM, and is found widely distributed among other nonrenal tissues such as colon, duodenum and bronchial epithelium.   The crude RTE preparation has also been crossreactive with RTE in rats, thereby illustrating that the antigen is not species-specific.   The purified RTE antigen is "kidney-specific" and not crossreactive with any other tissues.   The immunochemical and physicochemical properties of the antigen are different from those of GBM and TBM. The mobility of RTE in electrophoresis is in the alpha region, while GBM is in the beta and TBM in the gamma regions.   For the purpose of elution of these 3 antigens on DEAE cellulose column, various conditions existed for each—RTE in 0.7 M KCl, pH 6.3, GBM in 0.3 M NaCl, pH 7.2, and TBM in 0.12 M, pH 8.0 [56, 57].   The molecular weight of the RTE antigen is greater than that of human albumin while GBM and TBM molecular weights are smaller.

RTE antigen is usually demonstrated in the urine of normal subjects as well as of patients.   The immunochemical properties of RTE antigen in normal urine specimens very closely resemble those of crude RTE preparation.   Antiserum against normal urine RTE can also stain the target tissues of the kidney, duodenal epithelium, colonic epithelium and bronchial epithelium by immunofluorescence.   Chromatography on Sephadex G-200 of RTE antigen in normal urine shows antigenic activity in the first peak in similar patterns to that of crude RTE preparation.

Another RTE associated component is demonstrated in the urine of 5 cases of membranous nephropathy.   The antigen is eluted in the third peak on Sephadex G-200 column in which human IgG has been eluted simultaneously.   The result shows that the antigen has a molecular weight less than that of RTE antigen in normal specimens and is similar to the molecular weight of purified RTE antigen.   Therefore the immunochemical qualities of the RTE antigen in urine of patients resemble those of purified RTE antigen.   The antiserum against this antigen in urine stained only RTE in sections of some kidney but not any other organs.   The antiserum also stained the depositions on the GBM of some diseased kidney.   Therefore, these findings strongly suggest that the antigen could participate in the immune complexes on the GBM of patients.   We speculate from these results that the RTE antigen in urine might originate from the cicuiation, renal tubular epithelial cells, or from the immune complexes on the GBM following their dissociation.

Moreover, we consider that the detection and characterization of the RTE antigen in patient's urine is useful as an initial screening test to aid in the diagnosis of membranous glomerulonephritis.

RTE antigen has also been detected in the serum of a patient with membranous nephropathy.   The circulating antigen is similar to the antigen in the patient's urine in regard to molecular weight.   This antigen in serum seems also to participate in the immune complex nephropathy.   The RTE antigen has also been successfully demonstrated in immune complexes on the GBM in 2 cases.   Similar studies in human disease have been reported by Naruse and his associates [42].

REFERENCES

1. Batzing, B.L. and Hanna, M.G., Jr.: Localization of endogeneous C-type virus in the glomerular basement membrane of aged AKR mice. *J. Immunol. 110*: 1189–1193, 1973.

2. Benacerraf, B. and McDevitt, H.O.: Histocompatibility linked immune response genes. *Science 175*: 273–279, 1972.

3. Bergstein, J. and Litman, N.: Interstitial nephritis with antitubular-basement-membrane antibody. *N. Engl. J. Med. 292*: 875–878, 1975.

4. Border, W.A., Lehman, D.H., Egan, J.D., Sass, H.J., Globe, J.E., and Wilson, C.W.: Antitubular basement membrane antibodies in methicilin-associated interstitial nephritis. *N. Engl. J. Med. 291*: 381–384, 1974.

5. Boss, J.H.: Observations on the species-nonspecificity of the human renal and placental basement membrane antigens. *Experimentia 19*: 517-518, 1963.

6. Boss, J.H.: Isolation of a potent nephrotoxic serum antigen preparation from rat heart. *Brit. J. Exp. Path. 46*: 630–634, 1965.

7. Burch, R.R., Pearl, M.A., and Sternberg, W.H.: A clinicopathological study of the nephrotic syndrome. *Ann. Intern. Med. 56*: 54–67 1963.

8. Costanza, M.E., Pinn, V., Schwartz, R.S., and Nathanson, L.: Carcinoembryonic antigen-antibody complexes in a patient with colonic carcinoma and nephrotic syndrome. *N. Engl. J. Med. 289*: 520–522, 1973.

9. Dixon, F.J., Vazquez, J.J., Weigle, W.O., and Cochrane, C.G.: Pathogenesis of serum sickness. *A.M.A. Arch. Path. 65*: 18–28, 1958.

10. Dixon, F.J., Feldman, J.D., and Vazquez, J.J.: Experimental glomerulonephritis: the pathogenesis of a labolatory model of human glomerulonephritis. *J. Exp. Med. 113*: 899–920, 1961.

11. Edgington, T.S., Lee, S., and Dixon, F.J.: Autologous immune complex nephritis induced with renal tubular antigen. I. Identification and isolation of the pathogenetic antigen. *J. Exp. Med. 127*: 555–572, 1968.

12. Germuth, F.G.: A comparative histologic and immunologic study in rabbits of induced hypersensitivity of the serum sickness type. *J. Exp. Med. 97*: 257–282, 1953.

13. Glassock, R.J., Edgington, T.S., Watson, J.I., and Dixon, F.J.: Autologous immune complex nephritis induced with renal tubular antigen. II. The pathogenetic mechanism. *J. Exp. Med. 127*: 573–588, 1968.

14. Goodman, M., Greenspon, S.A., and Krakower, C.A.: The antigenic composition of the various anatomic structures of the canine kidney. *J. Immunol. 75*: 96–104, 1955.

15. Henson, J.B. and Gorham, J.R.: Persistent viral infections, immunologically-mediated glomerulonephritis and arthritis, dysgammopathies. Aleutian disease of mink. *Amer. J. Path. 71*: 345–348, 1973.

16. Heymann, W., Gilky, C., and Salehar, M.: Antigenic property of renal cortex. *Proc. Soc. Exp. Biol. Med. 73*: 385–387, 1950.

17. Heymann, W., Hackel, D.B., Harwood, J., Wilson, S.G.F., and Hunter, J.L.P.: Production of the nephrotic syndrome in rats by Freund's adjuvant and rat kidney suspension. *Proc. Soc. Exp. Biol. Med. 100*: 660–664, 1959.

18. Hillyer, G.V., and Lewert, R.M.: Studies on renal pathology in hamsters infected with Schistosoma mansoni and S. japonicum. *Amer. J. Trop. Med. Hyg. 23*: 404–411, 1974.

19. Hiramoto, R., Jurandowski, J., Bernecky, J. and Pressman, D.: Precise zone of localization of anti-kidney antibody in various organs. *Proc. Soc. Exp. Biol. Med. 101*: 583–586, 1959.

20. Huldt, S.: Studies on experimental toxoplasmosis. *Ann. N. Y. Acad. Sci. 177*: 146–155, 1971.

21. Hyman, L.R., Colvin, R.B., and Steinberg, A.D.: Immunopathogenesis of autoimmune tubulointerstitial nephritis. I. Demonstration of differential susceptibility in strain II and strain XIII guinea pigs. *J. Immunol. 116*: 327–335, 1976.

22. Hyman, L.R., Steinberg, A.D., Colvin, R.B., and Bernard, E.F.: Immunopathogenesis of autoimmune tubulointerstitial nephritis. II. Role of an immune response gene linked to the major histoconpatibility complex. *J. Immunol. 117*: 1894–1897, 1976.

23. Iesato, K., Wakashin, M., Wakashin, Y., and Tojo, S.: Renal tubular dysfunction in Minamata disease. Detection of renal tubular antigen and beta-2-microglobulin in the urine. *Ann. Intern. Med. 86*: 731–737, 1977.

24. Jaffe, I.A., Tresen, G., Suzuki, Y., and Ehrenreich, T.: Nephropathy induced by D-penicillamine. *Ann. Intern. Med. 69*: 549–556, 1968.

25. Kajima, M. and Pollard, M.: Ultrastructural pathology of glomerular lesions in gnotobiotic mice with congenital lymphocytic choriomeningitis (LCM) virus infection. *Amer. J. Path. 61*: 117–140, 1970.

26. Katz, A. and Little, H.: Gold nephropathy. An immunopathologic study. *Arch. Path. 96*: 133–136, 1973.

27. Kay, C.F.: The mechanism of a form of glomerulonephritis. Nephrotoxic nephritis in rabbits. *Amer. J. Med. Sci. 204*: 483–490, 1942.

28. Kefalides, N.A.: Isolation and characterization of the collagen from glomerular basement membrane. *Biochemistry 7*: 3103–3112, 1968.

29. Krakower, C.A., and Greenspon, S.A.: Localization of the nephrotoxic antigen within the isolated renal glomerulus. *A.M.A. Arch. Path. 51*: 629–639, 1951.

30. Lambert, P.H., and Dixon, F.J.: Pathogenesis of the glomerulonephritis of NZB/W mice. *J. Exp. Med. 127*: 507–522, 1968.

31. Lehman, D.H., Wilson, C.B., and Dixon, F.J.: Interstitial nephritis in rats immunized with heterologous tubular basement membrane. *Kidney Internat. 5*: 187–195, 1974.

32. Lerner, R.A., Glassock, R.J., and Dixon, F.J.: The role of antiglomerular basement membrane antibody in the pathogenesis of human glomerulonephritis. *J. Exp. Med. 126*: 989–1004, 1967.

33. Lerner, R.A., and Dixon, F.J.: The induction of acute glomerulonephritis in rabbits with soluble antigens isolated from normal homologous and autologous urine. *J. Immunol. 100*: 1277–1287, 1968.

34. Lewis, M.G., Loughridge, L.W., and Phillip, T.M.: Immunological studies in nephrotic syndrome associated with extrarenal malignant disease. *Lancet 2*: 134–135, 1971.

35. Lowry, O.H., Rosebrough, N.J., and Farr, A.L.: Protein measurement with Folin phenol-reagent. *J. Biol. Chem. 193*: 265–275, 1951.

36. Maizel, F.J.V.: Acrylamide-gel electrophoresis by mechanical fractions: Radioactive adenovirus proteins. *Science 151*: 988–990, 1966.

37. Mancini, G., Carbonara, A.O., and Heremans, J.F.: Immunochemical quantitation of antigens by single radial immunodiffusion. *Immunochemistry 2*: 235–254, 1965.

38. McPhaul, J.J., Jr., and Dixon, F.J.: The presence of anti-glomerular basement membrane antibodies in peripheral blood. *J. Immunol. 103*: 1168–1175, 1969.

39. McPhaul, J.J., Jr. and Dixon, F.J.: Characterization of human anti-glomerular basement membrane antibodies eluted from glomerulonephritic kidneys. *J. Clin. Invest. 49*: 308–317, 1970.

40. McPhaul, J.J., Jr. and Dixon, F.J.: Characterization of immunoglobulin G anti-glomerular basement membrane antibodies eluted from kidneys of patients with glomerulonephritis. *J. Immunol. 107*: 678–684, 1971.

41. Morel-Maroger, L., Kourilsky, O., Mignon, F., and Richet, G.: Antitubular basement membrane antibodies in rapidly progressive poststreptococcal glomerulonephritis: report of a case. *Clin. Immunol. Immunopath. 2*: 185–194, 1974.

42. Naruse, T., Kitamura, K., Miyakawa, Y., and Shibata, S.: Deposition of renal tubular epithelial antigen along the glomerular capillary walls of patients with membranous glomerulonephritis. *J. Immunol. 110*: 1163–1166, 1973.

43. Oldstone, M.B.A. and Dixon, F.J.: Pathogenesis of chronic disease associated with persistent lymphocytic choriomeningitis viral injection. II. Relationship of the anti-lymphocytic choriomeningitis immune response to tissue injury in chronic lymphocytic choriomeningitis disease. *J. Exp. Med. 131*: 1–19, 1970.

44. Oldstone, M.B.A. and Dixon, F.J.: Lactic dehydrogenase virus-induced immune complex type of glomerulonephritis. *J. Immunol. 106*: 1260–1263, 1971.

45. Pascal, R.R., Koss, M.N., and Kassel, R.L.: Glomerulonephritis associated with immune complex deposits and viral particles in spontaneous murine leukemia. An electron microscopic study with immunofluorescence. *Lab. Invest. 29*: 159–165, 1973.

46. Porter, D.D. and Larsen, A.E.: Aleutian disease of mink: infectious virus-antibody complexes in the serum. *Proc. Soc. Exp. Biol. Med. 126*: 680–682, 1967.

47. Porter, D.D. and Porter, H.G.: Deposition of immune complexes in the kidneys of mice infected with lactic dehydrogenase virus. *J. Immunol. 106*: 1264–1266, 1971.

48. Scott, D.G.: A study of the antigenicity of basement membrane and reticulin. *Brit. J. Exp. Path. 38*: 178–185, 1957.

49. Shibata, S., Nagasawa, T., Miyakawa, Y., and Naruse, T.: Nephritogenic glycoprotein. I. Proliferative glomerulonephritis induced in rats by a single injection of the soluble glycoprotein isolated from homologous glomerular basement membrane. *J. Immunol. 106*: 1284–1294, 1971.

50. Shirai, T. and Mellors, R.C.: Natural thymocytotoxic autoantibody and reactive antigen in New Zealand Black and other mice. *Proc. Nat. Acad. Sci. 68*: 1412–1412, 1971.

51. Shwayder, M., Ozawa, T., Boedecker, E., Guggenheim, S., and McIntosh, R.M.: Nephrotic syndrome associated with Fanconi syndrome. Immunopathogenic studies of tubulointerstitial nephritis with autologous immune-complex glomerulonephritis. *Ann. Intern. Med. 84*: 433–437, 1976.

52. Steblay, R.W. and Rudofsky, U.: Renal tubular disease and autoantibodies against tubular basement membrane induced in guinea pigs. *J. Immunol. 107*: 589–594, 1971.

53. Sternlieb, I., Bennett, B., and Scheinberg, I.H.: D-penicillamine-induced Goodpasture's syndrome in Wilson's disease. *Ann. Intern. Med. 82*: 673–676, 1975.

54. Tung, K.S.K. and Black, W.C.: Association of renal glomerular and tubular immune complex disease and antitubular basement membrane antibody. *Lab. Invest. 32*: 696–700, 1975.

55. Vitetta, E.S., Baun, S., and Uhr, J.W.: Cell surface immunoglobulin. II. Isolation and characterization of immunoglobulin from mouse splenic lymphocytes. *J. Exp. Med. 134*: 242–264, 1971.

56. Wakashin, Y., Wakashin, M., Iesato, K., Narita, M., and Tojo, S.: Immunochemical and physicochemical analysis of urinary renal tubular antigen in human. *Jap. J. Nephrol. 17*: 929–940, 1975. (in Japanese with English abstract)

57. Wakashin, Y., Wakashin, M., Narita, M., and Tojo, S.: Immunochemical characterization and quantitation of the human glomerular basement membrane antigen from the urine of patients with glomerular diseases. *Contributions to Nephrol. 6*: 124–135, 1977.

58. Weigle, W.O. and Nakamura, R.M.: Perpetuation of autoimmune thyroiditis and production of secondary renal lesions following periodic injections of aqueous preparations of altered thyroglobulin. *Clin. Exp. Immunol. 4*: 645–657, 1969.

Chapter **8**

Clinical Implications of Masugi and Other Immunologically Induced Experimental Glomerulonephropathies

Masaaki OKADA and Hiroki TSUCHIDA

I. Introduction

One hundred years ago, Klebs [46] first used the term "Glomerulo-Nephritis" instead of "parenchymatous nephritis" and claimed that the main pathology of Bright's disease is seen in the renal glomeruli, not being present in the tubules. Subsequently, Marchiafava and Valenti [56] described another form of glomerular lesion; extracapillary proliferative type, and named "Glomerulo-Nephritis epithelialis" contrasting with "Glomerulo-Nephritis interstitialis" of Klebs'. Engel [21] reported "Glomerulitis adhesiva" to be one particular type of glomerulonephritis in 1901. Thus in the 19th century, the fundamental glomerular "inflammatory" changes of Bright's disease seemed to be firmly established (older literature on glomerular histopathology, see reference 24).

In 1914, great progress in nephrology was made by the close collaboration of a clinician (Volhard) and a pathologist (Fahr) [93] in understanding correlations between the clinical evolution and histopathology of glomerulonephropathies in man. The concept and classification by these investigators has greatly influenced the opinions of glomerulonephropathies of their successors, and even now many of their ideas about the disease appear to be valid.

In 1942, Ellis [20] published a superb contribution to the natural history of Bright's disease with two of his colleagues at the London Hospital. Their thorough observations on some 600 cases over a period of 20 years with 200 being studied histologically after death, resulted in an outstanding classification, particularly for the clinical field and to a lesser extent for pathologic anatomy. Ellis' original publication is, however, written in a rather abbreviated manner, and a more detailed description was made by Hadfield and Garrod [34] with many morphological illustrations. The uniqueness of this classification in comparison with that of Volhard and Fahr is that first, "diffuse" nephritis is clearly divided into two groups according to natural history and second, that they raised a serious question about the existence of "lipoid nephrosis" which was the main disease of "Nephrose" of Volhard and Fahr's classification, and they finally included it with their type 2 diffuse nephritis. As for the first point, until at that time, "diffuse" nephritis was thought to be a single disease implying that whatever etiological, clinical and pathological variations may exist, they are due to the operation of one or a series of closely related causes, e.g. variable clinical and histological presentations are due to variations in intensity of the initial inflammation. Ellis and his colleagues were opposed to this concept from a statistical point of view and claimed that "diffuse" nephritis is not a single disease but falls into at least two entirely distinct types. This gives rise to a serious question about the etiopathogenesis and what causes the difference between these two types of inflammatory Bright's disease. With regard to the second point, although they classified "lipoid nephrosis" into their type 2 diffuse nephritis, the term they used is apparently not the same one currently used as the synonym for nil disease or foot process disease, but seems to be a rather comprehensive term of conditions being characterized by the nephrotic syndrome with mild glomerular pathology including membranous nephropathy.

The situation of understanding human glomerulonephropathies has changed considerably over the last two decades. This is mainly due to the development of appropriate experimental models, rapid progress in immunology and the introduction of renal biopsy procedures. After the report of Iversen and Brun [41] demonstrating that the percutaneous renal biopsy procedure is safe and relatively simple, increasing numbers of renal biopsies have been performed all over the world. The renal biopsy has made it possible to study renal changes at an early stage and to follow the evolution and the clinicopathological correlation of the disease with time even in a single patient. In addition, frequent or routine application of electron microscopy and immunohistochemistry on the biopsied material has added new insights to the understanding of the etiology and pathogenetic mechanisms of human glomerulonephropathies. With the aid of these sophisticated weapons and close collaboration of clinicians and pathologists, it has gradually become apparent that there exist well defined clinicopathologic entities in glomerulonephropathies of man. Energetic efforts have made to elucidate whether each of these entities shares the same etiology and/or the same pathogenetic mechanism. To date, while a few glomerulonephropathies have implied their etiologies and/or pathogenetic mechanisms, a majority of the diseases remain far from a complete understanding. Consequently, various classifications of renal diseases have been proposed over the last 20 years or so. However, the result appears to be rather confusing. This seems to be largely due to the terminology admixed with different "levels" even in a single classification. As a rule, a renal disease can be explained by several "levels" or "dimensions" of the disease; etiologic factors, mediating or amplifying factors resulting in tissue injury, morphologic expression and clinical presentation. To avoid this type of confusion, it is of particular importance that one should clearly realize at what level the terminology used is operating [12].

Generalization of renal biopsy procedures aided by electron microscopic and immunohistochemical analyses has enabled us not only to grasp the actual and precise condition of the patient and to select appropriate therapeutic maneuvers, but also to approach etiopathogenesis of glomerulonephropathies affecting man.

A tremendous amount of information has been collected over the last two decades which has made it clear that most primary glomerular diseases and those associated with systemic disease appear to be derived from immunological mechanisms. With the aid of successful production of appropriate experimental models of glomerular diseases, it has become apparent that at least two fundamental immunological mechanisms are operative in human glomerulonephropathies; the immune complex disease and the anti-basement-membrane disease [17, 99].

Nevertheless, histopathologic expression of human glomerulonephropathies has several characteristic features irrelevant to these different immunological mechanisms. Furthermore, glomerular lesions unrelated to any immunological involvement on the basis of immunohistochemistry may show also a similar variety of features of glomerular histopathology.

II. Fundamental Histopathology of the Glomerulus

1. Ultrastructural cellular changes in quality

This is the least change *per se* and is particularly seen in the case of nil disease or foot process disease.   In this condition, the visceral epithelial cells are swollen with increased microorganellas exhibiting a prominent villous pattern of the cell surface.   The foot processes of the visceral epithelial cells show characteristic fusion over almost all the glomerular basement membrane losing their discrete interdigitations.   By light microscopy, these cells are seen to be swollen and stained basophilically.   These cellular alterations may be present in a variety of conditions with the nephrotic syndrome and appear to relate to the amount of protein excreted from the glomerular capillaries.   Another example of this type of change is swelling of the glomerular endothelial cells characteristically seen in cases of eclampsia and preeclampsia.

2. Cellular proliferation or hypercellularity

This is supposed to be the most fundamental change of glomerular "inflammatory" reactions and is seen in most cases of various types of glomerulonephritis.   Recently an argument has appeared about the origin of the proliferating cells, particularly the cells within the glomerular capillary tufts (endocapillary cells).   This will be duscussed elswhere in this book.

Extracapillary cell proliferation is less frequent as compared to endocapillary cell proliferation and is usually regarded as crescent formation.   A peculiar extracapillary cell proliferation has been reported as adenomatoid transformation or adenomatous metaplasia of parietal epithelial cells [62].

To evaluate glomerular hypercellularity, one must keep in mind that the thickness of the section greatly influences the intensity of this change [44, 72].

3. Exudative change

By definition, exudation means escape and deposition of blood components into the tissue outside of the vessel.   This term, however, usually indicates infiltration of white blood cells into the mesangial area mostly accompanied with stasis of the same cells within the glomerular capillary lumens.   A rather particular use of this term has been applied in cases of diabetic glomerulosclerosis to indicate the deposition of proteinaceous materials in the glomerular tufts and along the capsular basement membrane without cellular elements.

4. Changes in quantity of the intercellular matrix

a. Mesangial matrix

Mesangial matrix increase may be seen in many conditions.   Its extreme example is centrilobular nodule formation seen in cases of diabetic glomerulosclerosis and of lobular glomerulonephritis.   A special form of mesangial matrix increase is circumferential mesangial interposition; extension of mesangial components toward the periphery of the glomerular capillary.   Mesangial matrix increase usually accompanies cellular proliferation, while in diabetic glomerulosclerosis, this proliferation is, as a rule, absent.

Decrease of the matrix is very rare.   Probably the only example of this is the case of intoxication by snake venom of Habu [77], in which it has been reported that the mesangial matrix is dissolved and the glomerulus becomes a huge sac filled with blood cells.

b. The glomerular basement membrane

Increase of the glomerular basement membrane is usually regarded as thickening and is observed most characteristically in cases of diabetic glomerulosclerosis. In this condition, the glomerular basement membrane is thoroughly and smoothly thickened. Membranous nephropathy [19, 74] (epi- or extramembranous glomerulonephritis) including a membranous type of lupus nephritis and possibly malarial nephropathy [95, 101], is another form of the glomerular basement membrane thickening. In this condition, by electron microscopy, the smooth and delicate appearance of the glomerular basement membrane changes into a comb shaped structure with multiple projections (spikes) parpendicular to the original basement membrane toward the epithelial aspect holding proteinaceous deposits in between. With time, a thin layer of the basement membrane is newly formed at the base of the visceral epithelial cells giving an impression of a ladder-like appearance or a moth-eaten structure of the basement membrane. At this stage, the proteinaceous deposits are incorporated into the thickened glomerular basement membrane.

Destruction of the glomerular basement membrane is currently described in a variety of human glomerulonephropathies [86]. Focal and complete destruction of the glomerular basement membrane may be observed particularly in cases of extracapillary proliferative glomerulonephritis [64, 65] (Fig. 8-1).

Rarefaction of the glomerular basement membrane is characteristically seen in Alport's syndrome [39]: The lamina densa of the glomerular basement membrane is made up of layers of very thin membranes and the glomerular basement membrane itself shows irregularity in thickness.

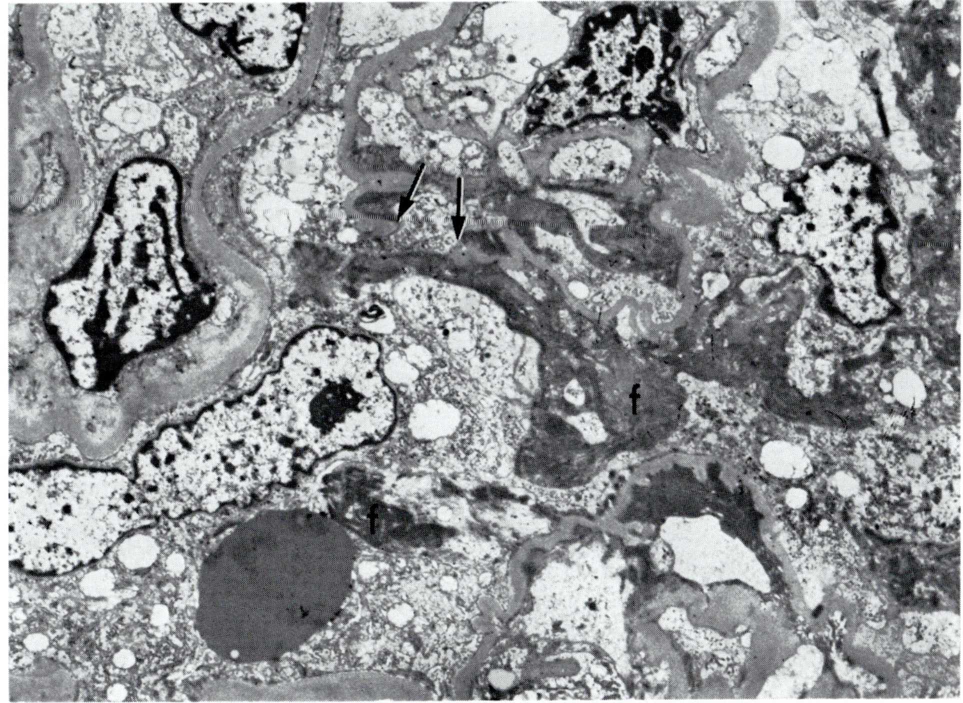

Fig. 8-1 A GBM break (arrows) with fibrillar fibrin (f) in the urinary space. Goodpasture's syndrome.

5. Deposition or existence of unusual substance

Amyloid nephropathy is one of the typical examples of this change.   In this condition, electron dense fine fibrillar material deposits first in the mesangial area, and then extends toward the peripheral walls of the glomerular capillary.   Lipid droplets have been observed to exist in the glomerulus particularly in the epithelial cells in Fabry's disease. Plasma proteins, supposedly unrelated to immunological mechanisms, are seen in various portions of the glomerulus in such conditions as diabetic glomerulosclerosis (exudative lesion) and focal glomerulosclerosis of the idiopathic nephrotic syndrome or focal hyalinosis [32, 76].

It must be attributed to the recent progress of renal pathology that the precise location and the presumed composition of the deposited materials have become clear not only in the conditions above mentioned but in various conditions of glomerulonephropathies.   The location of the unusual deposited substances is commonly described ultrastructurally.

a. The subepithelial aspect

Large subepithelial dome-shaped electron dense deposits (humps) have been described particularly in cases of acute poststreptococcal glomerulonephritis and less frequently in cases of nephropathies due to syphilis [10, 37, 104] and bacterial endocarditis [31]. These deposits are supposed to represent immune complexes by immunohistochemical techniques.   However, the antigens have not yet been detected with certainty within the humps [103].   More small electron dense subepithelial deposits are seen in such conditions as lupus nephritis, membranous nephropathy, malarial nephropathy [95, 101] and occasionally in membranoproliferative glomerulonephritis.   These deposits are also thought to represent immune complexes.

b. The intramembranous aspect

The intramembranous deposits are characteristically seen in a special form of membranoproliferative glomerulonephritis; dense deposit disease or membranoproliferative glomerulonephritis with intramembranous dense deposits [6, 28, 33, 42, 54].   The electron dense deposits are located within the lamina densa of the glomerular basement membrane, capsular basement membrane and tubular basement membrane as well.   They usually do not contain any immunoglobulins but components of complement.   This condition will be discussed later.   Small and occasional intramembranous deposits may be observed in various conditions.   However, one can not be certain whether the deposits are definitely within the glomerular basement membrane or are subepithelial or subendothelial deposits seated deeply in the glomerular basement membrane having been cut obliquely.

c. The subendothelial aspect

The subendothelial deposits may be observed in a variety of conditions.   Examples of this type of deposit are "wire-loop" lesion of lupus nephritis and eclampsia and preeclampsia.   In the former condition, deposits contain DNA and anti-DNA, while in the latter, deposits are composed of plasma proteins particularly fibrin-fibrinogen substances.

d. The mesangial area

The mesangial cells are believed to have phagocytic activity in the physiologic condition. Therefore, in various pathologic conditions, substances may be observed within phagolysosomes of the cytoplasm.   Apart from these intracytoplasmic substances, electron dense materials outside of the cytoplasm, intermingled with the mesangial matrix in some instances, are observed.   These electron dense materials are usually referred to as mesangial deposits.   The mesangial deposits are seen in most cases of glomerulonephritis and are particularly prominent in membranoproliferative glomerulonephritis, lobular glomerulonephritis, IgA nephropathy and lupus nephritis.

6. Disorganization of glomerular structure

There is not full agreement among pathologists whether this structural change is the consequence of inflammation or inflammation *per se* in the strictest sense.   Nevertheless, this change is serious to the particular glomerulus since the change disturbs the circulation in the glomerulus resulting more or less in the loss of function of the nephron.   This change affects the glomerular supporting system; glomerular and capsular basement membranes and mesangial components, taking place in Bowman's space (crescent), between a part of Bowman's capsule and a part of the glomerular tufts (capsular adhesion) or within the glomerular tufts.

Crescents are multi-layered proliferations of the extracapillary cells (mostly parietal epithelial cells) with basement membrane like materials in between.   Later, fibroblastic and/or fibrocytic cells replace epithelial cells resulting in fibrotic crescents adhering and incorporating the glomerular tufts.   Massive proliferation of the extracapillary cells not only compresses the glomerular tufts but also obliterates the urinary pole of Bowman's capsule giving rise to a complete loss of the glomerular function as a filtering system. Therefore, a large number of crescent formations in the section indicates a poor prognosis for the patient, aroviding the term of rapidly progressive glomerulonephritis [38] or malignant glomerulonephritis [85].   Capsular adhesions are seen in most cases of "chronic" glomerulonephritis in varying amounts.   The impact of this change to the particular glomerulus is apparently less severe as compared to that of crescents, since this change usually involves a part of the capillaries of a glomerulus (local or segmental involvement).

It is highly probable that the morphogenesis and sequence of events of disorganization are as follows: At first, destruction of the glomerular basement membrane and/or mesangial matrix takes place (Fig. 8-2, 8-3) and is followed by an inflammatory process with cellular accumulation and an influx of plasma proteins including fibrin-fibrinogen substances.

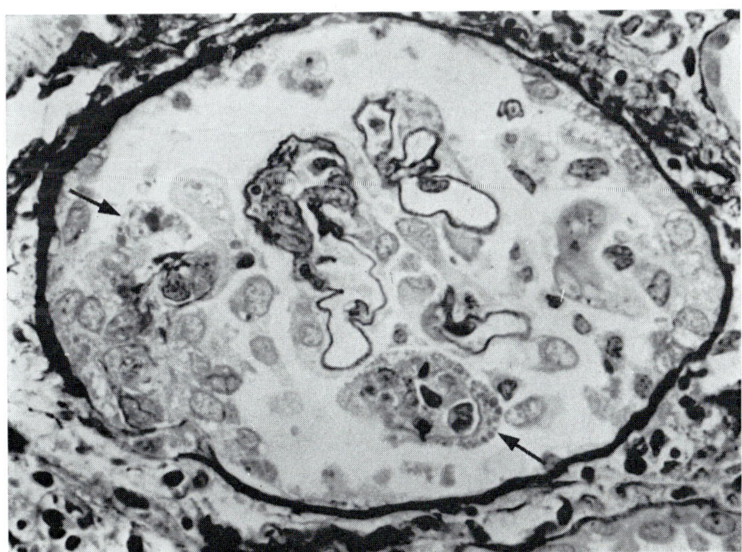

Fig. 8-2   Somewhat tangential cut of a glomerulus demonstrating extracapillary proliferation leading to crescent formation. Note droplets in podocytes cytoplasm (arrows). Lupus nephritis. PASM-H&E stain. This finding appears somehow to relate to ultrastructural lytic or destructive changes of the GBM as seen in Fig. 8-3. The droplets in the podocyte's cytoplasm undoubted correspond to ultrastractural phagolysosomes.

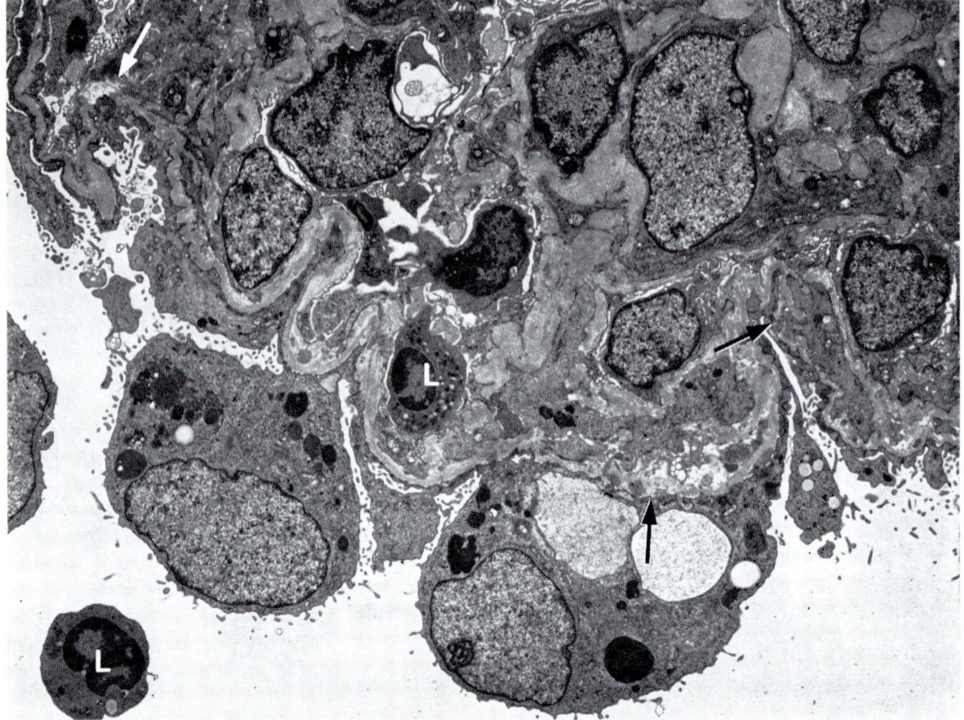

Fig. 8-3 A part of the capillary tuft exhibiting swollen podocytes with phagolysosomes and foci of destructive or lytic changes of the GBM (arrows). Endocapillary proliferation and infiltrating polymorphonunclear leukocytes (L) are seen. Chronic and active glomerulonephritis of undetermined etiology.

Second, a process of repair occurs characterized by proliferation of cells and increase of intercellular substances including collagen fibers, scleroprotin and/or basement membrane like materials.   Thus the process of glomerular disorganization is considered to be a defensive reaction to the destructive lesion, because, although the glomeruli fail to recover their original function resulting in scar formation followed by a granulating process, the glomeruli presumably make every effort to minimize the structural damage.

7. Necrosis

Necrosis in the strict sense is apparently the most severe change being characterized by death of glomerular intrinsic cells.   This change may be observed in a variety of conditions such as collagen diseases, malignant nephrosclerosis and embolic type glomerulonephritis.   Thrombotic or embolic processes resulting in a rather acute ischemia of the tufts play an important role in this change.

III. Analogy of Nephropathies between Human's and Experimental Animal's

Accumulation of a large amount of information gained from clinico-pathologic studies on patients with various glomerulonephropathies and successful production of appropriate experimental models of glomerulonephritis by means of immunological procedures have contributed considerably to a better understanding of human glomerulonephropathies.

Through these investigations, human glomerulonephropathies, primary or associated with systemic diseases, may be divided into several groups according to their presumptive pathogenetic mechanisms as suggested by McCluskey [59]:

1. Immunologically mediated glomerulonephropathies.
   a. Immune complex disease.
   b. Anti-glomerular basement membrane antibody disease.
2. Glomerulonephropathies presumed to be mediated by immunological mechanisms.
3. Glomerulonephropathies unlikely to be related to immunological mechanisms.

1. Immunologically mediated glomerulonephropathies

a. Immune complex disease

One of the most typical examples of immune complex disease may be acute poststreptococcal glomerulonephritis (Fig. 8-4). The onset of this disease is usually abrupt after a latent period of a few weeks following on infection with certain strains of group A hemolytic streptococci, and is characterized by such clinical presentations as dark urine, edema, features of circulatory disturbances as well as hypertension and azotemia in the more severe cases.

Serological studies on acute poststreptococcal glomerulonephritis show increased titers of antistreptolysin-O, antistreptokinase and antihyaluronidase in a good proportion of patients implicating the existence of antibodies against components of the organism in the circulation. However, all the patients exhibiting increased titers of these serological parameters do not necessarily develop glomerulonephritis, and some of those who fail to develop increased titers of these parameters exhibit glomerulonephritis. In fact, it has been reported that there is a tendency of frequent occurrence of completely curable, transient glomerulonephritis in those who demonstrate higher titers of serological parameters than those who have the lower titers [51].

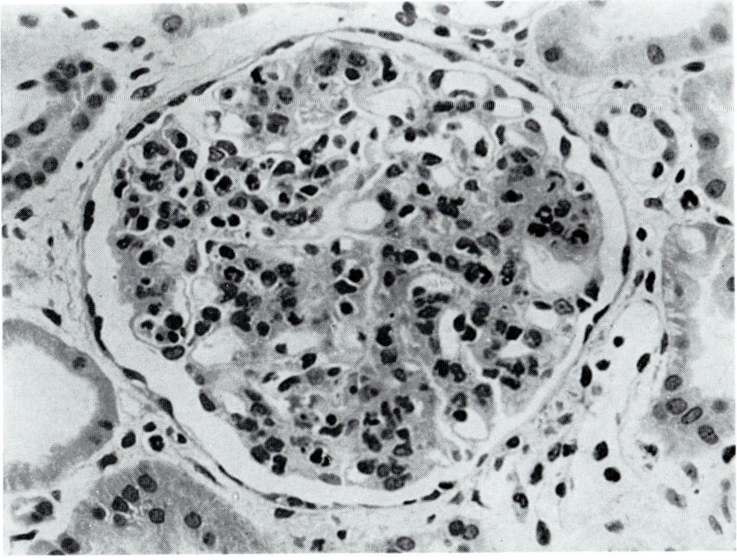

Fig. 8-4 Moderate endocapillary proliferative and marked exudative glomerulonephritis, diffuse and global, consistent with acute post-streptococcal glomerulonephritis. H&E stain.

Serum complement levels are usually depleted during the active phase of the disease and tend to return to the normal range within a few weeks. This phenomenon has been described in a patient with this disease without apparent abnormal urinary findings [40].

The morphological expression of acute poststreptococcal glomerulonephritis is characterized by diffuse and global endocapillary proliferative and exudative glomerular lesions with an accentuated lobular pattern of the glomerular tufts in most instances (Fig. 8-4). The glomerular basement membrane of the peripheral capillaries are not thickened and have a thin and delicate appearance with special stains for the basement membrane, while with well fixed and properly cut thin sections, one can observe small acidophilic dots outside of and along the glomerular basement membrane. By electron microscopy, aside from proliferative and exudative changes seen by light microscopy, characteristic electron dense subepithelial deposits (humps) are observed (Fig. 8-5,8-6). These humps correspond almost undoubtedly to the acidophilic dots seen by light microscopy. Exudated polymorphonuclear leukocytes are sometimes prominent in the glomerular tufts and occasionally come to an intimate contact with the glomerular basement membrane from which the endothelial cell cytoplasm has already been stripped off. With immunohistochemistry, immunoglobulins and complement components are observed in a finely granular pattern along the capillary wall and to a lesser extent in the mesangial area of the glomerulus (Fig. 8-7). A coarse granular or a "lumpy-bumpy" as well as an interrupted linear pattern of immunoglobulins and complement components along the glomerular capillary wall can also be seen. The difference of these immunohistochemical presentations is considered to be that of either histological expressions or clinical stages or both of the two, rather than different disease processes [87].

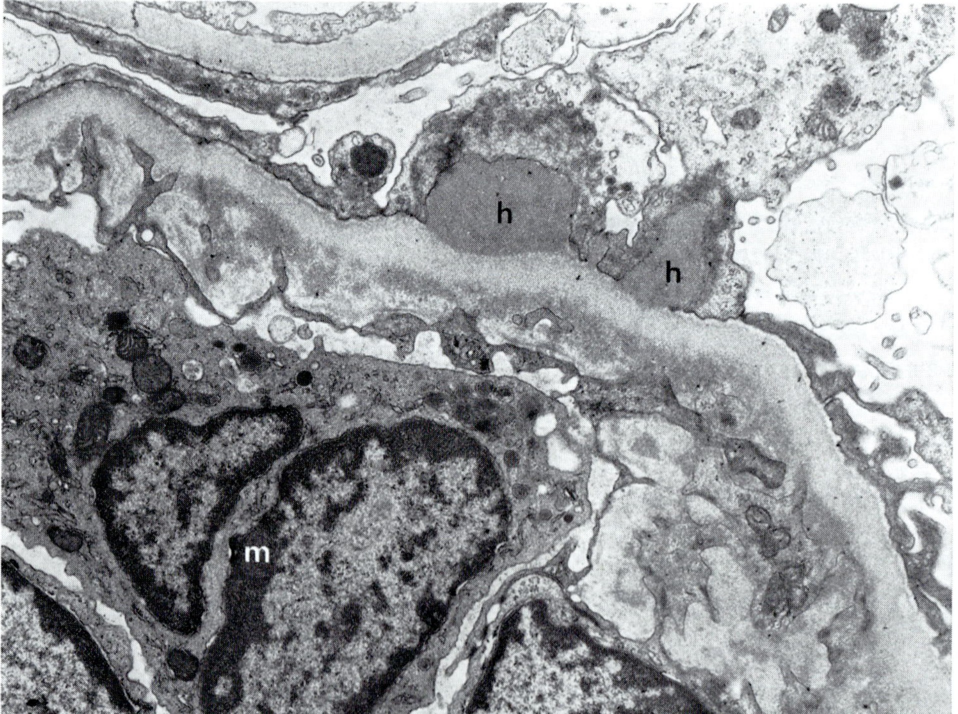

Fig. 8-5 Tow humps (h) with some subendothelial electron dense deposits. Note an emigrant cell (m) in
the capillary lumen. Acute poststreptococcal glomerulonephritis.

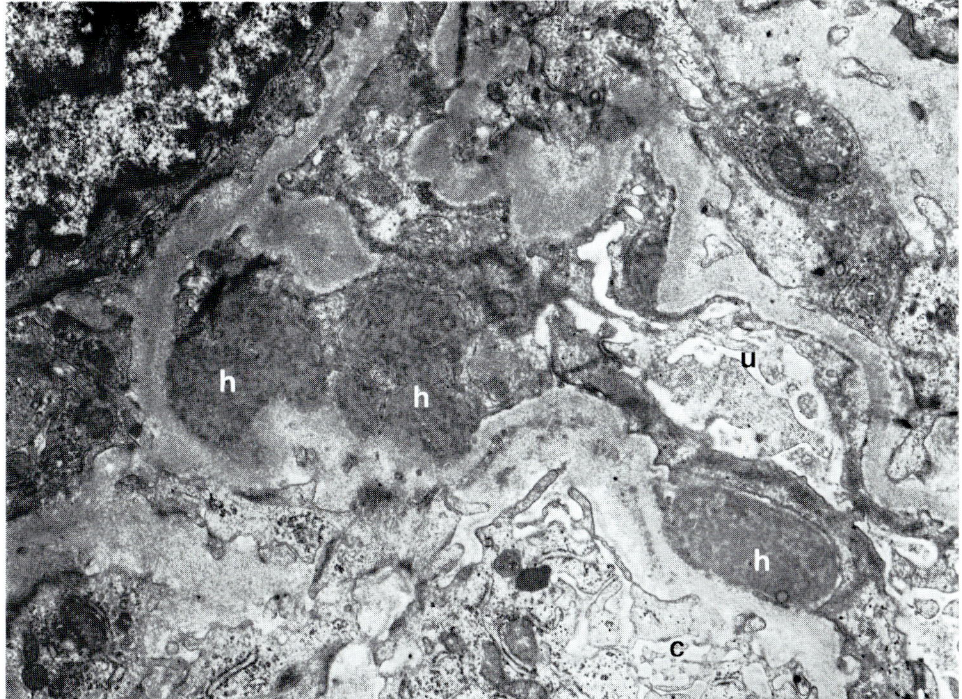

Fig. 8-6 Several atypical humps (h) with mottled appearance. Acute glomerulonephritis superimposed on cirrhosis of liver. c: capollary lumen, u: urinary space. Whether these atypical humps represent different etiopathogeneses as compared to typical poststreptococcal glomerulonephritis is unknown.

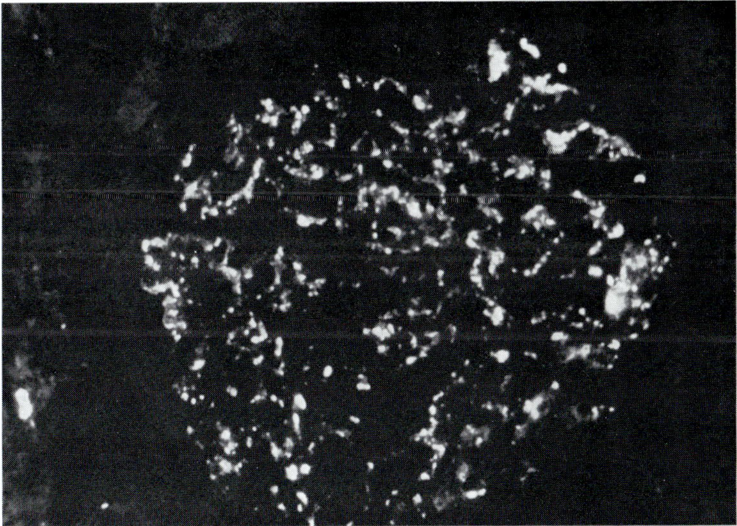

Fig. 8-7 Widely distributed granular fluorescence in acute poststreptococcal glomerulonephritis. Anti-C3 staining.

Clinical presentations and morphological expressions including electron microscopy and immunohistochemistry of acute poststreptococcal glomerulonephritis are surprisingly close to those of acute "one shot" serum sickness type experimental glomerulonephritis. In the first place, the latent interval between onset of glomerulonephritis and streptococcal infection corresponds well to the time interval between the onset of renal lesion and the administration of foreign proteins in the experimental animal. Second, serum complement levels fluctuate concomitantly with the onset of the renal lesion in both acute poststreptococcal glomerulonephritis and this type of experimental glomerulonephritis. Third, glomerular pathology in both humans and experimental animals is almost identical by light, electron and immunohistochemical microscopy including its evolution. Thus there is substantial evidence indicating that acute poststreptococcal glomerulonephritis is initiated and mediated by the same pathogenetic mechanisms through which acute "one shot" serum sickness type glomerulonephritis is produced in experimental animals. However, there appear to be several points that need to be clarified.

The first point is the antigen(s) responsible for acute poststreptococcal glomerulonephritis. The antigen(s) has been demonstrated to exist only occasionally in the glomerulus by immunohistochemistry [12, 103]. The immunohistochemical pattern against components of nephrotoxic organisms seems to be different from that of immunoglobulins and complement components showing a mixture of mesangial and peripheral granular pattern. Humps, that are considered to represent immune complex deposition, usually do not contain any antigen(s) and this has been confirmed by immunoelectron microscopy [103]. The explanation for this is that the determinant(s) of the antigen(s) in humps have been completely covered by host's immunoglobulins and complement components, so that no binding sites have been left for the specific antiserum against the streptococcal antigen(s). Second is with regard to the complement profile. Acute "one shot" serum sickness type experimental glomerulonephritis has been known to show depressed complement levels from Clq to C9; circulating immune complexes activate Clq first, then the whole complement cascade is activated via the classical pathway. On the other hand, acute poststreptococcal glomerulonephritis is reported to show the serum complement profile composed of depressed C3 and the following distal components, while remaining early components are relatively within normal range [48]. In addition, properdin, a key factor for activation of an alternate pathway of the complement system is also found in the glomeruli [48] and depleted in the serum of patients [61]. Third, the quantity of the antigen(s) responsible for glomerular lesions in experimental serum sickness nephritis is considered very large in comparison with that of acute poststreptococcal glomerulonephritis, while glomerulonephritis resulting from administration of anticancer horse serum is comparable in amount to that in experimental acute nephritis, and is reported to be fatal [15]. What causes the difference between acute poststreptococcal glomerulonephritis and acute "one shot" type serum sickness in man is not known. The existence of cryoglobulins in the glomeruli of acute poststreptococcal glomerulonephritis is another factor to be elucidated [30].

Glomerulonephropathy associated with SLE (lupus nephritis) is an example of immune complex type nephritis. In this condition, it has been said that DNA as the antigen and antiDNA form complexes in the circulation and deposit in the glomeruli [1, 59]. However, only complexes resulting from DNA anti-DNA do not neccessarily indicate that whole etiopathogenesis, but probably much more complicated etiopathogeneses intermingled with DNA mediated complexes play a role in producing glomerular lesions in this condition [12]. Panem et al. [69] reported in vitro and in vivo evidence indicating that C-12 virus plays an important role for the etiopathogenesis in lupus nephritis.

Histopathology of lupus nephritis is characterized by a wide variety of elemental morphologic features described earlier in this chapter. By light microscopy, lupus nephritis may be divided into three or four representative forms of glomerular changes [58], essentially normal, focal or diffuse proliferative glomerulonephritis and (epi)membranous glomerulonephritis (Fig. 8-8). The proliferative lesion in lupus nephritis seems to have a tendency for a focal and local or segmental distribution by light microscopy even in diffuse lupus nephritis in which focal and local or segmental exaggeration of involvement is apparent. Characteristic features having been described in lupus nephritis such as the wire-loop lesion, hematoxylin bodies and karyorrhexis are mostly observed in this diffuse proliferative form of lupus nephritis. The membranous form of lupus nephritis is indistinguishable from idiopathic membranous glomerulonephritis or membranous nephropathy by light and electron microscopy and even by immunohistochemistry.

Virus like microtubular structures and a finger print like appearance of electron dense deposits have been, in addition, reported. Properdin is also present in the glomerulus of lupus nephritis by immunohistochemistry.

Experimental models that closely resemble human SLE are those of naturally occurring disease of NZB and NZB/NZW mice. Rabbits receiving prolonged sensitization of foreign proteins exhibit immunological and histopathological features that closely resemble human SLE. This is described elsewhere in this book.

A recent investigation searching for circulating immune complexes in the serum of patients with acute glomerulonephritis and SLE using polyethylene glycol and labeled C1q has shown that C1q bound immune complexes were found in a majority of patients (28 of 35 cases of acute glomerulonephritis and 46 of 71 cases of SLE) [35].

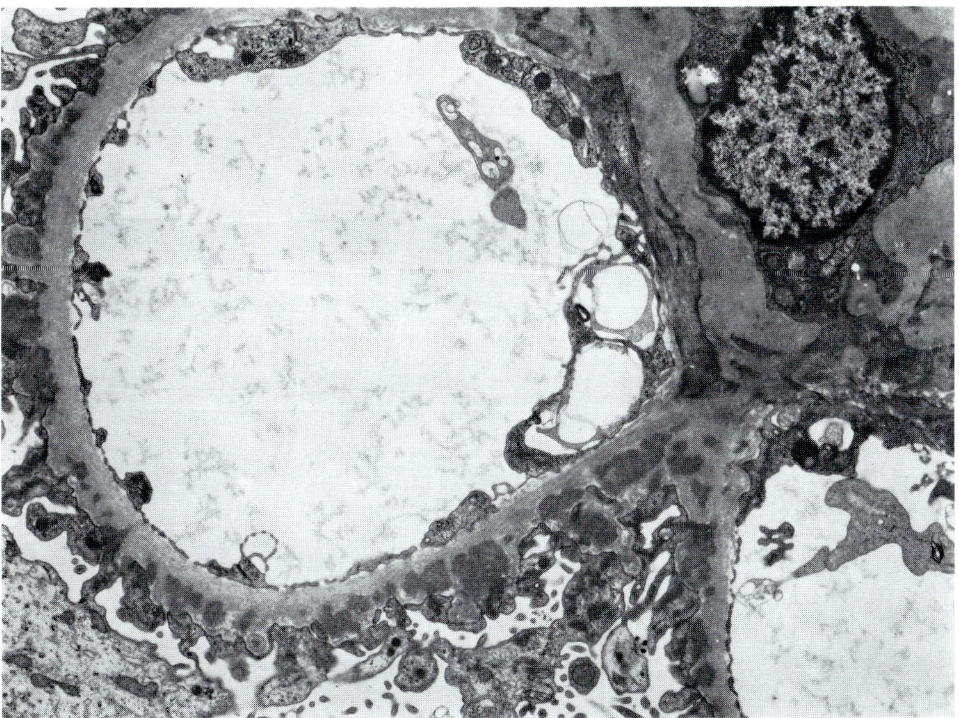

Fig. 8-8 Regular subepithelial deposits with spike-formation. The capillary lumens are well patent. A membranous form of lupus nephritis.

Membranous nephropathy is a well established clinicopathologic entity [3, 19, 26, 29, 74]. Clinical onset is insidious and when clinical presentations are apparent, patients usually present a nephrotic syndrome. In general, the disease progresses slowly with deterioration of renal function, increase of serum urea nitrogen and hypertension in some.

The morphological expression is highly characteristic. Glomerular pathology in this condition is characterized by the presence of electron dense deposits at the subepithelial aspect of the glomerular basement membrane and the lack of cellular response; no hypercellularity and in particular no exudation in glomeruli. The subepithelial deposits are, in general, smaller than humps and much more densely and regularly distributed over the entire glomerular basement membrane. The deposits contain immunoglobulins and complement components implicating immune complex deposition by immunohistochemistry (Fig. 8-9). Perpendicular projections of basement membrane like material (spikes) to the original glomerular basement membrane are seen in between these electron dense deposits by electron microscopy or by light microscopy with sections stained to demonstrate the basement membrane.

With the progress of the disease, the spikes become fused at the most distal point from the original glomerular basement membrane by a layer of newly formed basement membrane. The electron dense deposits originally situated at the subepithelial aspect are thus incorporated into the enormously thickened glomerular basement membrane. At the same time the deposits change their texture; they may be electron dense as have been, they may become electron lucent with granular stippling or coarse granular in appearance. Thus the disease was thought to be an irreversible condition terminating in uremia. However, recent studies have shown that with appropriate therapy, or even without therapy in some cases, the disease can regress with complete recovery clinically as well as morphologically [3].

The morphological expression including electron microscopy and immunohistochemistry is very close to the experimental model of "chronic" serum sickness type nephritis and that of Heymann's autologous immune complex nephritis. In both experimental models, immune complexes deposit at the subepithelial aspect of the glomerular basement mem-

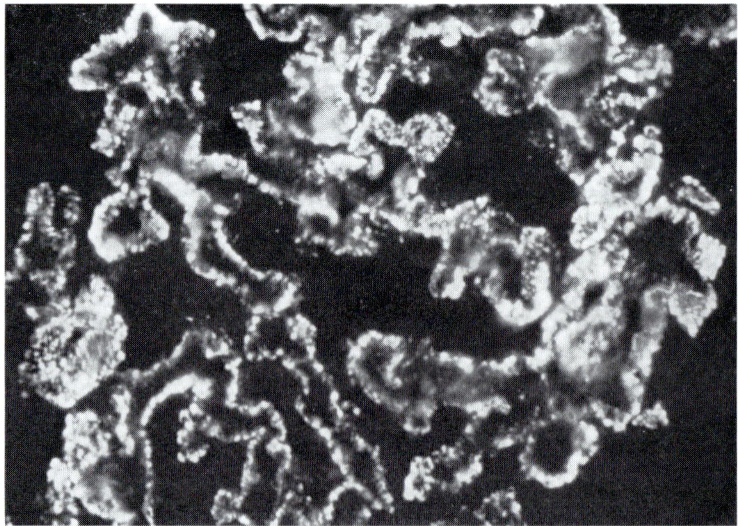

Fig. 8-9   Regular granular deposition of IgG along the capillary wall. Membranous nephropathy.

brane to give essentially the same features as human membranous nephropathy by electron microscopy and immunohistochemistry. In those experimental models, antigens (foreign proteins or components of homologous tubular epithelial cells) are detected in the same pattern as immunoglobulins and complement components in the glomeruli. Thus membranous nephropathy has been believed to be a typical example of immune complex nephritis in man because of the analogy gained from those experimental models. Search for antigens in this condition has not yet been fruitful. Only isolated reports have demonstrated antigens in a few instances of this condition. Those are Australian antigen [11, 14], tumor related antigens [50, 52, 94] and heavy metals as the hapten [74].

b. Anti-glomerular basement membrane antibody disease

Glomerulonephropathy mediated by anti-glomerular basement membrane antibodies should be defined only by the detection of antibodies specifically directed to the glomerular basement membrane either in the eluted immunoglobulins from diseased glomeruli or from the circulation of the patient.

In practice, the immunohistochemical patterns of immunoglobulins and complement components of this type of glomerulonephropathy exhibit so characteristically a delicate, continuous "linear" appearance that this immunohistochemical appearance has been appreciated to indicate anti-glomerular basement membrane antibody mediated glomerulonephropathy (Fig. 8-10).

A typical example of this type of glomerulonephropathy is seen in Goodpasture's syndrome [5]. Patients suffering from this syndrome show rapidly progressive renal lesions and severe hemorrhagic pulmonary involvement. Renal pathology is characterized by either focal glomerulonephritis in less severely affected instances or diffuse extracapillary proliferative glomerulonephritis (Fig. 8-11) in most instances. Electron dense deposits are not observed in the glomeruli with electronmicroscopy, while with immunohistochemistry, a characteristic linear pattern of immunoglobulins and complement components is demonstrated. Immunoglobulins eluted from the glomeruli of the patients react not only to the normal glomerular basement membrane but also to the normal alveolar basement membrane of the lung. This anti-basement membrane activity is also found in the serum of the patients. Thus the etiopathogenesis of this syndrome is considered to be the autologous anti-basement membrane antibodies against both glomerular and alveolar basement membranes.

Although the mechanism by which anti-basement membrane antibodies are formed in man is unknown, two explanations can be considered; a) endogenous basement membrane materials somehow become altered or released and acquire antigenic properties to the host, b) exogenous agents bearing similar antigenic determinants to basement membrane materials produce antibodies cross-reactive to the basement membrane.

Reports regarding epidemics of Goodpasture's syndrome related to hydrocarbons [4] and influenza [70, 100] could support a hypothesis related to the first explanation above that exposure of the alveolar basement membrane to hydrocarbons or influenza virus could alter the alveolar basement membrane resulting in formation of anti-basement membrane antibody(ies) cross-reactive with the glomerular basement membrane.

With respect to the second explanation, althought the possibility that in certain conditions antibodies against streptococcal or other antigens can cross-react with the glomerular basement membrane has been suggested [45, 89], further evidence is needed to support this hypothesis.

Some cases of primary glomerulonephropathies classified clinically as rapidly progressive glomerulonephritis and pathologically as diffuse extracapillary proliferative glomerulonephritis show a characteristic linear immunohistochemical pattern of immuno-

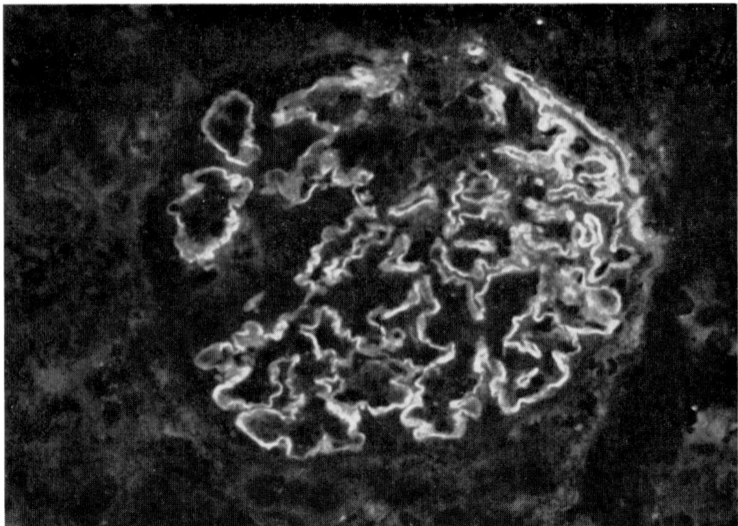

Fig. 8-10   Linear staining of IgG. Goodpasture's syndrome.

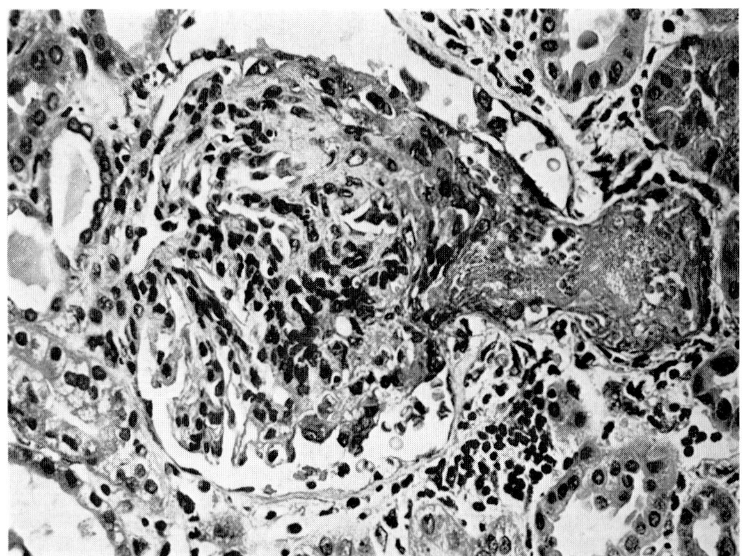

Fig. 8-11   Early crescent formation. Note cellular debris and fragmented RBC's at the urinary pole. The glomerular capillary tufts are compressed by somewhat segmental extracapillary proliferative processes. Good pasture's syndrome. H&E stain.

globulins and complement components identical to that seen in the renal glomeruli in Goodpasture's syndrome.   Results of elution studies on diseased glomeruli are also similar to those of Goodpasture's syndrome as far as the anti-glomerular basement membrane antibody activity is concerned [49, 84].   Thus the etiopathogenesis in certain cases of idiopathic rapidly progressive glomerulonephritis is considered to be the same as glomerulo-nephropathy of Goodpasture's syndrome, i.e. autologous anti-glomerular basement membrane antibody(ies).

However, not all diseases or conditions that show glomerular localization of immuno-globulins and complement components in a linear pattern by immunohistochemistry indicate definitely that anti-glomerular basement membrane antibodies play a role in glo-merular lesions.   An example of this case is seen in certain cases of diabetic glomerulo-sclerosis in that a typical linear localization of immunoglobulins is sometimes observed by immunohistochemistry [97].   Immunochemical analyses, however, have failed to demon-strate anti-glomerular basement membrane antibodies play a significant role in this condi-tion [97].   What causes these linear localizations of immunoglobulins is not known.

2. Glomerulonephropathies presumed to be mediated by immunological mechanisms

This group includes a majority of glomerulonephropathies that can be seen in practice as either the primary lesion or associated with systemic diseases.   Possible immunological pathogeneses in these conditions are suggested mostly by immunohistochemical analyses of the glomeruli.   In general, there are immunoglobulins and complement components in glomeruli, whereas antigens are not found.   Glomerulonephropathies of this group include such clinicopathologic entities as IgA nephropathy, membranoproliferative glo-merulonephritis with subendothelial deposits and glomerulonephropathies associated with such systemic diseases as anaphylactoid purpura, rheumatoid arthritis, polyarteritis nodosa and Wegener's granulomatosis.

Membranoproliferative glomerulonephritis with subendothelial deposits is a distinct clinicopathologic entity characterized clinically by the nephrotic syndrome and progressive deterioration of renal function despite intensive chemical therapy.   Pathologically, it is characterized by moderate to severe endocapillary proliferative glomerulonephritis toge-ther with diffuse and global circumferential mesangial interposition (Fig. 8-12) giving a sense of almost global thickening of the glomerular capillary wall with H&E stained sections

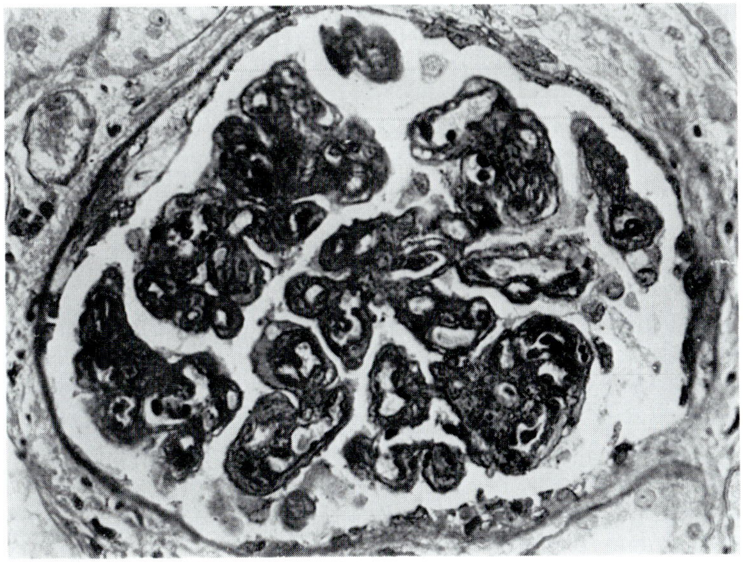

Fig. 8-12 Membranoproliferative (mesangiocapillary) glomerulonephritis with subendothelial deposits. Note fairly global double contour of the GBM. PAS stain.

in a fairly diffuse manner.   With electron microscopy, aside from the pathologic features seen by light microscopy, marked increase of mesangial matrix and frequent electron dense deposits situated at the subendothelial and mesangial aspects are characteristic findings. With immunohistochemistry, these deposits contain immunoglobulins and complement components as well as fibrin-fibrinogen substances.   Because of the presence of immuno-globulins and complement components in glomeruli, the pathogenetic mechanism of this condition has been thought to be mediated by immunological mechanisms, particularly by immune complexes.   However, antigens responsible for this condition have not yet been found with certainty.   Only suggestive antigens (Schistosoma and its components) have been reported recently from upper Egypt [22].

On the other hand, the presence of persistent hypocomplementemia seen in a majority of patients with this condition has given rise to a serious question about its etiology.   The complement profile of the serum of this persistent hypocomplementemia is characterized by depletion of C3 and the remaining later components, while early complement components remain within normal range [13, 48, 96].   In addition, the presence of a factor (C3NeF) being able to activate the complement system via an alternate pathway in the serum of the patients suggests depleted complement levels to be mainly due to complement activation via an alternate pathway [63, 96, 98].   To support this idea or hypothesis, frequent relapse of this glomerulonephropathy have been reported in grafted kidneys [27, 78, 105].

A special form of membranoproliferative glomerulonephritis is the one named lobular glomerulonephritis.   This is characterized pathologically by marked accentuation of a lobular pattern of the glomerular tufts with frequent centrilobular acellular nodule forma-tion in a fairly diffuse and global fashion.   Characteristic mesangial circumferential inter-position seen in membranoproliferative glomerulonephritis with subendothelial deposits is not prominent in this form of glomerulonephritis.   Careful clinicopathologic studies with sequential renal biopsies have revealed that both diseases show essentially the same clinical presentations and immunohistochemical features, and the only difference between these two diseases is a histological expression.   However, this histological difference may not be a fundamental one in view of the fact that both histological characteristic expressions can be observed alternatively in sequentially biopsied tissues from the same patient.   There-fore, it is highly possible that the difference seen in the sections appears only to relate to a reaction of mesangial cells to inflammatory stimuli [55].

Another particular morphologic entity of membranoproliferative glomerulonephritis is glomerular basement membrane dense deposit disease or membranoproliferative glomerulonephritis with intramembranous dense deposit [2, 6, 28, 33, 54] (Fig. 8-13). Morphologically, the most characteristic change of this entity is deposition of electron dense homogeneous materials not only within the glomerular basement membrane, but in the glomerular capsular basement membrane as well as in the renal tubular basement membrane in a ribbon like fashion (Fig. 8-14).   Of interest, these deposits always contain complement components with only occasional immunoglobulins [33].   Neither centrilo-bular nodules nor circumferential mesangial interposition are prominent in this case.   The clinical presentations are generally similar to typical membranoproliferative glomerulone-phritis, while persistent hypocomplementemia is always associated with this particular condition which typical membranoproliferative glomerulonephritis does not neccessarily exhibit [13, 96].   Recent studies have suggested that this persistent hypocomplementemia is mainly due to the increased catabolic rate of serum C3 and the deposition of complement components in the kidney is the result of an alternate pathway activation of the complement system thus introduced [66, 71].   The pathogenetic mechanism by which membrano-proliferative glomerulonephritis is brought about is thus controversial at the present time.

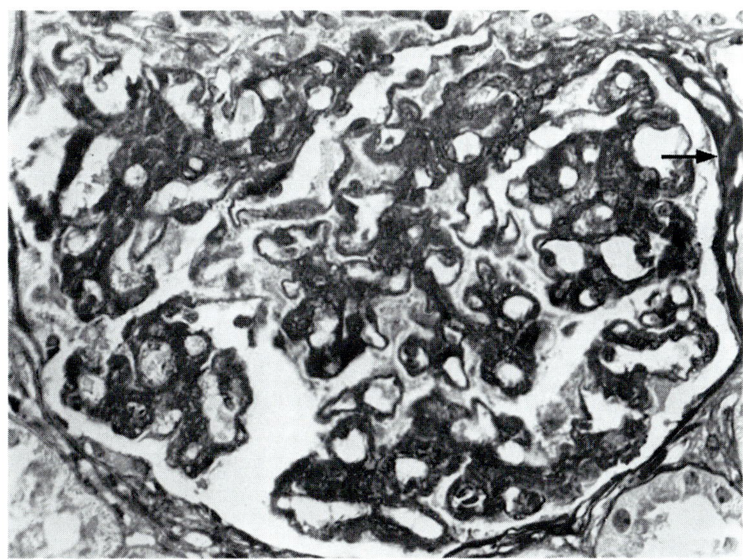

Fig. 8-13 Membranoproliferative glomerulonephritis with intramembranous dense deposits (MPGN with IMDD). PAS stain. Note irregular thickening due to deposits along the capillary wall and Bowman's capsule as well (arrow).

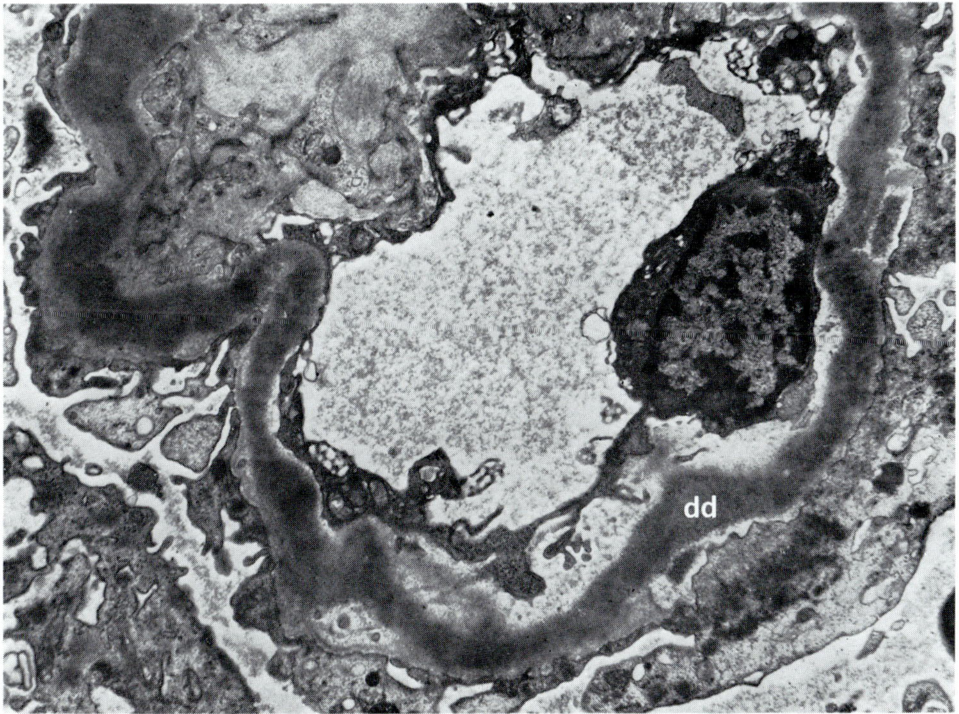

Fig. 8-14 MPGN with IMDD. Irregularly thickened GBM with intramembranous dense deposits (dd).

This is partly due to the lack of investigation at early stages of this condition and partly due to the complexity in the mechanism of this type of nephritis.

IgA nephropathy is one of the typical examples of this category. This condition was first described by Berger and Hinglais [7] in 1968 and subsequently by many others [16, 25, 53, 60, 83, 90, 91, 106]. It is characterized by diffuse and global localization of IgA as a predominant immunoglobulin usually together with less intense IgG and complement components in a mesangial pattern by immunohistochemistry (Fig. 8-15). By light microscopy, a focal and segmental form of glomerulonephritis has been described as the dominant renal pathology [7, 16, 91], while diffuse and global glomerular lesions do occur and this is the usual renal pathology of this condition in our own experience (Fig. 8-16). In any instance, renal pathologic alterations in general are mild and normal renal tissue may even be seen in this condition. Ultrastructurally, the characteristic finding is electron dense deposits confined to the mesangial area beneath the glomerular basement membrane and to some extent at the subendothelial sapect of peripheral capillary loops (Fig. 8-17). Electron dense deposits outside of the glomerular basement membrane (subepithelial aspect) have not been observed. The glomerular basement membrane itself is thin and delicate and is well preserved.

Clinical presentations are characterized by recurrent hematuria and/or persistent light proteinuria in a majority of patients with benign and very slowly progressive impairment of renal function, while a small proportion of the patients exhibit impaired renal function, hypertension, nephrotic syndrome or even renal insufficiency. The fact that not a small number of patients experience upper respiratory infection or loin pain just before the apparent clinical manifestations and that the presence of immunoglobulins and complement components in the glomeruli suggests the possibility of immune complexes playing a significant role in this condition.

IgA is known to play a particular role at the mucus membrane where IgA is dimerized by a secretory component [88]. However, in our own experience, no secretory component was found in the glomeruli of IgA nephropathy of 37 patients so tested by the indirect immunofluorescent technic [67]. McCoy et al. [60] also reported that a secretory

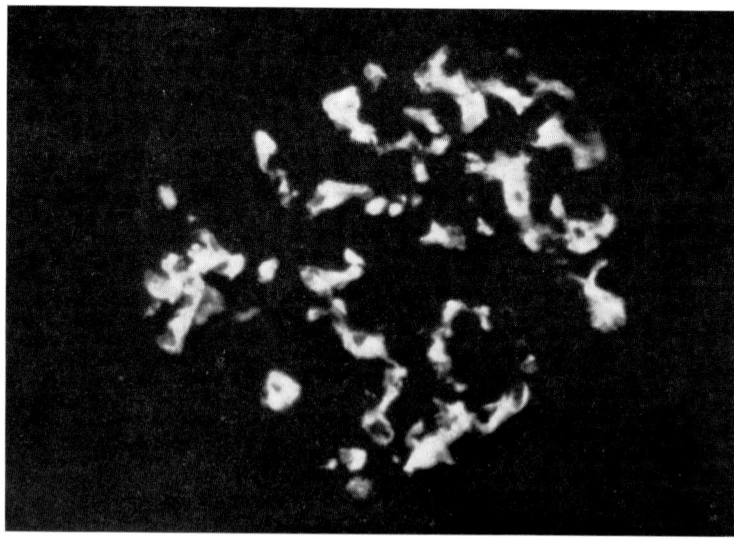

Fig. 8-15 Mesangial IgA deposition.

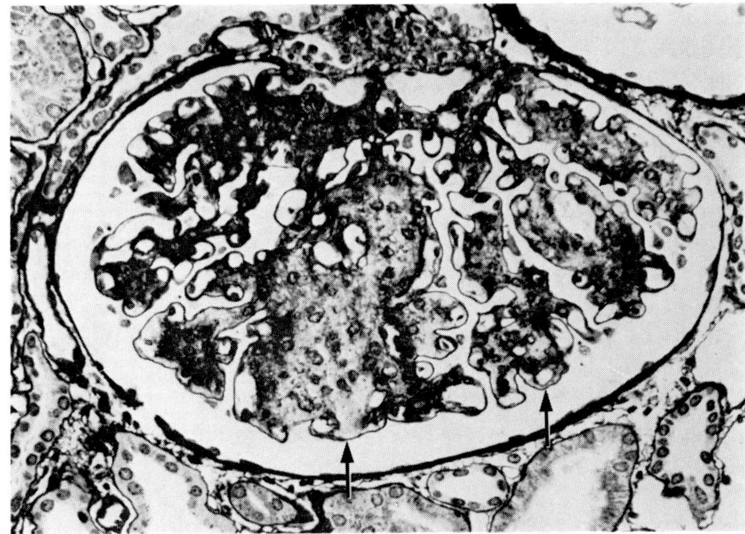

Fig. 8-16 Large mesangial deposits in IgA nephropathy. Occasional subendothelial extension of the deposits is also seen (arrows). PASM-H&E stain.

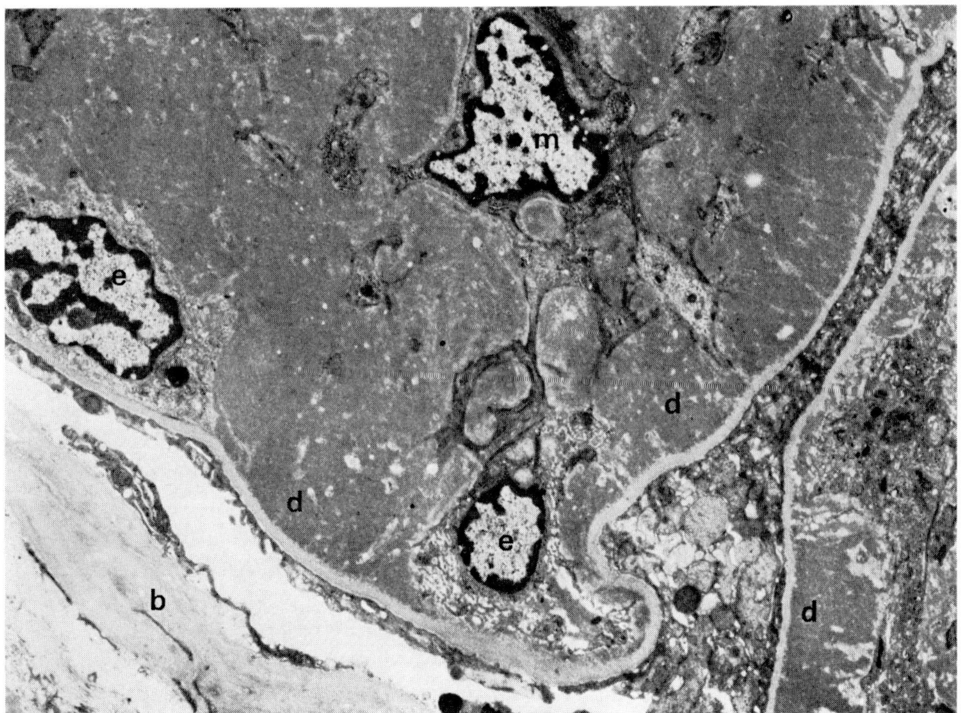

Fig. 8-17 Massive mesangial electron dense deposits with some locating at the subendothelial aspect (d). b: Bowman's capsule, e: endothelial cell, m: mesangial cell. IgA nephropathy, the same case as Fig. 8-16.

component of IgA was only weakly positive in a minority of their patients with IgA nephropathy and concluded that it is unlikely that the secretory IgA played a significant role in this condition. IgA participating as the antigen in this condition is also unlikely bacause in a considerable number of patients IgA was the only immunoglobulin demonstrated in the glomeruli. In addition, Lowance et al. [53] were unable to demonstrate any antibody activity in the patients' sera including an anephritic one. Therefore, it is likely that deposited IgA in the glomerulus is the consequence of immune complexes formed either in the circulation or within the mesangium, the circulating type IgA being the antibody. Recent reports from France have further suggested the possibility of autoantibody activity of IgA against components of the mesangium in view of the fact that IgA nephropathy tends to be transmitted to the grafted kidney [8, 9]. Currently, we have experienced a family of 4 of whom 3 are affected by IgA nephropathy in a similar but rather peculiar glomerular pathology [68]. This family has a densely involved nephropathy-prone pedigree on the maternal side (10 of 21) implicating the influence of some genetic factors playing a role in this particular condition.

This category includes the vast majority of such patients seen in practice. However, lack of appropriate experimental models corresponding to this category of human glomerulonephropathies has made it difficult to elucidate the pathogenetic mechanisms or etiopathogeneses. Shibata et al. [79, 80] reported production of an experimental nephritis characterized by a mesangial pattern localization of IgG and complement components in rats with a single injection of isologous or heterologous glycoprotein or glycopeptide. Mauer et al. [57] also reported production of a mesangial immune complex type glomerulonephritis using a complex experimental procedure such as transplantation and mesangial phagocytic activity. However, the pathology of these experimental models does not fit well with either membranoproliferative glomerulonephritis or IgA nephropathy in view of the lack of circumferential mesangial interposition or participation of IgA as a predominant immunoglobulin in the glomeruli of the experimental animals.

3. Glomerulonephropathies unlikely to be related to immunological mechanisms

Lipoid nephrosis (nil disease, foot process disease) is perhaps one of the typical examples of this category. The disease usually affects children and young adults with the typical nephrotic syndrome; massive proteinuria mostly of a well selective type, hypoalbuminemia, generalized edema, hyperlipemia and lack of other nephritic factors such as hematuria and hypertension. Renal function is well preserved and a majority of patients respond well to steroid therapy.

Light microscopy reveals only prominent glomerular visceral epithelial cells and increased PAS positive hyaline granules in the proximal tubular epithelial cells. By electron microscopy, the glomeruli are generally well preserved only showing swollen visceral epithelial cells with marked villous configuration of the cytoplasm. The most characteristic feature is extensive fusion of visceral epithelial cell foot processes over the glomerular basement membrane hence the name of foot process disease. By immunohistochemistry, usually no staining against immunoglobulins and complement components as well as fibrin-fibrinogen substances is observed, though faintly linear staining of immunoglobulins along the capillary wall has been reported in cases of this condition [36]. Some cases of this condition show polycyclic recurrence or exacerbation of the syndrome and further isolated cases have been reported to exhibit recurrence or exacerbation of the syndrome in association with exposure to grass pollen [102] implicating reaginic hypersensitivity playing a role.   However, so far studies on the possibility of IgE playing a particular role in this condition have not been proved [12, 75].   To date it seems to be a general consensus among the nephrologists that lipoid nephrosis is the result of other mechanisms than immunological ones and is probably a consequence of metabolic disorders of the glomerular basement membrane resulting in an increased permeability particularly to low molecular proteins and that extensive epithelial foot process fusion over the glomerular basement membrane is the result of this increased permeability rather than the cause of the disease.

Other glomerulonephropathies that may be included in this category are glomerular lesions of malignant nephrosclerosis, nephropathies associated with genetically transmitted diseases such as Alpot's syndrome, Fabry's disease and certain forms of congenital nephrotic syndrome.

IV. Mediators Participating in Glomerular Pathology and Conclusion

As has been written, the morphological expressions of glomerular diseases are largely irrespective of whether they are caused by immunological mechanisms or not.   It is then possible to say that the actual process by which tissue damage resulting in morphological expressions of the glomerular disease is brought about is nonspecific.   Indeed, experimental studies revealed that with coagulopathy only, one can produce a variety of glomerular lesions [81] and that the administration of Warfarin can greatly reduce morphological expressions of Masugi nephritis [92].

Among human glomerulonephropathies, focal glomerulosclerosis with the nephrotic syndrome is possibly brought about by coagulation processes [18], because the nephrotic syndrome itself is considered to be a hypercoagulable state [43, 47].   Glomerular lesions of malignant nephrosclerosis are characterized by proliferation of glomerular intrinsic cells with thrombotic and necrotic features of glomerular tufts with or without polymorphonuclear leukocytic exudation.   However, immunological pathogeneses have not yet been demonstrated to play a significant role in this condition.   Consequently, it is reasonable to believe that coagulation processes can produce or at least accelerate glomerular "inflammatory" changes and that coagulation processes can be triggered not only by immunological mechanisms but also by other ones.

The complement system is one of the important systems by which tissue injuries are brought about.   This system consists of 9 main components and associated factors. Activation of this system leads to cytolysis through its cell-bound factors and is responsible for such events as immune adherence, anaphylatoxin release and attraction of polymorphonuclear leukocytes through its soluble factors released into surrounding tissue [23, 66]. The complement system can be activated through either the classical or the alternate pathways [23].   Classical complement activation occurs when IgG and/or IgM related antigen-antibody complexes are formed anywhere in the circulation or in situ in certain organs such as in the kidney.   A portion of the antibody, forming antigen-antibody complexes, undergoes some alteration which enables antigen-antibody complexes to activate the first component of the complement.   Thus all the complement components are activated until C9 results in cytolysis.   In addition, alternate complement activation may be generated through the classical complement activation at the level of C3.   In the course of these complement activations, various soluble factors capable of generating such functions as phagocytosis, immune adherence, anaphylatoxin generation, neutrophil chemotaxis, histamine release, neutrophil chemotaxis and stabilization are liberated.   All of those functions are responsible for tissue damage and are essential to inflammation.

The alternate pathway activation of complement components is initiated at the level of

C3 without participation of early complement components; C1, C4 and C2. Activation of C3 by this pathway can be triggered by various substances such as lipopolysaccharides, aggregated IgA, IgE and even colloidal particles. Once C3 is activated, the following complement components (C5–C9) are sequentially activated irrespective of initiating mechanisms, in other words, activation of late complement components is a nonspecific phenomenon and is independent from initiating mechanisms whether or not they are immunological.

Recent studies on the complement system and coagulation mechanisms have revealed that these two systems interact intimately with each other and are assumed to have a major responsibility for actual tissue damage resulting in morphological inflammation and functional disturbance [73]. However, further detailed explanation about the interrelationship of these two systems will not be described here, because it is far beyond the aim of this book and is still in an early stage of investigation. The role of these mediators to the clinical and morphological manifestations of experimentally induced glomerulonephropathies in animals by means of immunological mechanisms has been reviewed briefly describing three systems of injury; complement and polymorphonuclear leukocyte-independent injury, complement and polymorphonuclear leukocyte-dependent injury and fibrin-fibrinogen-dependent process [82]. These systems of injury are expressed differently from species to species depending upon the animal used implying that mediators may behave differently in different species of animals, so that every facet of these system of injury should be considered in human glomerulonephropathies.

In any events, mediators and macromolecules participating in inflammation resulting in actual tissue damage are very important in view of the fact that recent advances in therapeutic maneuvers of glomerulonephropathies have been largely achieved in the field of anticoagulant and antiinflammatory drugs.

Advances and better understanding of various human nephropathies over the past 20 years or so have been tremendous because of the introduction and general application of percutaneous renal biopsy technics, successful production of appropriate experimental models and rapid progress in immunology together with the application of such sophisticated methods as electron microscopy, immunohistochemistry and radioimmunoassay.

It is certain that a vast majority of human nephropathies are mediated through immunological mechanisms, particularly of the immune complex type. However, responsible antigens are detected in an only small number of cases and in the majority of cases are left in the presumed stage. Therefore, it is important not only to maintain efforts to elucidate responsible antigens, but also to clarify mediators, macromolecules and their interactions participating in the actual tissue damage leading to clinical and morphological manifestations of nephropathies. Because there are now many reasons to believe that an initial immunological phenomenon can very well be followed by secondary local, nonspecific phenomena in which we have a possible explanation as to why the disease continues after the immunological process can no longer be identified [35].

In addition, more attention should be given to the host's state or condition in terms of immunology, coagulation, complement as well as other factors that are able to influence the intensity and the character of inflammation. Of course, many of these factors could very well be under the genetic control. However, the possibility of acquired conditions under which these factors may behave differently is also considered in human beings as suggested by experimental animals. This is clearly stated elsewhere in this book.

241

REFERENCES

1. Agnello, V.: The immunopathogenesis of lupus nephritis. *In* Hamburger, J., Crosnier, J., and Maxwell, H.M. (eds.) *Advances in Nephrology*, Vol. 6, 119–136, Year Book, Chicago, 1976.

2. Antonie, B. and Faye, C.: The clinical course associated with dense deposits in the kidney basement membranes. *Kidney Int. 1*: 420–427, 1972.

3. Bariéty, J., Druet, P., Lagrue, G., Samarcq, P., et Milliez, P.: Les glomérulopathies "extra-membraneuse" (G.E.M.). Étude morphologique en microscopie optique, électronique et en immunofluorescence. *Path. Biol. 18*: 5–32, 1970.

4. Beirne, G.J. and Breennan, J.T.: Glomerulonephritis associated with exposure to hydrocarbon solvents, mediated by antiglomerular basement membrane antibody. *Arch. Environ. Health 25*: 365–369, 1972.

5. Benoit, F.L., Rulon, D.B., Theil, G.B., Doolan, P.D., and Watten, R.H.: Goodpasture's syndrome. A clinicopathologic entity. *Amer. J. Med. 37*: 424–444, 1964.

6. Berger, J. et Galle, P.: Dépôts denses au sein des membranes basales du rein. Étude en microscopies optique et électronique. *Presse Med. 71*: 2351–2354, 1963.

7. Berger, J. et Hinglais, N.: Les dépôts intercapillaries d'IgA-IgG. *J. Urol. Nephrol. 74*: 694–695, 1968.

8. Berger, J., Noël, L.H., and Yaneva, H.: Contribution of immunofluorescence to the study of graft lesions. *In* Giovannetti, S., Bonomini, V., and D'Amico, G. (eds.) *Proceedings of the VIth International Congress of Nephrology*, Florence 1975, 736–739, Karger, Basel, 1976.

9. Berger, J., Yaneva, H., Nabarra, B., and Barbanel, C.: Recurrence of mesangial deposition of IgA after renal transplantation. *Kidney Int. 7*: 232–241, 1975.

10. Bhorde, M.S., Carag, H.B., Lee, H.G., Potter, E.V., and Duena, G.: Nephropathy of secondary syphilis. A clinical and pathological spectrum. *J.A.M.A. 216*: 1159–1166, 1971.

11. Brzosko, W.J., Krawczyński, K., Nazarewicz, T., Morzycka, M., and Nowoslawski, A.: Glomerulonephritis associated with Hepatitis-B surface antigen immune complexes in children. *Lancet 2*: 477–482, 1974.

12. Cameron, J.S.: Bright's disease today: The pathogenesis and treatment of glomerulonephritis. *Brit. Med. J. 4*: 87–90, 160–163, 217–220, 1972.

13. Cameron, J.S., Glasgow, E.F., Ogg, C.S., and White, R.H.R.: Membranoproliferative glomerulonephritis and persistent hypocomplementemia. *Brit. Med. J. 4*: 7–14, 1970.

14. Combes, B., Stastny, P., Shorey, J., Eigenbrodt, E.H., Barrera, A., Hull, A.R., and Carter, N.W.: Glomerulonephritis with deposition of Australia antigen-antibody complexes in glomerular basement membrane. *Lancet 2*: 234–238, 1971.

15. De La Pava, S., Nigagozyan, G., and Pickren, J.W.: Fatal glomerulonephritis after receiving horse antihuman-cancer serum. *Arch. Intern. Med. 109*: 391–399, 1962.

16. de Werra, P., Morel-Maroger, L., Leroux-Robert, C., et Richet, G.: Glomérulites a dépôts d'IgA diffus dans le mésangium. Etude de 96 cas chez l'adulte. *Schweitz. med. Wschr. 103*: 761–768, 797–803, 1973.

17. Dixon, F.J.: The pathogenesis of glomerulonephritis. *Amer. J. Med. 44*: 493–498, 1968.

18. Duffy, J.L., Cinque, T., Grishman, E., and Churg, J.: Intraglomerular fibrin, platelet aggregation, and subendothelial deposits in lipoid nephrosis. *J. Clin. Invest. 49*: 251–258, 1970.

19. Ehrenreich, T. and Churg, J.: Pathology of membranous nephropathy. *In* Sommers, S.C. (ed.) *Pathology Annual*, Vol. 3, 145–186, Appleton-Century-Crofts, New York, 1968.

20. Ellis, A.: Natural history of Bright's disease. Clinical, histological and experimental observations. *Lancet 1*: 1–6, 34–36, 72–76, 1942.

21. Engel, H.: Glomerulitis adhesiva. *Virch. Arch. path. anat. Physiol. 163*: 209–226, 1901.

22. Ezzat, E., Hafeeze, R., Tohamy, M., Ata, S., and Omar, A.H.: Mesangiocapillary glomerulonephritis in Upper Egypt and its relation to chronic bacterial and parasitic diseases. *VIth International Congress of Nephrology*, Florence 1975, Abstract No. 307.

23. Fearon, D.T., Ruddy, S., Knostman, J.D., Carpenter, C.B., and Austen, K.F.: The functional significance of complement. *In* Hamburger, J., Crosnier, J., and Maxwell, M.H. (eds.) *Advances in Nephrology*, Vol. 4, 15–35, Year Book, Chicago, 1974.

24. Fichera, G. und Scaffidi, V.: Beitrag zur pathologischen Histologie der Glomeruli. *Virch. Arch. anat. Physiol. 179*: 63–96, 1904.

25. Finlayson, G., Alexander, R., Juncos, L., Schlein, E., Teague, P., Waldman, R., and Cade, R.: Immunoglobulin A glomerulonephritis, a clinicopathologic entity. *Lab. Invest. 32*: 140–148, 1975.

26. Forland, M. and Spargo, B.H.: Clinicopathological correlations in idiopathic nephrotic syndrome with membranous nephropathy. *Nephron 6*: 498–525, 1969.

27. Galle, P., Hinglais, N., and Crosnier, J.: Recurrence of an original glomerular lesion in three renal allografts. *Transplant. Proc. 3*: 368–370, 1971.

28. Germuth, F.G. Jr., and Rodoriguez, E.: Class II immune complex deposit disease in humans: Laminal glomerulonephritis. *In:* Germuth, F. G. Jr. and Rodoriguez, E: *Immunopathology of the Renal Glomerulus*, 107–112, Little, Brown, Boston, 1973.

29. Gluck, E.C., Gallo, G., Lowenstein, J., and Baldwin, D.S.: Membranous glomerulonephritis. Evolution of clinical and pathologic features. *Ann. Intern. Med. 78*: 1–12, 1973.

30. Grupe, W.E.: IgG-β1C cryoglobulins in acute glomerulonephritis. *Pediatrics 42*: 474–482, 1968.

31. Gutman, R.A., Stricker, G.E., Gilliland, B.C., and Cutler, R.E.: The immune complex glomerulonephritis of bacterial endocarditis. *Medicine 51*: 1–25, 1972.

32. Habib, R. and Gubler, M.: Focal sclerosing glomerulonephritis. *In* Kincaid-Smith, P., Mathew, T.H., and Becker, L.E. (eds.) *Glomerulonephritis*, 263–278, John Wiley & Sons, New York, 1973.

33. Habib, R., Gubler, M., Loirat, C., Maiz, H.B., and Levy, M.: Dense deposit disease: A variant of membranoproliferative glomerulonephritis. *Kidney Internat. 7*: 204–215, 1975.

34. Hadfield, G. and Garrod, L.P.: Bright's disease. *In: Recent Advances in Pathology*, 5th ed., 278–303, Churchill, London, 1947.

35. Hamburger, J., Bach, J.F., Hinglais, N., Noel, L.H., and Digeon, M.: Reflections on the classification of glomerulonephritis. *In* Giovannetti, S., Bonomini, V., and D'Amico, G. (eds.) *Proceedings of the VIth International Congress of Nephrology*, Florence 1975, 49–59, Karger, Basel, 1976.

36. Hatano, M. and Yoshizawa, N.: Lipoid nephrosis. in *18th Annual Meeting of Japanese Society of Nephrology: Classification of Primary Glomerular Disease*, Osaka, Japan, 42–47, 1975.

37. Hellier, M.D., Webster, A.D.B., and Eisinger, A.J.M.F.: Nephrotic syndrome: A complication of secondary syphilis. *Brit. Med. J. 4*: 404–405, 1971.

38. Heptinstall, R.H.: Rapidly progressive glomerulonephritis. *In:* Heptinstall, R.H.: *Pathology of the Kidney*, 2nd ed., 371–391, Little, Brown, Boston, 1974.

39. Hinglais, N., Grünfeld, J.P., Tronconis, L., and Bois, E.: Ultrastructural lesions of the glomerular basement membrane in hereditary chronic nephritis. *In* Hamburger, J., Crosnier, J., and Maxwell, M.H. (eds.) *Advances in Nephrology*, Vol. 3, 133–152, Year Book, Chicago, 1974.

40. Hoyer, J.R., Michael, A.F., Fish, A.J., and Good, R.A.: Acute poststreptococcal glomerulonephritis presenting as hypertensive encephalopathy with minimal urinary abnormalities. *Pediatrics 39*: 412–417, 1967.

41. Iversen, P. and Brun, C.: Aspiration biopsy of kidney. *Amer. J. Med. 11*: 324–330, 1951.

42. Jenis, E.H., Sandler, P., Hill, G.S., Knieser, M.R., Jensen, G.E., and Roskes, S.D.: Glomerulonephritis with basement membrane dense deposits. *Arch. Path. 97*: 84–91, 1974.

43. Kendall, A.G., Lohmann, R.C., and Dossetor, J.B.: Nephrotic syndrome. A hypercoagulable state. *Arch. Intern. Med. 127*: 1021–1027, 1971.

44. Kincaid-Smith, P. and Hobbs, J.B.: Glomerulonephritis. A classification based on the significance of vessel lesions. *Med. J. Austral. 2*: 1397–1403, 1972.

45. Klassen, J., Elwood, C., Grossberg, A.L., Milgrom, F., Montes, M., Sepulveda, M., and Andres, G.A : Evolution of membranous nephropathy into anti-glomerular-basement-membrane glomerulonephritis. *New Engl. J. Med. 290*: 1340–1344, 1974.

46. Klebs, E.: *Handbuch der pathologischen Anatomie*. I Band, Zweite Abtheilung, 644–647, August Hirschwald, Berlin, 1876.

47. Lange, L.G., Carvalho, A., Bagdasarian, A., Lahiri, B., and Coleman, L.G.: Activation of Hageman factor in the nephrotic syndrome. *Amer. J. Med. 56*: 565–569, 1974.

48. Lewis, E.J., Carpenter, C.B., and Schur, P.H.: Serum complement component levels in human glomerulonephritis. *Ann. Intern. Med. 75*: 555–560, 1971.

49. Lewis, E.J., Cavallo, T., Harrington, J.T., and Cotran, R.S.: An immunopathologic study of rapidly progressive glomerulonephritis in the adult. *Human Path. 2*: 185–208, 1971.

50. Lewis, M.G., Loughridge, L.W., and Philips, T.M.: Immunological studies in nephrotic syndrome associated with extrarenal malignant disease. *Lancet 2*: 134–135, 1971.

51. Lewy, J.E., Salinas-Madrigal, L., Herdson, P.B., Pirani, C.L., and Metcoff, J.: Clinicopathologic correlations in acute poststreptococcal glomerulonephritis. A correlation between renal functions, morphologic damage and clinical course of 46 children with acute poststreptococcal glomerulonephritis. *Medicine 50*: 453–501, 1971.

52. Loughridge, L.W. and Lewis, M.G.: Nephrotic syndrome in malignant disease of non-renal origin. *Lancet 1*: 256–259, 1971.

53. Lowance, D.C., Mullins, J.D., and McPhaul, J.J. Jr.,: Immunoglobulin A (IgA) associated glomerulonephritis. *Kidney Internat. 3*: 167–176, 1973.

54. MacDonald, M.K.: Dense deposit disease: A subgroup of membranoproliferative glomerulonephritis, identified by electron microscopy. *In* Kincaid-Smith, P., Mathew, T.H., and Becker, E.L. (eds.) *Glomerulonephritis*, 515–530, John Wiley & Sons, New York, 1973.

55. Mandalenakis, N., Mendoza, N., Pirani, C.L., and Pollak, V.E.: Lobular glomerulonephritis and membranoproliferative glomerulonephritis. A clinical and pathologic study based on renal biopsies. *Medicine 50*: 319–355, 1971.

56. Marchiafava e Valenti: Della glomerulo-nefrite scharlatinosa: Studi clinic ed istologici. *Atti dell'Academia Medica di Roma*, Anno I (1875–1876), Fasc. 1: 198–211, 1877.

57. Mauer, S.M., Sutherland, D.E.R., Howard, R.J., Fish, A.J., Najarian, J.S., and Michael, A.F.: The glomerular mesangium. III. Acute immune mesangial injury: A new model of glomerulonephritis. *J. Exp. Med. 137*: 553–570, 1973.

58. McCluskey, R.T.: Lupus nephritis. *In* Sommers, S.C. (ed.) *Pathology Annual*, Vol. 5, 125–144, Appleton-Century-Crofts, New York, 1970.

59. McCluskey, R.T.: Immunologic mechanisms in renal disease. *In* Heptinstall, R.H. (ed.) *Pathology of the Kidney*, 2nd ed., 273–317, Little, Brown, Boston, 1974.

60. McCoy, R.C., Abramowsky, C.R., and Tisher, C.C.: IgA nephropathy. *Amer. J. Path. 76*: 123–144, 1974.

61. McLean, R.H. and Michael, A.F.: Properdin and C3 proactivator: Alternate pathway components in human glomerulonephritis. *J. Clin. Invest. 52*: 634–644, 1973.

62. McPherson, D.J.: Metaplasia of renal glomerular capsular epithelium. *J. Clin. Path. 16*: 220–222, 1963.

63. Michael, A.F. and McLean, R.H.: Evidence for activation of the alternate pathway in glomerulonephritis. *In* Hamburger, J., Crosnier, J., and Maxwell, M.H. (eds.) *Advances in Nephrology*, Vol. 4, 49–66, Year Book, Chicago, 1974.

64. Min, K.W., Györkey, F., Györkey, P., Yium, J.J., and Eknoyan, G.: The morphogenesis of glomerular crescents in rapidly progressive glomerulonephritis. *Kidney Internat. 5*: 47–56, 1974.

65. Morita, T., Suzuki, Y., and Churg, J.: Structure and development of the glomerular crescent. *Amer. J. Path. 76*: 349–368, 1973.

66. Müller-Eberhard, H.J.: The complement system and nephritis. *In* Hamburger, J., Crosnier, J., and Maxwell, M.H. (eds.) *Advances in Nephrology*, Vol. 4, 3–13, Year Book, Chicago, 1974.

67. Okada, M. and Tsuchida, H.: A clinicopathologic study on patients with asymptomatic hematuria/proteinuria. With special reference to Berger's nephropathy (in Japanese). *Report to the Ministry of Health and Welfare Chronic Nephritis (Renal Insufficiency) Research Committee*, 56–59, 1976.

68. Okada, M., Tsuchida, H., and Yamamoto, S.: Familial IgA nephropathy characterized by a peculiar glomerular pathology (in Japanese). *Report to the Ministry of Health and Welfare Chronic Nephritis (Renal Insuficiency) Research Committee*, in press.

69. Panem, S., Ordóñez, N.C., Kirstein, W.H., Katz, A.I., and Spargo, B.H.: C-type virus expression in SLE. *New Engl. J. Med. 295*: 470–475, 1976.

70. Perez, G.O., Bjornsson, S., Ross, A.H., Amato, J., and Rothfield, R.: A mini-epidemic of Goodpasture's syndrome. *Nephron 13*: 161–173, 1974.

71. Peters, D.K. and Williams, D.G.: Complement and mesangiocapillary glomerulonephritis: The role of complement deficiency in glomerulonephritis. *In* Hamburger, J., Crosnier, J., and Maxwell, M.H. (eds.) *Advances in Nephrology*, Vol. 4, 67–78, Year Book, Chicago, 1974.

Index